DOGS & HUMAN HEALTH

The New Science of
Dog Therapy & Therapy Dogs

Milena Penkowa, M.D., Ph.D., DMSc

BALBOA.
PRESS
A DIVISION OF HAY HOUSE

Balboa Press books may be ordered through booksellers or by contacting:

Balboa Press
A Division of Hay House
1663 Liberty Drive
Bloomington, IN 47403
www.balboapress.com.au
1 (877) 407-4847

Print information available on the last page.

ISBN: 978-1-4525-2902-8 (sc)
ISBN: 978-1-4525-2903-5 (e)

Balboa Press rev. date: 05/29/2015

CONTENTS

AUTHOR INFORMATION

Dr. Milena Penkowa, MD, PhD, DMSc (born 1973) is a neuroscientist and medical doctor living in Copenhagen, Denmark.

She graduated as a medical doctor (MD) at the University of Copenhagen, where most of her scientific research has been conducted. She began as a neuroscientist in 1993, graduated as MD in 1998, and by 2009 she was professor of neuroprotection at the University of Copenhagen. She has authored > 115 scientific publications and contributed to 15 innovations including novel drug compounds, medical devices and diagnostic tools. She also holds two doctoral degrees, the PhD (obtained in 2001) and the Doctor of Medical Sciences (DMSc) (obtained in 2006) at the University of Copenhagen. By December 2010 she left the University and founded a private company "Hjerneeksperten" (www.hjerneeksperten.dk) that is an expert center for neuroprotection, neurorehabilitation and development. At Hjerneeksperten she provides expert second opinions and personalized solutions within medicine, health care, rehabilitation and neuroprotection.

She applies dog-assisted therapy professionally as she is joined every day by her certified therapy dog Snubbi, a male English field trial (FT) cocker spaniel (seen on the photos and the cover). Snubbi excels at detecting cancer tissue, though most of the time, he assists in the functional rehabilitation of brain injured patients.

Besides her interest in neuroscience and therapy dogs/dog therapy, Milena loves to watch Formula One racing, listening to Metallica, and to go hunting together with Snubbi.

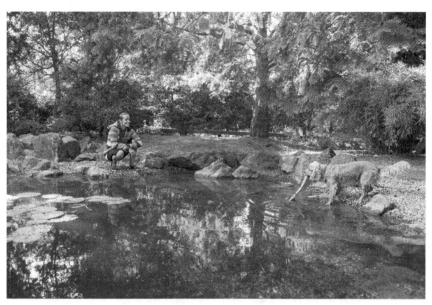

Dogs are great companions for exploring the outdoors,
finding adventures and having fun.

AUTHOR'S NOTE

This book describes dog therapy and how dogs improve human health and survival, but the book cannot replace a visit to your doctor. The contents of the book cannot be used to make a diagnosis or replace conventional treatment, it is meant as a supplement to aid your conventional health-care program.

While the content of the book may benefit the majority, it will not be applicable to each and every individual case and will not necessary explain why professional medical advice, examination, and treatment plans are recommended for any specific purpose and/or personal health matters.

Neither the author nor the publisher will accept any kind of liability for any personal or canine injury, damage, or loss derived from the misuse of information in this book.

FOREWORD BY DR. MARC BEKOFF

Dr. Milena Penkowa's new book *Dogs & Human Health* reveals how and why human health and well being are influenced by the presence of a dog. Instead of relying on cute anecdotes, her book is based on a wealth of scientific experiments showing how dogs (as compared to placebos) influence the human brain, mind, behavior, and various bodily functions. This is what makes this book different from many others, as it translates scientific data into inspirational everyday language in order to share medical discoveries with people who would otherwise not have access to the latest research. Dr. Penkowa's goal is to share knowledge, educate, arouse, inform, and entertain readers.

As most people around the globe know of cases in which a pet dog rescued his or her owner's life or discovered a yet unidentified cancer in a person, there is a growing demand for solid scientific placebo-controlled information on this subject. Thus, a book that explains the results of medical research studies to non-professional readers including dog owners (guardians) is very much needed. *Dogs & Human Health* does just that and more, as it seeks to provide readers with scientific explanations for the highly popular and touching 'doggy anecdotes' that flood the Internet and other media, including global TV.

To achieve Dr. Penkowa's goals, *Dogs & Human Health* describes scientific studies that have demonstrated how a dog's company prevents diseases and the need for pain-killers, sleeping pills, and anti-allergic medications, as dog exposure improves human health, happiness, and resilience when compared to placebo interventions like a robotic pet, a fake toy dog, or a live pet other than a dog. What's more, being exposed to a dog increases patients' survival rates from cancer and after a heart attack, stroke, and other severe medical conditions. And, this is why the health care industry has implemented therapy dog visits for both inpatients, whether they are in hospital, nursing homes, or any other health care institution. Another good reason to involve dogs in the health care sector is their ability to reduce pain as well as the severity of immune system disorders such as allergies, asthma, and dermatitis in both children and adults.

Dogs also reduce the burden of epilepsy, Alzheimer's and Parkinson's diseases, and in addition, dog exposure increases functional recovery after cancer, stroke, and brain injuries. Moreover, a furry friend may also ameliorate the burden of many psychiatric and developmental disorders such as depression, anxiety, post-traumatic stress disorder (PTSD), schizophrenia, and autism spectrum disorders. Our coping ability with life's challenges such as loneliness, distress, bereavement, cancer, trauma, or chronic diseases can be positively transformed if a friendly dog accompanies us.

Dr. Penkowa is careful to note that dogs do not necessarily cure different ailments, but rather they help people heal and get back to a more normal life. Our long and shared history with dogs and the ways humans and dogs shaped one another's behavior provide a starting place as to why dogs became, second to none, so adept in responding to humans, reading our emotions, and helping us heal from myriad medical disorders. While some people might quibble with some of Dr. Penkowa's conclusions, the care with which she approaches the 'hot' topic of dog-mediated therapy is much welcomed, and I hope her book enjoys a broad and global audience. As Dr. Penkowa writes, "Though some might dislike the thought of being diagnosed with cancer by a wet nose, one shouldn't underrate the brainpower attached to that nose and its amazing ability to distinguish right from wrong."

Marc Bekoff
Boulder, Colorado

ACKNOWLEDGMENTS

To my fellow doctors and medical scientists who night and day take care of suffering, fear, pain, and chronic diseases sometimes with a courage and passion not often seen in other professions. I hope they will implement the contents of this book and promote the message to their wards and boards, as we all need to strive for better lives for all of us.

Yet, this book would not have been made without the star of all therapy dogs, my beloved, brilliant, and uniquely intelligent English cocker spaniel named Snubbi.

The truth is that Snubbi taught me just *how much* dogs can do ... and beyond. Moreover, he taught me things about patients' resilience and the human mindsight that are beyond the traditional curriculum applied at medical universities. So, by combining my academic knowledge and scientific background with canine insight, certain keys to a better, more healthy, and happier life emerge, and so naturally I am eager to share all of it with you.

To conclude, this book is also for my beloved parents and sister.

I am thankful to photographer Hanne Paludan Kristensen (www.hpkristensen.com) because she has granted me permission to use her photos.

CHAPTER 1

The Perfect Match

Life brings good and bad times to all of us, and not knowing when disaster strikes seems to be the human condition. In life's storms or fortune, pets offer an island of relief that brings us carefree joy in the moment. Pets make us smile and unwind, no matter how fragmented life may seem.

If you have ever had a dog, you already know the magic bond. If you've never had dogs, you should know it is a life-changing experience you can look forward to because dogs make you feel good, and you will be surprised at just how many ways a dog can enhance your health, happiness, liveliness, and resilience.

Humans and dogs teamed up so long ago that no one remembers when or where. While most people know how we have altered dog breeds with time, very few know how dogs altered us.

In fact, canines did more to us than we will ever be able to artificially breed into them. Being top predators of the Ice Age, they gave prehistoric humans access to protein-rich meat from prey animals. The dietary shift from vegetarian to omnivore ignited vast metabolic changes, and most importantly it induced the growth spurt of our brain, which set off our neurobiological development and ultimately brought us matchless thinking skills (cognition) (Driscoll & Macdonald, 2010; Howard, 2006; Olmert, 2009). Thanks to dogs (who smell, hear, and sense the world better than us) our ancestors could concentrate on sophisticated cognitive functions like language and calculation. In that regard, dogs made us become *Homo sapiens*.

Thousands of decades later modern dogs are not just great companions but are also still providing us great biological benefits. Science supports the conclusion that having a dog improves your physiological and psychological health, particularly by boosting your heart, brain, and immune system. Man's best friend also turns out to be a secret weapon in the fight against diseases, as dogs sniff their way to identify cancer (Marcus, 2012b). Being accompanied by a furry friend also ameliorates the course of dementia, cardiac attack, depression, allergies, elevated blood pressure (hypertension), asthma, and malignant tumors just to mention a few examples from a long list of diseases (Marcus, 2011; Penkowa, 2014). By noticing the subtle biochemical changes that occur in the human body, dogs are known to notify their owners before a seizure or when blood sugar drops to dangerous levels (hypoglycemia) (Fine, 2010; Penkowa, 2012; Rooney et al., 2013; Wells, 2011).

These amazing achievements, all of which make the dog look like some sort of medical expert, can be traced back to the dog's evolutionary past, which is closely intertwined with our own. Hence, dogs' extraordinary senses became finely attuned, while canines back in the Ice Age got more and more adjusted to human company (Miklósi, 2007). In fact, our common history holds the key as to why dogs outperform all other animals in terms of human-directed awareness, behavior, affection, sensitivity, loyalty, and bonding. In other words, to find out why the dog became man's best friend (and therapist), we have to turn our attention toward our ancient past.

Man's Oldest Friend

The earliest documented apelike humans (genus *Homo*) lived four to eight million years ago in the great African forests (Larsen, 2003; Wood, 2010). In a lengthy process of change, they evolved into our prehistoric ancestors (hominins), who appeared during the Paleolithic period (2.6 Mya - 10.000 years before present (BP)). Rather early in this period, the Ice Age climate changes made us leave a tree-dwelling life in the great forests in order to enter the open savanna around 1.8 Mya BP as upright, walking hominin, the *Homo erectus* (Haeusler et al., 2012; Wood, 2010). Much later, approximately a hundred to two hundred thousand years ago, the first members of *Homo sapiens* (i.e., modern mankind) emerged (Schleidt & Shalter, 2003; Shipman, 2011).

However, the modern human species did not get here all by itself. Since prehistoric times we have traveled the globe together with canines, initially the gray wolf (*Canis lupus*) and later on the dog (*Canis lupus familiaris*), which is a domesticated subspecies of the wild wolf (Miklósi, 2007; Olmert, 2009). Though nobody knows for sure when the wolf-to-dog transition happened, molecular genetic DNA analyses indicate that the dog emerged 135,000 to 145,000 years ago (Vilà et al., 1997,1999; Wayne & VonHoldt, 2012).

Accordingly, modern man and his best friend evolved together more than a hundred thousand years BP, which makes the dog the first domesticated animal on earth (Driscoll & Macdonald, 2010; Larson et al., 2012; Ostrander & Wayne, 2005; Zeder, 2012). Since ancient history, our ancestors and canines have interacted and mutually influenced each other's survival, biological fitness, and behavior. That is why our development is best described as co-evolution (Olmert, 2009; Schleidt & Shalter, 2003). And there's one more thing. Prehistoric cooperation with canid hunters or early wolf-dogs likely resulted in the transformation that gave rise to our successful human lineage just as the lack of cooperative wolf-dogs likely have contributed to the extinction of the Neanderthals (Shipman, 2010,2015). Hence, the ancestors of modern humans extensively used early wolf-dogs for hunting, safeguarding, tracking/alerting, and protection of campsites or food resources, but Neanderthals didn't.

From Wolf to Woof

After some initial debate, scientists now agree that today's dog is a descendant and subspecies of the gray wolf. In terms of genetics, the dog's DNA sequence is practically identical to the whole genome of the wolf, as only a few distinct genes separate the wild from the domestic animal (Case, 2008; Vilà et al., 1997; VonHoldt et al., 2011; Wayne & Ostrander, 2007; Wayne & VonHoldt, 2012). Yet their size, shape, behavior, and in particular tameness and trainability are tremendously and obviously different, as one (the dog) is born tame, trainable, and trustful of people with an inborn desire to stay close to us, while the other (the wolf) is wild, rather distrustful of people, not very trainable, and has no obvious desire to stay close to us (Miklósi, 2007). Moreover, the offspring of a tamed or trained wolf is born wild, no matter how tamed or trained the parent is. The differences between dogs and wolves are hardly explained by their negligible DNA variation. So where did they come from?

The answer lies in their remarkably different ways of decoding the DNA into molecules, in particular within the brain (Albert et al., 2012; Saetre et al., 2004). Therefore, wolves and dogs behave as different as humans and apes.

The lessons learned are that a species' DNA sequence provides a genotype, but it does not necessarily have much to do with the same species' phenotype, behavior, or mind-set. Another lesson learned from genetic research is that as the human brain underwent major adaptive changes, the dog brain advanced by leaps and bounds during our co-evolution as well (Ostrander & Wayne, 2005). In fact, those genes that separate dogs from wolves are mainly genes involved in brain structure and functions (Axelsson et al., 2013). Consequently scientific discoveries regarding conditions of the brain or mind are in many regards applicable to both humans and dogs (Awano et al., 2009; Hare & Woods, 2013; Ostrander & Beal, 2012; Parker et al., 2010).

What may come as a bigger surprise are the recent findings from research using functional MRI scans, an imaging method that shows the brain structures and how, when, and why brain cells are activated and fire signals within specific regions of the brain. As described by independent researchers, the dog's brain cells, cognitive responses, mental activation pattern, and emotional reactions are comparable to those of the human brain (Andics et al., 2014; Berns, 2013; Berns et al., 2012,2014; Coren, 2000,2004; Grimm, 2014; Hare & Woods, 2013; McConnell, 2007; Overall, 2011). According to this, the brain and mind of both dogs and humans respond in similar ways to positive and negative events just as they are comparable with regards to their composition and physiology, including the state of neurons (nerve cells), molecular biology, and biochemistry. For the very same reason all those psychoactive medications, mind-altering pharmaceuticals, and brain-targeting drugs that are used by your medical doctor work not only in us humans but also in our dogs, in whom most if not all of these compounds were originally tested before they went to market.

Our mounting insight into the canine brain and mind ought to transform the way we think of and treat dogs, as these critters are likely among the most underestimated species on earth. At its core, we share more than anyone ever thought of, whether we look at the past or present, and perhaps this is why man and his best friend have always made -and still make- such a perfect match.

In Each Other's Pocket

Our ancestors benefitted greatly from canine predatory skills as well as their prosocial traits, which conveyed to humans tremendous advantages in terms of survival, growth, and progress (Miklósi, 2007; Olmert, 2009).

Prehistoric wolf packs were the apex predators at the very top of the food chain, as they reigned the Pleistocene when the upright running apes (*Homo erectus*) entered the open lands of the savanna. As the two species gradually adapted to the sight of each other, the first hesitant beginnings of a developing relationship had started, and in many regards it represents a major milestone in human history (Derr, 2012; Olmert, 2009; Ostrander & Wayne, 2005; Shipman, 2010).

Exactly when mutual bonds were established between us is not precisely defined, but numerous archaeological findings of canine and human remnants placed together at prehistoric sites indicate that our coexistence with wolves is at least four to five hundred thousand years old, which is much older than *Homo sapiens* (Galibert et al., 2011; Miklósi, 2007; O'Haire, 2010; Schleidt & Shalter, 2003; Smith, 2004). The fossils were found in quite different places, including France, Russia, England, Spain, and Northern China, which indicates that even the very early human-canine alliance must have preexisted for quite a while because of their geographical dissemination. This is supported by a study published in 2009 in which new data were obtained from the Peking man (*Homo erectus pekinensis*), who represents a prehistoric group of upright humans deriving from Northern China (Shen et al., 2009). The study found that the Peking man lived 770,000 years ago, which is hundreds of thousands of years earlier than many previously believed. The most interesting part, though, is that these early ancestors lived in close contact with wolves as indicated by fossil remains (Messent & Serpell, 1981; Serpell, 1996).

Accordingly, the first contact between Paleolithic canines and our early forbears was likely initiated much earlier than anyone thought (Serpell, 1996; Shipman, 2010). This notion is supported by scientists who judge the very first interactions between *Homo* and wolf to have occurred at the time when apelike humans left their tree-dwelling life in the forest and in an upright position walked out on the open grasslands (Burton, 2009; Olmert, 2009; Pante et al., 2012; Plummer, 2004; Schleidt & Shalter, 2003).

It follows that the human-canine contact was made in the earliest subdivision of the Paleolithic period (very early Stone Age), as it likely goes back to at least 1.8 million BP (Olmert, 2009; Shipman, 2010). In that case it was most likely the prehistoric clade *Homo erectus* who paved the way for modern man's dog.

This is in agreement with recent scientific reports describing a socially responsible and intrepid behavior of *Homo erectus*, as it appears that human relatives took good care of injured or fragile individuals (Haeusler et al., 2012).

But would these early humans dare to approach the mighty wolves? If one may choose between all the animals present on the steppe, why pick the most dangerous one, the one who instinctively would enjoy us for his dinner? To answer this, let's have a closer look at the very nature of wild wolves and humans, including their survival strategies, which in the end might explain how we truly fell in love. As detailed here, human predecessors were likely not responsible for the contact or the opening of domestication.

Meet and Greet

Wolves are not exactly animals who would make for good pets in many people's eyes; however, in contrast to popular beliefs, wolves are in fact highly social by nature, and within a pack each member acts amiably toward each other, including the pups (Miklósi, 2007; Olmert, 2009).

The wolf's strongest personality trait is its aptitude for social and emotional bonding with other individuals as observed when the pups are just a few weeks old. They show distress when they are separated from familiar pack members while they display relief and joy when the pack reunites. This ability is the foundation of their strong pack behavior, the unit of wolf society (Serpell, 1996).

Consequently wolves collaborate closely and act in a coordinated manner when they perform their routines, including attacking and killing larger prey, during which each individual knows exactly what the other pack members are doing, when it will happen, where and to which prey animal, etc. Not only do they share the prey and available food sources, but they also share the risks during the hunt. As another example of their highly social nature, wolves collaborate in order to carry heavy items that are too big for any single individual to bear, and they also provide food for the needy family members staying put in the den. Hence, pack members not participating in the hunt, such as pups, dams, or fragile animals, are fed by the strong ones who are able to hunt down more prey and feed on it before they return to the den, where they regurgitate in order to share a meal (Schleidt & Shalter, 2003).

These examples reflect the social, flexible, and considerate behavior of wolves, and within a pack they are emotionally attached to one another as well. Likewise, in case of any threat to the pack, intrusion of territory by other animals, or even if a close kin fails to comply with the pack structure, wolf behavior can readily shift to attack, lacerate, drive off, or even kill the target (Olmert, 2009; Schleidt & Shalter, 2003).

In fact, it is a widely held belief that wolf pack behavior is a rigidly organized dominance hierarchy centered around an alpha pair that supposedly dominates the subordinate pack members; however, this does not meet the terms of noncaptive wolves living in the wild. Nor does it apply to dogs (van Kerkhove, 2004). Hence, investigations of social order, attachment, and behavior within wild wolf packs disagree with the popular perception of dominance hierarchies (Olmert, 2009; Serpell, 1996; Schleidt & Shalter, 2003).

Accordingly, wolves' team spirit, their collaborative awareness, and their fair sharing of risk within the pack remain unmatched by any other mammalian predator, including the big cats, and that's why the Pleistocene wolf went all the way to the top of the food pyramid. In fact, wolves applied a smart and cooperative strategy as they did not specialize highly as hunters unlike the big cats. Wolves kept a full repertoire of prey animals, allowing them to choose between their possible targets, and in so doing, the wolfy dinner party was guaranteed all year round.

The only species that rivals the wolves' social, flexible, and cooperative behavior is our own. In fact, the closest approximation to wolf pack behavior is found in humans. Humans are able to exhibit highly social, empathetic, mutually caring, considerate, and ethical behaviors (Olmert, 2009; Schleidt & Shalter, 2003). When canine pups are raised by humans, the aptitude of both species for social and emotional bonding is particularly evident. The fact that humans are the only species that interacts and lives together with other predator species might somehow reflect the way by which our ancestors avoided becoming the predator's next meal at dinnertime.

In the Wild

Even though wolves form highly social pack structures, they were unlikely to consider hominins as anything but an easy target for a nice meal, and yet our ancestors were able to stick around. There are a number of reasons for this, and one is that wolves are naturally shy in approaching humans. They usually run off, even when they don't have to (Miklósi, 2007; Olmert, 2009). Moreover, very early humans were able to make and use stone tools, a talent characterizing our species for approximately 2.6 million years (Shipman, 2010,2011). Even more important, our earliest ancestors knew how to use fire for heat and light, a capacity that scientists consider as the most decisive in terms of evolutionary advantage and survival of our species (Burton, 2009; Wrangham & Carmody, 2010). Hence, the acquisition of fire led to fire-based weapons, allowing the hominin a self-defense against hungry predators, a terrestrial lifestyle, and control of temperature and light-dark cycles. By these critical changes, hominins were able to stay safe, warm during nights, and grounded in the middle of the open savanna, which was otherwise populated with a range of predators like wolves, hyenas, lions, saber-toothed big cats, and leopards.

As directly evidenced by archaeologists, early humans used their stone tools for processing abandoned carcasses and old bones left by satisfied predators (Pante et al., 2012). Whatever remained after the hunting carnivores' initial feast could therefore be accessed by scavenging hominins, and by means of flaked stone tools, they broke the bones in order to munch marrow and its fats as they ate the partially defleshed carcass. Thereby, the human diet no longer consisted of vegetables, forest plants, and fruits only. Once in a while these human foragers now obtained some leftover flesh, fats, and marrow (Larsen, 2003; Plummer, 2004).

However, it could take days of searching before they found the next scraps, and simultaneously they could on a distance watch the mighty wolf packs indulging in large game and freshly killed ungulates (Schleidt & Shalter, 2003). To our disadvantage, humans lacked the physical strength, speed, predatory killer instinct, fangs, and claws needed to conquer big animals, and so if the hominins were to feed more often on animal food sources, let alone freshly killed game, they would have to come up with another strategy. Meanwhile, time passed while a future strategy simmered, and our ancestors could not do much but grow envious of the wolves' instinctive tracking and successful hunting of prey.

Then again, one unique gift of *Homo* was about to change the picture. Our ancestors went from knowing fire to becoming able to tame, control, and light their own fire, whereby they took a tremendous step forward that completely transformed our evolution, physiology, self-esteem, and the environment. Hence, the taming of fire was a requirement for the ability to cook our food. As explained below, this is perhaps the most important step in evolution of today's mankind and dogs (Axelsson et al., 2013; Plummer, 2004; Wrangham & Carmody, 2010).

On the open grasslands tubers and roots were accessible, and if cooked, they could yield enough nutritional value to constitute an essential part of the calorie requirement. This reflects the huge evolutionary benefits derived from cooking in terms of ingestion, energy availability, net nutritional gain, and the energy expenditure needed for digestion and uptake of nutrients, vitamins, and minerals (Wrangham & Carmody, 2010). Accordingly, while our ancestors could not match the wolf packs regarding the hunting of big game, the early humans could at least get going by their cooking over fire, and once in a while they would likely scavenge and find a piece of carrion or leftover bones to add to their vegetarian food sources. The bones were rich in marrow fats, and by use of their stone tools, hominins could extract and take nourishment from the bone marrow (Olmert, 2009).

Hominins' food preparation and cooked scraps naturally attracted scavenging animals, particularly those that were less afraid of humans, and among them the canids (Axelsson et al., 2013; Driscoll & Macdonald, 2010). This trait reflects canine nature since they are not only predators but also efficient and opportunistic foragers nourishing on an omnivorous diet (Plummer, 2004; Schleidt & Shalter, 2003).

The most tolerant, opportunistic, and/or adaptable individuals would be the first to arrive at such dumpsites, where they found a new and commensal opportunity of feeding on fall-back foods or on human waste (feces) at the edge of the hominins' campfire, which eventually may have provided a refuge for a subset of these canids (Olmert, 2009; Zeder, 2012).

Hence, our ancestors' camps would by coincidence provide approaching wolves with cooked or digested foodstuff, which would allow them to eat and metabolize much larger diets plus more than double the intestinal digestion of nutrients, vitamins, and trace elements (Case, 2008; Herculano-Houzel, 2012; Schleidt & Shalter, 2003). In fact, cooking of foods enables an individual to rapidly ingest its entire daily caloric requirement, which saved both time and energy demands for digestion and reduced the risk of infection from microbes. Thus, thanks to our ancestors' cooking of foods, a subgroup of wolves got to maximize their fitness, chance of survival, thriving, and reproduction rates. These canid loiterers had found a suitable, opportune source of benefits (Wrangham & Carmody, 2010).

By exploiting this new niche, subgroups of wolves likely instigated the process of domestication by following an opportunistic pathway that made them become more and more used to being around humans and vice versa (Derr, 2012; Olmert, 2009). The proto-domestic lifestyle with its shift in diet, metabolism, and behavior led to genetic and molecular adaptation. Gradually changes would also surface in terms of morphology, smaller body size, and phenotypic appearance (such as type and color of coat, floppy ears, high-held tail, etc.). Thereby, the canine loiters likely paved the way for the impending wolf-to-dog transition, though the full details behind the process of domestication remain largely unknown (Derr, 2012;

Driscoll & Macdonald, 2010; Fogle, 1990; Olmert, 2009; Serpell, 1996; Zeder, 2012).

Moreover, when canine scavengers find such a new niche, it leads to reproductive isolation from the self-sufficient, truly wild wolf packs, whereby the canine dichotomy separating the "doggish wolves" versus the "wolfish wolves" had set out (Case, 2008; Driscoll et al., 2009). Hence, the wolf-to-dog transition was not as much a result of early humans' intentional intervention as it was a matter of canine-human interplay as both species exploited our ecological niche—Paleolithic campsites (Derr, 2012; Driscoll & Macdonald, 2010; Schleidt & Shalter, 2003).

Though the new niche resulted in the ability of proto-dogs to digest and nourish from starch, grains, and carbohydrates—a trait that particularly differentiate the dog from its wolf ancestor—these transitional canines would still require substantial amounts of high-protein food from prey (Axelsson et al., 2013; Case, 2008; de Godoy et al., 2013). Hence, the majority of these wolf-to-dog canines would still go hunting like their wild conspecifics, and so in the role of trailing scavengers their human neighbors got easier access to the killed prey or at least its remains, whereby our ancestors got to eat nourishing meat, marrow, fats, flesh, viscera, and make use of skin (Driscoll et al., 2009; Olmert, 2009; Schleidt & Shalter, 2003). The result of these changing eating habits was that both dogs and humans became omnivorous, feeding on animals, vegetables, and grains. The optimum diet of both species has ever since contained a mix of proteins, fats, and carbohydrates (Axelsson et al., 2013; de Godoy et al., 2013).

The proto-dogs gradually developed other convenient utilities, such as becoming alarm guards in the form of barking sentinels in case undesired animals, invaders, or nomadic strangers approached at night (Fogle, 1990; Serpell, 1996). Those individual canines who excelled at such tasks would likely get rewarded by receiving some extra scraps from our cooking, while their less skilled conspecifics were more likely chased off or perhaps even killed.

This coexistence between humans and canines provided both with benefits and reciprocal interactions, which undoubtedly were facilitated by the highly social nature of both species. They would gradually develop closer bonds, mutual trust, and attachment, which all facilitated our rising companionship (Zeder, 2012).

As for the human proactive influence and direct impact upon the dog's anatomy (in some cases malformation), this process came much later with targeted breeding interventions directed by our request for different skills, behaviors, appearances, sizes, neoteny, color, and temperament (Case, 2008; Driscoll & Macdonald, 2010; Driscoll et al., 2009; Fogle, 1990; Schleidt & Shalter, 2003; Serpell, 1996). In that regard, humans have certainly influenced today's different dog breeds, but it was an act made possible only after the ancient canines had gained access to our lives and hearts.

However, it is not as important which species initially made contact to the other or who domesticated who since the most imperative is the fact that our eternal bond, attachment, and friendship were established.

The First Kiss

When the very first *bona fide* contact was made is difficult to know, but as both humans and wolves are social opportunists, some valuable and specific benefits for both parts had to be present for a rewarding and lasting relationship to develop. Undoubtedly the ancestral humans had the perfect motive, as they lacked access to freshly killed game and ungulates, which were an easy kill for the daunting predators on the open grasslands, namely the wolf packs (Driscoll & Macdonald, 2010; Olmert, 2009). For our part the wolves must have seemed to be the most attractive collaborators since wolf packs were the top predators of Eurasia and were able to track down and kill migrating herds of prey animal. At this early point in evolution our primitive ancestors were only starting to transform from vegetarian ape-man to premodern human walking the open lands of the savanna. At this point hominins were an easy-to-kill target for the predators reigning over the open plains, and yet these prehistoric humans were also badly in need of an easy-to-get meal (Olmert, 2009; Schleidt & Shalter, 2003). So wolves were the most brilliant partners in terms of gaining a proper protein-rich and fleshy daily meal.

Once hominins got used to having canines close to their nomadic encampments, some of the pups were undoubtedly taken as pets. For each generation that was influenced by our ancestors, the proto-dogs became socialized to humans, and so the selection pressure toward tamable, trainable, or otherwise suitable individuals had begun (Driscoll et al., 2009; Olmert, 2009; Shipman, 2010,2011). When desired behavior traits became the target of selection for several generations, the path to domestication was laid.

One example of this selection process is the dog's barking, which is used for many different purposes and is a frequent if not daily characteristic of many dogs while it is a rare feature of wolves (Coren, 2000,2004; Fogle, 1990; Yin & McCowan, 2004). Likewise, by our interference with canine feeding and breeding, we have enhanced other basic characteristics in order to augment some specifically desired traits in our dogs, which thereby have differentiated into diverse breeds with assorted functions such as hunting, guarding, and herding (Case, 2008; Driscoll et al., 2009; Serpell, 1996).

The point is, when the first contact was established between these two highly social species, a perfect match had been made (Olmert, 2009; Schleidt & Shalter, 2003).

Just Watching

Both before and during the time when the wolf-to-dog transitional canines established their proto-domestic lifestyle, our ancestors would still need to watch carefully the wolf behavior and its potential threat since even the most doggish wolves were still more wolf than dog. After all, it took a long time for them to become even remotely tame.

By watching also the hunting skills of the predatory wolf packs, hominins learned what it takes, if they were to kill large game themselves, while on a more practical level their scrutiny would reveal where to forage for scraps of carcasses and/or skeletons. By watching also the preys' behavior before and during the hunt, our ancestors learned what would work or fall short in terms of survival and hunting strategies. By merely watching the Pleistocene daily shows, these human antecedents slowly found their way to become one day the most powerful species known in history. Hence, while we were watching the fascinating yet threatening animals, our brain and senses received important inputs, whereby modern humans' highly developed visual system and attentional focus were founded (Olmert, 2009; Shipman, 2010). Certainly these human pioneers did not just stare and glare without a purpose, as their early observational studies likely contributed also to the development of human vocalization leading to one of our most distinct characteristics, the use of symbolic behavior and verbal communication (Shipman, 2010). By the ability to convey important facts to relatives, humans could share vital information on potential dangers and pitfalls with regards to the surrounding predators, potentially poisonous foods, and/or how to best survive throughout the day on the open savanna. According to this, the tireless watching of animals have likely contributed to the evolutionary development of symbolic language, which are hallmarks of the human species (Olmert, 2009; Shipman, 2010,2011).

If our ancestors' watching of animals gave humans an evolutionary advantage, one would expect it to precipitate in our sensory or visual biology and behavior. Indeed, it was recently published that the human brain contains a subset of neurons (brain cells) that selectively and specifically respond to the sight of animals (Mormann et al., 2011). This study, which was performed by a multinational group of scientists, revealed that the human brain readily activates these animal-specific neurons even when animals are only seen in photographs, which reflects how our brain is specialized for processing visual information regarding animals.

The animal-specific neurons within the human brain are found on the right side of the brain (right hemisphere) in a structure called amygdala (in Greek, almond). Amygdala is an almond-shaped mass controlling our emotional behavior, alertness, and arousal (Howard, 2006; Kandell et al., 2013). Accordingly, it is not surprising that also today dogs can easily catch our attention and make us look at them, while our thoughts are distracted from whatever we were doing simply because citizen canine walks by.

The brain's responsiveness to the sight of animals is independent from the observer's emotional condition, which likely reveals how important animals have been during our history. Hence, we are both adapted and dedicated to looking at canines. This behavior obviously makes sense in terms of prehistoric survival since any salient animal could be either predator or potential prey.

In fact, humans react quicker, earlier, and more precisely to the sight of an animal as compared to the times when they see nonanimal objects such as vehicles, tools, buildings, and plants (New et al., 2007). Despite their current utility level, motor vehicles can not attract our attention as fast and accurate as animals can, even though we are taught how dangerous traffic can be throughout life. Hence, our visual monitoring and attention levels are clearly more tuned to our ancestral roots in the wild than they are to modern societies' city life.

According to this, the early hominins were not *just watching* when they rambled the savanna in a world of wild animals. They were rather observing in order to develop an innate, instinctive radar system that inevitably brings into focus any canine popping up in the surroundings.

This is supported by the insight into another highly specialized brain function, namely empathy, which relates to the mirror neurons of the mammalian brain (Rizzolatti, 2009). The mirror neurons are both involved in our own motor actions and in the recognition or mental mirroring of the same actions performed by others (Cattaneo & Rizzolatti, 2009). The mirroring is not restricted to motor or voluntary actions, as emotional states are also recognized in others as well as they are felt within. Therefore, we have the ability to sympathize with another human being or feel what he or she feels, and so the mirror neurons are basically the foundation of empathy, social understanding, and kinship. Moreover, the mirror neuron system is the root of human mind-reading abilities and empathy (qualities often described as *theory of mind*), by which we are able to predict what other individuals feel, wish for, think, intend to do, what they hide from us, or what they are about to do. This ability is of vital importance for any social species since its survival relies on the capacity to understand others' intentions, emotions, and behavioral repertoire (Reid, 2009; Udell & Wynne, 2011; Udell et al., 2010, 2011). Dogs also hold mirror neurons in their brains, and so we are not the only species to emotionally decode other individuals and possess empathy (Bekoff, 2007; Hare et al., 2002; Silva & de Sousa, 2011; Udell et al., 2011). Hence, both man and dog are capable of feeling empathy, sympathy and to decode each other, and accordingly, man and dog naturally form a strong social bond with each other.

Milena Penkowa, M.D., Ph.D., DMSc

It Takes a Canine to Become Sapient

The *Homo sapiens'* brain is amazingly big relative to body size and even more so when compared to all other known animal species, including all the ancestral humans paving the way for modern man (Howard, 2006). One of the biological reasons for the brain's evolutionary growth spurt was the fact that the human diet changed from a vegetarian one to one with high-protein foods (prey animals), a change we owe to our canine associates and their hunting skills, which granted us access to large game, including ungulates and a variety of prey (Olmert, 2009).

The benefits associated with feeding on meat and fats were huge in terms of cellular metabolism, growth, and differentiation (Larsen, 2003; Milton, 2003). Accordingly, hunger for calorically rich foods that are high in fat and proteins became positively selected, and that's why humans also today still crave for these kinds of high-calorie snacks.

As human nutrition and metabolism changed, so did our brains, which expanded greatly in size and complexity, leading to the sapient version known as the modern human brain.

Hence, the transformation from vegetarian to omnivore is one of the most important steps in the evolution of modern mankind, as the animal-based protein-rich meals derived from successful hunting of game made our brains grow so that we could completely outperform all the extinct human lineages, including the Neanderthals (Larsen, 2003; Schleidt & Shalter, 2003).

Accordingly, the domestication of the gray wolf (i.e., the rise of man's best friend) is a prerequisite that brought our human lineage vast benefits during evolution. In that regard, dogs shaped and tuned the human race, and in fact, without our canine partner and the domestication, we would likely not have been us.

It Takes a Human to Become a Pet

With the big and highly complex brain, one would expect *Homo sapiens* to show some yet unseen resourcefulness already in ancient times. In fact, this was the case at least some fifteen-thousand-years ago, since humans at that time kept different dog types (or precursor breeds) as shown by means of excavations (Larson et al., 2012; Miklósi, 2007; Schleidt & Shalter, 2003; Serpell, 1996). Hence, at least three distinct types of dogs were living in Scandinavia around eight thousand years ago (Henriksen et al., 1976), and by that time many more distinct breeds were likely present at other central sites.

At the same time our early antecedents also kept dogs as pets (Miklósi, 2007; Serpell, 1996). This notion comes from the discovery of numerous ancient dog burials as well as from the excavation of up to twelve-thousand-year-old human graves, which were found to also contain the skeleton of a dog lying next to the human remains (Morey, 2006). Hence, an old burial place in Northern Israel that dates back to 12,000 BP contained a human being who was buried together with a puppy (Davis & Valla, 1978). The buried person was found with one arm around the dog, who was an approximately five-month-old puppy, and this mortuary practice indicates that the deceased person had an affectionate pet-like relationship with the dog (O'Haire, 2009; Serpell, 1996). As detailed by Miklósi (2007), other ancient human graves have been found to contain dog remains, including one in Germany that dates back to 13,000 BP in which the dog was buried as part of a human double grave.

In fact, the finding of intact animals inside human graves is rather common, and canine entombments are known from all over the globe just except the Antarctica (Maher et al., 2011). While it is a common human practice to bury different species, the dog is absolutely at the head of the pack, as it outnumbers all other animals in terms of burial together with humans, and only dogs are regularly found in a direct association with the human skeleton, indicating an intimacy that reflects the close bond between man and dog. Since genetic studies indicate that domestication began much earlier than these burials, we are likely to see in the future the discovery of older human-dog interments that may well appear on any major land mass that has been populated by people.

Consequently ancient humans found the needed time and resources to feed extra mouths of individuals who most likely did not pay off in terms of hunting or herding, which reflects that dogs already in the Ice Age provided other values across the species, most likely friendship, loyalty, and affection as evidenced by the many globally distributed burials of dogs along with humans (Miklósi, 2007; Morey, 2006).

On the other hand, dogs may well serve as both a pet, companion, and worker as seen today where they are readily both family and hunting dogs, as to why some of the ancient pet dogs may well have provided their own food.

Humans have kept this relationship strong since millions of people around the world keep dogs, though the way we keep them shows gigantic differences for better or worse. Many dogs are simply a household pet left home alone all day, while the luckiest ones get to live as companion dogs, as they accompany humans most of the time. Whether they belong to one or the other group or something in between, modern dog owners spend billions on their pets (Grimm, 2014). Today's dogs are treated more and more like small furry humans. Dogs have their own fitness centers, hairdressers, groomers, kindergartens, etc., a tendency likely reflecting that we have taken the dog into our most private lives, including our beds at night, and so we prefer our dog to be just as clean and well-groomed as we are.

Independent from how humans behave around their pets, dogs haven't been equally obsessed with outer looks, appearances, or what to buy. Instead, dogs have taken the opportunity to observe us, see our different cues and emotions in order to recognize certain behavioral patterns (Fogle, 1990; Horowitz, 2010; Olmert, 2009). In fact, they did so in much the same way ancestral hominins watched, observed, and learned from the Pleistocene's predatory canines. In a way dogs seem to have grabbed their chance and developed an ability to decode and predict human behavior, emotions, and intentions (Horowitz, 2010; Penkowa, 2012; Smith, 2004).

The Perfect Match

The connection between the genera *Homo* and *Canis* represents a very long, mutual, and fascinating history. Not only did this connection provide our ancestors with advantageous hunting and survival skills, but it also paved the way for companionship, bonding and social skills (Olmert, 2009; Schleidt & Shalter, 2003; Smith, 2004). As suggested by paleoanthropologist Pat Shipman of Penn State University, the human-canine connection has for at least 2.6 million years played a crucial role in the shaping of the human species, including some of our most distinguished traits (e.g., the development of spoken language, fine tools, and symbolic behaviors) (Shipman, 2010,2011,2015). In her writings and books, Dr. Pat Shipman sets forth a theory stating that the human-canine connection is basically what makes us human.

According to this, human adaptation and evolution are closely connected to the domestication of man's best friend. Or in other words, the dog civilized us.

In fact, studying dog development, behavior and socialization provides us with knowledge of not only the dog but also of our own species (Geerdts et al., 2015; Grimm, 2014; Hare & Woods, 2013). Given that dogs evolved for living in a human niche, studies of dogs' social cognition provide information also with regards to the development of modern man. Accordingly, the way puppies mature and behave toward us as they grow into adult dogs provides an excellent homologous mammalian model for the development of social behavior in human children.

> Research into dog evolution keeps informing us about our own history as exemplified by DNA sequencing of ancient dog remains from Alaska and Latin America, by which it emerges that European colonists systematically have avoided breeding of the Native American dogs (Leonard et al., 2002).

The human-animal connection also discloses our emotional codevelopment by means of the reciprocal interaction and social relationship between at first Paleolithic wolves and ancestral humans and later between dog and man. In fact, building a close bond with another animal species is exceptional for humans, as no other mammal is consistently willing to nurture in the wild a different species, especially not a predator.

The human-canine connection resulted in simultaneous shaping and development of both species, resulting in the dog's amazing senses (e.g., the dog's sense of smell), while we developed complex cognitive skills allowing us to become the most powerful species on earth (Horowitz, 2010; Serpell, 1996; Smith, 2004).

Thanks to our canine companions, we did not ourselves need to find the speed, muscle strength, fangs, claws, or olfactory expertise required to trail and kill big game just as we did not need the ability to smell danger at a distance in order to alert and safeguard settlements, at least not when we were accompanied by canines. This is why the human species had the opportunity to grow an amazingly big and advanced brain rather than developing a powerful snout (Herculano-Houzel, 2012; Howard, 2014; Serpell, 1996; Smith, 2004).

Likewise, since canids in general were superior hunters, sentinels, and companions, they had developed brilliant sensory skills, such as their sense of smell, which outperforms any other living creature or mechanical apparatus in terms of sniffing, tracking, detecting, herding, stalking, sensing, and finding a target (Driscoll & Macdonald, 2010; Fogle, 1990; Overall, 2011; Schleidt & Shalter, 2003; Udell & Wynne, 2008).

In view of that, humans and dogs have developed and differentiated by means of reciprocal interactions, and so our coevolution has been tremendously rewarding in terms of becoming a complete and complementary unit. Or in other words, nature and time have worked their way to create the perfect match. Since then, the bonds between man and his dog have been documented in numerous ways and several times.

One thing experienced by most if not all affectionate dog owners is the dog's unconditional affection and loyalty along with its empathetic ability to sense how we feel.

Accordingly, humans are drawn toward their dogs, and we remain willing to spend huge amounts of money, time and efforts on them, even if the utilitarian profit to some people may appear to be somewhat missing. On the other hand, dogs do return a great deal, and often they return much more than the owner gives. Science supports the long-held supposition that dogs enhance our well-being, health, longevity, and the coping with disease. In this regard, dogs provide so much more to their owners than the other way round, no matter how much money people like to spent on their dog.

How Old Are We?

Though the first domesticate in history is the dog, its origin remains uncertain. The scientific literature on this subject is divergent, which is due to the fact that scientists used two highly different approaches. Each one has yielded highly different conclusions (Larson et al., 2012). One approach uses archaeological studies of fossils (bones) with regards to skeletal morphology. (Archaeologists look for ancient bones based upon an idea of what ancient dogs may have looked like, even if nobody really knows.) These data points indicate that dogs (as defined by presumed size and a morphology that is different from those of wolves) have been around humans for at least thirty-three thousand years (Galibert et al., 2011; Germonpré et al., 2009,2012; Ovodov et al., 2011). However, it is not possible to say how many other dog bones the Earth saw. Nor does anyone know how much older such yet unidentified fossils might be. Besides, the likelihood of finding such evidence decreases with time as they either come to nothing or are buried deeper and deeper. Finally it is close to impossible to distinguish small wolves from domesticated dogs by looking at their remnant bones. Besides, dog domestication did almost certainly take place at multiple geographical sites at different times in history. That's why the archaeologist can only show us a sort of fossil snapshot relating to its particular location. Yet archaeology has indeed shed light on the fact that dogs originated, evolved, and were domesticated much earlier than anyone would have guessed.

The other scientific approach uses phylogenetics comprising molecular techniques to analyse genetic DNA including the entire genome. These methods showed that man's best friend is a great deal older, as the domesticated dog emerged as a distinct species earlier than a hundred years ago, and the best estimate suggests dogs emerged 135,000 to 145,000 years ago (Larson et al., 2012; Ostrander & Wayne, 2005; Vilà et al., 1997,1999). Hence, DNA analyses propose that dogs originated much earlier than archaeology indicates. The major point here is the dog's gene pool since it contains some species-specific DNA mutations that create the dog's genetic diversity. This diversity is much bigger than anyone would possibly find, in case dogs originated at the time proposed by archaeology (Vilà et al., 1997,1999). DNA data are limited by the fact that they are based on the DNA of modern pet dogs, by whom evolutionary, genetic events are being extrapolated, after which they are compared to the wolf. Accordingly, both methods used are limited, and so the origin of dog domestication is still not settled.

However, the described divergence might also have other logical explanations since scientists generally agree that dogs' domestic behavior preceded morphological changes and size reduction (Miklósi, 2007). The currently known bodily differences between dog and wolf were unlikely to have emerged in the beginning, during which crossbreeding of wolves and dogs may also have countered major phenotypic divergence (Sablin & Khlopachev, 2002). This is supported by descriptions of Sioux Indians who came to America thirty thousand years ago and whose dogs have the size and shape of wolves (Maximilian, 1906). In effect, for the first 100,000 to 125,000 years of our common history, we lived a highly active, nomadic life as hunters. That's why Ice Age dogs looked somewhat like their wild relatives (Larson et al., 2012; Ostrander & Wayne, 2005; Vilà et al., 1997). In contrast, when humans settled down as agriculturists around ten to fourteen thousand years ago, our common lifestyle significantly changed, and we favored a less wolfish, more doggish appearance for man's best friend (Larson et al., 2012).

Another facilitator of the changes in dog looks was the human interference of breeding, which resulted in selection pressure and led to certain behaviors and looks (Fogle, 1990; Ostrander & Wayne, 2005; Serpell, 1996). This intervention saw its first wave when humans settled as agriculturalists and occurred even more so in the last two hundred years. Hence, most of today's different breeds (more than four hundred) emerged during the nineteenth century, although at least three distinct dog phenotypes were recorded at the eight-thousand-year-old Svaerdborg site in Denmark (Henriksen, 1976; Miklósi, 2007).

Accordingly, ancient fossils are hardly suitable for identifying a bone's species-specific origin, and it is even less suitable for defining the time of origin of the domestic dog (Larson et al., 2012; Ostrander & Wayne, 2005; Vilà et al., 1997,1999). Nevertheless, it leaves us with an idea of dogs originating as an independent species about the time when *Homo sapiens* emerged. As explained in chapter 1, it is hardly a coincidence that man and his best friend appeared around the same time in our evolutionary past (Case, 2008; Driscoll & Macdonald, 2010; Schleidt & Shalter, 2003; Shipman, 2010).

CHAPTER 2

Who Needs Dr. Phil When We Have Dr. Fido?

Modern Life of Ancient Critters

Dogs make us smile, but did you know they are also good for your health? Science has shown how dogs convey a range of physical and psychological health benefits to humans. You don't even have to own dogs yourself. You only have to spend a little time with a friendly dog before your body and mind respond with lowered stress hormones and reduced blood pressure along with an increased release of mood-elevating molecules.

If you don't own a dog, it takes on average fifteen minutes of petting someone else's dog before the health effects can be measured, and if you are the lucky owner of a dog, they occur many times faster (Cole et al., 2007; Odendaal, 2000; Odendaal & Meintjes, 2003).

Even the scientists have been puzzled, as research revealed the dog's ability to modify human biology, including the hormones in your blood stream, immune defense systems, and mind-altering chemicals released within your brain (Hare & Woods, 2013; Marcus, 2011,2013a; Oyama & Serpell, 2013; Payne et al., 2015; Penkowa, 2012). Maybe science is telling us that our furry friends are not only man's best friend but also man's most health-promoting friend. The number of disorders that can be ameliorated by a dog's company is growing as shown by mounting medical researchers. Just to mention a few, there is evidence of dogs reducing

23

not just mental problems like depression, post-traumatic stress disorder (PTSD), and anxiety but also diseases of the heart and vascular system, cancers, allergies, dementia, and pain (Beetz et al., 2012b; Engelman, 2013; Marcus, 2012a,b; Penkowa, 2012; Shiloh et al., 2003; Wells, 2007; Walsh, 2009a,b). However, most of us choose to get a dog for other reasons, such as friendship, fun, and devotion. As we are learning more and more about their surprising effects, you shouldn't be surprised to see patients or disabled individuals getting dogs for their specific health-boosting magic.

Another benefit is the absence of side effects as we normally see when one is taking pharmaceuticals, and dogs also lack the ability to cause drug addiction and substance abuse. However, if you have a dog, you are most likely to experience a kind of withdrawal or feel the pain of loss, as one sad day you have to say good-bye to your furry friend.

The fact that a dog's life is much shorter than ours is the dark side of the bond. If you want to read a most gripping example of this loss, I can think of no better example than Dr. Patricia B. McConnell's book titled *For the Love of a Dog*. It is in fact a must-read for any dog owner who'd like to know also what dogs are thinking and doing when we—as we often do—once again fail to communicate with them. On top of this, McConnell shares her own personal story. And watch out! It might bring out tears or break your heart as it did mine. Nevertheless, this book is about the dog's ability to heal our hearts as well as our brains, minds, and body parts.

Make Your Choice

To me, dog therapy and therapy dogs combine my major interests—medicine, science, and canines. Medicine and brain research have been my area of expertise for decades, while the canine part emerged in 2010 due to the arrival of Snubbi, a male English FT cocker spaniel who did nothing less but change my life, not just on the personal level but on a professional one as well.

Snubbi is the one who showed me the therapeutic power of canines, as he opened my eyes to something that was certainly not part of the academic curricula in Denmark. But thanks to him, some very important aspects have been added to my professional life as a doctor since Snubbi taught me the difference between being treated and being healed. Certainly, your physician can provide a treatment by means of medical or surgical procedures, but to be healed, we need something more. As doctors, we handle injuries based upon pharmaceuticals and surgery, but that doesn't necessarily heal you or make you feel whole again. However, this is what our four-legged friends do.

In fact, this fundamental difference in human versus canine skills is also reflected in those early stages before people are diagnosed with diseases—let's say with cancer since we medical doctors can only detect a tumor when it has grown big enough to be found on a scanning image, while dogs are able to sniff their way to a nascent cancer as early as eighteen months before it can be detected by the scanner (Marcus, 2012b, Millan, 2011; Penkowa, 2012).

Think about it. The training of a cancer-detecting dog will cost approximately two thousand dollars, and it will be able to detect very early cancers, such as those in the breast (by smelling breath samples) and prostate cancers (by smelling urine samples). Not all but quite a lot of mammograms, painful biopsies, and invasive procedures could be spared. The science behind this is what this book is about. Mounting scientific reports point to why and how our interacting with dogs leads to more joyful and healthier lives not only for the dog's owner but for the entire household (Engelman, 2013; Fine, 2010; Penkowa, 2014).

One Man's Tall Is Another Man's Small

Our view of the dog is rooted in cultural traditions, and so the dog is considered a member of the family in some cultures, while Fido is part of the diet in other cultures. In modern societies dogs are very popular and in general highly appreciated for their unconditional love, loyalty, health-promoting effects, and ability to perform various tasks that no other species can perform. Dogs are all over popular media, such as TV, which is being flooded by dog behavior programs that have become global hits among the viewers despite the fact that they are slammed by scientists and vets for being built on self-taught philosophies (Bradshaw et al., 2009). One of the prominent myths surrounding these shows claims that domestication of the dog changed only the superficial traits of the wolf, and so it is said the owner's interaction with the dog needs to be in line with some alleged manners of wolf society. It follows that dogs are persistently trying to dominate the household, and so it is said dogs should be put in their place by means of hierarchy, which basically means instructing owners to go through doors first, eat before the dogs, and never allow the dogs to lead the walk. However popular this concept may be among TV viewers, this concept isn't supported by knowledge or facts, and in reality, our understanding of wolf pack behavior in the wild is very limited. Besides, it is subject to changes (Fogle, 1990; Hare & Woods, 2013). In fact, though dogs and wolves are comparable in terms of genetics, they are quite the opposite in terms of behavior toward humans (Miklósi, 2007; Serpell, 1996). Hence, displaying strong hierarchy or dominance as a supposed dog-training method is unlikely to change a dog's perception of humans (Bradshaw et al., 2009; McConnell, 2007).

Another self-taught myth promoted by popular media claims that problem behaviors among dogs are rooted in their lack of jobs or purposes in life and this is why they purportedly would redirect all their excess energy into other (destructive) activities. Eventually dogs develop problem behaviors that are—so it is argued—best corrected by means of the owner asserting a strong hierarchy.

Though I am fully aware that the previously mentioned issues may collide with popular belief, the time has come for a change. Today's dogs are far from deprived of meaningful jobs. They obviously fulfill important tasks. In other words, humans are not the only ones who have advanced since the Ice Age. In fact, our dogs have adapted too, as they have complied with the needs of modern man living in a modern world.

It is true though that traditional hunting and herding are no longer widespread duties assigned to dogs, or at least only a small fraction go hunting with their owners. However, life's purpose and profession have certainly not vanished for today's dogs, as they have moved on to the health-care business (Fine, 2010; Marcus, 2011; Oyama & Serpell, 2013; Penkowa, 2012; Walsh, 2009a,b).

If you want to better understand dogs, be understood by them or successfully communicate with your dog, I urge you to read Dr. Patricia B. McConnell's eye-opening books: *The Other end of The leash* and *For the Love of a Dog* or visit her webpage [http://www.patriciamcconnell.com/] for more.

Mutts on a Mission

The human-dog bond is a much-studied field among psychologists, vets, behaviorists, anthropologists, dog trainers, and ethologists, not to mention dog owners all over the globe. The bond contains the mutual benefits and relationship between humans and dogs, and in fact, it goes far beyond the traditional notion of the dog acting loyal and loving in order to be fed by the owner, who gets company and gets to feel loved. But is that all? A free lunch in trade for devotion? Of course not. There is so much more to the bond than the free lunch.

The rather uncomplicated nature of the human-dog bond makes it stronger than most human-human relationships. Dogs don't have politics, and they don't expect you to put them through college and buy their first car. Nor do they act dishonest, vengeful, and unforgiving as people might do. Impressively dogs act in their very nature and without any self-help books, personal trainers, or coaching. It turns out that we are prone to love dogs because of their incessant humanity, something that's frequently lacking from our own species. Another aspect to the bond is the fact that we and canines are highly social species with an inborn inclination to biophilia, whereby other living creatures instinctively appeal to us (O'Haire, 2010; Serpell, 1996).

Humans naturally approach and intermingle with other animals, a behavior rooted in our ancient brain chemistry, whereby we can relax in each other's company, and in dogs we found the perfect match, which is why we naturally bond (Olmert, 2009).

Consequently people's lives are utterly enriched by having dogs, and most owners consider them to be loyal, loving sources of security and emotional support (McConnell et al., 2011; Walsh, 2009a). Certainly human-animal attachment, friendship, and mutual dependency have remained intact since the Ice Age, although everything else in society has changed dramatically.

Don't Just Survive—Thrive

Dogs follow humans all over the globe and in any climate or condition. Dogs love us whether we are homeless or live in a mud hut or mansion, which reflects just how flexible and unconditioned the dog's mind is. In fact, besides the human species, dogs are among the most successful animals in terms of geographical spreading on earth, as dogs are found anywhere you can find human beings. Their adaptability and their unparalleled devotion explain their evolutionary success, not to mention the fact that dogs are far from running out of meaningful jobs. In fact, as described in this book, dogs have rather climbed up the chain of command, as they got themselves into one of modern society's most demanding segments, namely the health-care sector. Today's dogs are just as important for human survival as their ancestors were back in the Ice Age. While our human forebears needed them for hunting (food sources) and protection (staying alive), modern humans need dogs to rescue us from the hazards of modern lifestyles, provide resilience, and reduce the burden of diseases. Dogs represent our best chance of staying sane and sound, as they provide modern man with an oasis of harmonious well-being and a lifeline to healthiness and happiness (Marcus, 2011; Penkowa, 2012; Serpell, 1996; Walsh, 2009a,b; Wisdom et al., 2009). Luckily we learned more about this in the past decade than we did in the previous millennium, and we know that the therapeutic and health-promoting effects of dogs are needed more than ever since modern man is being challenged like never before, whether on a personal, emotional, professional, marital, or psychosocial level.

To modern city dwellers, dogs provide a stable link to the natural world and remind us of our roots in a forgotten past, and their unconditional devotion nurtures our social brain (O'Haire, 2010; Olmert, 2009).

Many people have ended in a position where coping skills and assertiveness do not come as easy as we'd wish for, as evidenced by the frequency of suicides, depression, stress disorders, loneliness, anxiety, and a range of other health problems, not to mention drug addiction, divorce rates, violence, and crimes. Hence, many people feel lost—that is, unless we find ourselves some kind of reliable anchor. Undoubtedly being such an anchor is a tough job, one not meant for anybody to fulfill.

In previous times it would likely have been the vicar or family doctor who offered consolation, while today people search for other ways to be comforted. The medical staff members we encounter in today's hospitals are primarily taking care of physical injuries and surgeries. That's why we have to look elsewhere if we are searching for a better quality of life or a wholesome feeling of harmony. This is precisely where the dog comes in. Dogs have a natural ability to soothe, relax, and comfort not only those in need but all of us (McConnell et al., 2011; Sakson, 2009; Shubert, 2012a; Walsh, 2009a; Wood et al., 2007). Like no other, dogs are able to make us smile, forget our troubled minds, and burst into laughing at their playful behavior, and they even enjoy doing it time after time. In fact, science supports that free, imaginative, and unstructured play (playing like kids) is tremendously important for the human brain to develop normally, stay on top and for us to grow emotionally, socially, and intelligently (Howard, 2014). And who else but our furry friends can make us laugh and engage in play every day? Next time you need to get those worries off your chest, find some dogs, as they will be happy to share as much of their time as you want.

According to this, modern dogs certainly have a very important job. As explained in the following chapters, dogs endow their owners with meaningful social and emotional support. While science showed that humans facing serious conditions like heart attacks, cancers, brain damage, or HIV/AIDS fare significantly better with dogs, it has also become clear that healthy people can benefit from owning dogs (Friedmann & Son, 2009; Marcus, 2011; Oyama & Serpell, 2013; Penkowa, 2012).

Pet Planet

When you look at them, those dogs are very smart. A great deal of today's dogs managed to substitute a health-supporting or therapeutic role with their previous role in hunting or herding food sources. No matter how you put it, dogs are playing an indispensable role in our lives, and accordingly, we can't live or won't do without them.

This is reflected in the number of dogs living on the planet, which is estimated to contain at least 525 million canines according to Dr. Stanley Coren, a professor of psychology at the University of British Columbia and author of the brilliant blog "Canine Corner," which is hosted by *Psychology Today*. His statements are supported by the American Pet Products Association (APPA) in Scarsdale, New York, which announced that more than 78 million dogs are currently living in US households. In the United States alone, there are at least fifty thousand therapy animals, and more than fifteen thousand canines are part of law enforcement (Grimm, 2014).

When all types of companion animals are considered, nearly 67 percent of American households own at least one pet, and among them cats and dogs are the most common (de Godoy et al., 2013).

Dr. Stanley Coren further estimates that Western Europe holds approximately forty-three million pet dogs, the biggest dog populations located in France (8.8 million), Italy and Poland (7.5 million each), and the United Kingdom (6.8 million). Russia and Ukraine have at least seventeen million dogs, and South America, Asia, and Africa have equally large dog populations. The latter continents do not provide reliable statistics though, and since they also contain unusually high numbers of strays, wild dogs, unowned dogs, and unregistered dogs living with people, a total of 525 million dogs worldwide is likely an understatement.

From Happy to Crappy

The majority of the world's population is now living in a city, and we are facing an era of megacities in the foreseeable future (Lederbogen et al., 2011). As a result, most of us live among concrete walls, high-rise blocks, traffic, and asphalt, whereas other wild species have been pushed into their urban equivalent, the zoos—that is, if they have not gone extinct (Serpell, 1996). Accordingly, our biophilic roots are neglected. Consequently our lifestyle is nothing like the one our ancestors knew out on the open fields, and despite that we are surrounded by crowds of people, we are touched by none.

This should also be taken quite literally since sensory reciprocities, knowing touch and how to be touched, are not what they used to be. Modern people have to a large degree substituted the computer's digital universe for the real-life experience of face-to-face contact. In other words, we have become *Homo digitalis et metropolis*. This development does not always agree with our social nature, as it deprives us of natural sensations, such as physical and tactile contact (being touched) as well as the sight and smell of other individuals with whom we can exchange airborne pheromones, the molecules providing us with social clues and interconnectedness. Sensory deprivation prevents us from feeling connected and fulfilled as part of a social group, and all the while we get more and more isolated (Olmert, 2009).

This tendency was reinforced as we stopped depending on one another the way we used to. In fact, many households rely on robots and machines instead of human hands, and so relational experience and touch decrease even further. The result is a lack of social interactions, depriving modern people of the reciprocal feeling of being truly needed by others, and likewise the feelings of caring for others and being cared for are challenged.

People in the growing megacities are facing an increasing lack of affiliation or contact with the natural world, and considering our biophilic roots, it is not surprising that more and more urbanites are losing their sense of cohesion.

Consequently big city living makes people feel alienated, psychologically dispossessed, stressed, and lonely (O'Haire, 2009; Olmert, 2009). In fact, researchers are able to demonstrate how city life and urban upbringing change specific stress-sensitive brain regions like the limbic system and in particular the amygdala. That's why the brain's processing and coping with stress, social threats, and defeat are disturbed in metropolitans relative to the findings in control subjects from the countryside (Lederbogen et al., 2011). This finding underscores that modern life has changed us and left its footprint in our brain tissue. At least this is the case for urbanites, who are more likely than rural people to develop mental diseases like anxiety, depression, and schizophrenia.

In fact, urbanization causes a general shift in the burden of diseases from acute, transient infections to chronic, noninfectious diseases, and it also brings an array of health problems, including stress, obesity, pollution, feelings of alienation, mental and social dysfunction (Howard, 2014; Valavanidis et al., 2013).

Maybe It's Just Stress

How many times have you heard your family members or doctors say, "Maybe it's just stress" when you tell them about your aches, exhaustion, or other ailments?

Instead of writing it off as being "just stress" we need to rethink the condition. Stress is not just some subjective feeling of having too much to do in a modern world. Stress is a bodily hazard, and when left unmanaged, it may cause premature aging and deterioration of every cell inside your body leading to reduced resistance to disease (Howard, 2006; Servan-Schreiber, 2011; Stankiewicz et al., 2013). Consequently chronic stress leaves you more susceptible to infections, inflammation, cancer, chronic pain, neuropsychiatric, and cardiovascular disorders (Howard, 2014; Wilson & Sato, 2014). In other words, stress takes its toll on your health, as it affects organs ranging from your brain, mind, and heart to your immune system. Stress makes us more susceptible to diseases, including cancer, and it reduces survival rates in those who have already developed cancer (Servan-Schreiber, 2011; Stankiewicz et al., 2013).

According to this, stress-related problems cause no less than three-quarters of visits to the doctor's office, and generally most people today are burdened by health problems that can be ascribed to stress impacts (Servan-Schreiber, 2011).

Knowing that stress triggers a cascade of physical changes, we need to take stress more seriously. Having said that, we should also point out that there are different levels of stress. Hence, mild stress is not the problem. In fact, mild stress can even make us better, so it isn't always bad. For instance, a little splash of pressure because of a work deadline can ignite a burst of energy and creativeness just as the adrenaline released during emergency situations can make us run faster. The problem is the relentless daily bouts of stress that many people put up with for economic reasons, careers, marriages, kids, etc. In that case the ongoing, chronic, or perhaps even skyrocketing stress won't just lead to high blood pressure or heart attacks. It will twist your brain, mind, and behavior while it counteracts your immune system and makes way for cascades of transformations that ultimately may drive the development of cancer (Stankiewicz et al., 2013; Wilson & Sato, 2014). How each of us reacts to or copes with stress is mainly decided by our lifestyles, childhood exposures, past experiences, attitudes, and genetics. This combination of nature and nurture is connected by means of epigenetics, which denotes the actions of regulatory proteins that bridge environmental input with the behavior of our chromosomes. Hence, our genes do not rely only on their underlying DNA sequence but also on the so-called epigenetic modulation of their activity (D'Urso & Brickner, 2014; Meng et al., 2015). In other words, the behavior of your genes doesn't depend only on your specific DNA sequence, since the genes are regulated by epigenetic factors. Moreover, epigenetics is influenced by your lifestyle and diet, and in the end, this machinery plays a critical role in health and disease.

Epigenetics refers to the biological processes performed by proteins inside the cell nucleus whereby heritable changes in the activity of our genes will occur, even though the specific sequence of DNA remains unchanged. Hence, epigenetic changes alter the way our cells make use of our genome—that is, which genes are turned on or off at a given time. All the while the inbred architecture of those genes (i.e., their DNA sequence) remains the same (D'Urso & Brickner, 2014; Meng et al., 2015). Epigenetic modulation of our genes' behavior is influenced by our lifestyle and can last throughout life. That is why they can be passed on to multiple generations of cells despite the fact that they are not put on display if you get your DNA sequenced.

Consequently we dynamically respond to our daily environment and lifestyle (diet, pets, exercise, smoking, marriage, sleep, friendships, meditation, adventures, fun, etc.) by adapting the activity of our DNA, and this is why each person becomes a genetic product formed by daily behaviors, choices, habits, and surroundings. It is not only a matter of our genetic or biological adaptation to life in general. It is also a matter of how resilient we are or can become in order to resist mutations, cellular damage, abnormalities, and/or cancer-promoting events. Hence, by our daily lifestyle and how we live our lives, we can influence our odds with regards to long-term health and disease (Meng et al., 2015).

In this regard, one of the most important hazards to avoid is chronic stress, and so we all have to eliminate our major stress triggers or work hard to improve our ability to wisely cope with stress, be it due to school/college, starting a new job, getting married or divorced, experiencing loss, or any other life event.

From Crappy to Happy

Vulnerable city dwellers need support from someone who is always loyal, caring, and available, and this is where our dogs come in. A dog represents a link to nature and lets us know that we are indispensable and never left alone (Beck & Katcher, 1983; Woods et al., 2007). Accordingly, people and in particular those with a city background are much more prone to consider their dogs not only as family members but also as their furry children. The reason is that dogs enrich us physically, psychologically, socially, and emotionally. That is why we seek their company (Grimm, 2014; Hare & Woods, 2013; Penkowa, 2014). It turns out that some doctors have known for ages how dogs improve people's mood, behavior, and psychosocial well-being (Johnson et al., 2002; Serpell, 1996; Walsh, 2009a,b).

From early on these effects were ascribed to the way dogs provided man with unconditional friendship, devotion, and a feeling of safety. Dogs also prevent us from feeling alone and miserable (Fine, 2010; O'Haire, 2009; Rossetti & King, 2010).

The plain act of being a dog's caretaker or serving as the one who feeds and walks him or her evokes the feeling of cohesiveness and daily contentment, whereby dogs represent a solid contrast to the digital world of cyberspace (Beck & Katcher, 1983; McConnell et al., 2011; McNicholas et al., 2005; Serpell, 1996). At least we have yet to see dogs trying to reach us by sending e-mails, and for that reason dogs are also our guarantee for being touched and having someone to touch (Miller, 2010; Smith, 2004). In fact, our tactile sense (the sense of touch) is the first sensory ability we attain as human beings, and in terms of social interaction and development, touch represents our very first way of communicating with others. In support of this, research shows how touching can be more accurate than talking as a mean for emotional communication (Chillot, 2013; Dunbar, 2010; Gallace & Spence, 2010). Tactile interaction such as holding, stroking and petting, is the key to social bonding, attachment, affiliation, and strengthening of relationships not only with our dog but also with other people (Beetz et al., 2012b; Feldman, 2012). In fact, research shows that our perception of comforting support and its soothing effect upon our minds and bodies can be determined by the amount of physical contact (touch) that we exchange, and this is not only true in adults. It also applies to insecure children (Beetz et al., 2012a). However, not many people will guarantee you gentle touches and snuggles as much and as sweet as your dog. That is why a dog's presence in some regards has been deemed superior to human company in terms of providing the most helpful emotional and psychosocial support (Beck & Katcher, 1983; Beetz et al., 2012a,b). In other words, dogs know touch and how to be touched.

The calming and stress-buffering effect of a dog's company is to a large degree mediated by our tactile contact (touching), and this fact reflects that humans are social by nature. So we are rewarded by means of brain biochemistry every time we touch another living being (Cheshire, 2013; Beetz et al., 2012b; Smith, 2004). Without touch, the brain of human babies fails to develop and function normally. We need physical affection and tactile inputs in order to survive the first years of life. Touch is critical for our emotional system to develop (McConnell, 2007). However, many cultures have impaired our opportunity to touch one another. Luckily that does not include pets. Dogs in particular are perfectly tactile in that their soft fur and snuggly quotient make them superbly cuddlesome to us (Horowitz, 2010; Olmert, 2009; Smith, 2004). The kind of unconditional touch (not associated with any drawback, consequence, or price to pay) has the most calming effect upon the human mind. That is why petting a friendly naturally leads to vast emotional and psychosocial benefits (Beetz et al., 2012; Feldman, 2012; McConnell, 2007; Smith, 2004).

Both adults and children interacting with dogs get vast emotional, social, and psychological benefits because the dog offers social bonding also through its gaze, body language, sounds, facial and emotional expressions.

That is why dogs make us feel good and relaxed. In fact, dogs send us a daily message stating how much they love us, and this is exactly what dogs say best.

Perhaps it's the dog's capacity to make our lives seem happier and more meaningful that makes many of us want to spoil our pets and sometimes even soak them in luxury.

Realize This

According to the APPA (the American Pet Products Association), which collects a very comprehensive consumer research study of the behaviors and the buying habits of pet owners, we are spending more than ever on our dogs. By 2012, Americans were spending almost fifty-three billion on their pets, which was more than double the level seen fifteen years ago. The expenses do not include traditional necessities like food and vaccinations, as a market for luxury pet products has been rapidly rising along with the current movement toward the daily pampering of dogs. Hence, consumers can easily get a variety of luxury products, accessories (doggy bling), and sumptuous services that are designed specifically for dogs and extend far beyond any canine necessity, including massages, classical music sessions, aromatherapy, acupuncture, spa treatments, among others.

In line with this, the pet care industry has proven to be recession-resistant. Hence, while most markets have experienced major difficulties during the global crisis, the pet care industry did exceptionally well, according to APPA. Generally the expenditures for pet care, services, and products have been steadily rising also on a global scale.

In line with this, the world's largest pharmaceutical company, Pfizer, invested time and money to develop the first prescription medication (dirlotapide) for treating canine obesity (Klonoff, 2007). Their staff knows that pet owners are ready to spend big money on their dogs, financial crisis or not.

There's little doubt that dogs are increasingly cherished by modern people. This assertion is supported by a 7 percent increase in American dog owners. In total, the American population increased by only 2 percent in the same period, as reported by the APPA. Surveys support the fact that dog owners consider their furry companions family members. Most people are not ashamed to admit that they love and cherish their dogs more than any other critter (O'Haire, 2009; Walsh, 2009a; Wood et al., 2007). In the APPA's survey, no less than 16 percent of dog owners declared that their dogs' medical needs take priority over their own treatments if they had to choose one over the other.

On the surface some (who don't own dogs) might think the payback for the dog's owner is pretty small, but in fact, this is not the case. According to mounting scientific studies, dogs return a great deal and most likely even more than they are receiving from us (Grimm, 2014; Penkowa, 2012; Serpell, 1996). Hence, a dog's company provides us with significantly improved health and happiness. The physiological and psychological benefits have been observed not only in dog owners but also in those visited by friendly dogs, including the disordered or healthy people, such as hospitalized patients, outpatients, institutionalized people, residents of nursing homes, kids in school, prisoners, combat soldiers, or the worker in business and organizational settings (Beetz et al., 2012a,b; Fine, 2010; Grimm, 2014; Goodavage, 2012; Jeon, 2011; Knisely et al., 2012; Kotrschal & Ortbauer, 2003; Marcus, 2011; Miller, 2010; Oyama & Serpell, 2013; Penkowa, 2014; Serpell, 1996; Wells, 2007; Wisdom et al., 2009).

Pills, Potions, or Pets?

The best things in life are rarely novel to mankind. The idea that *dogs are good for us* is by no means a novel one. Even if the last two decades of canine research are best described as burgeoning, one of the most elegant proof-of-concept studies was published more than twenty-three years ago by Dr. James A. Serpell, who is a professor at the School of Veterinary Medicine at the University of Pennsylvania. In a prospective study, Dr. Serpell assessed the health conditions of people before and after they adopted either a dog or a cat. The study was designed to determine whether a pet could change the recipient's health status and reveal any potential differences in the outcome of owning either a cat or a dog. In other words, Dr. Serpell could compare the participants' health conditions before the pet acquisitions with the putative changes induced by the pets as he followed them for ten months after the pets' arrivals (Serpell, 1990,1991). While the cat-acquiring group served as an interesting control with regards to the dog-acquiring group, a third group without any pet adoption served as a basic control to be followed in the same period of time.

In the first month after the pet acquisition, both dog and cat owners reported highly improved health conditions, but only the dog owners sustained the health benefits in the long run (Serpell, 1990, 1991). Hence, the dog could convey sustainable, long-term, significant health benefits as determined by assessing thirty different aspects of general health (the thirty-item general health questionnaire) and twenty health problems, such as headaches, hay fever, pain, difficulty sleeping, constipation/indigestion, eye problems, back problems, nerve problems, colds/flu, fatigue, kidney or bladder problems, lack of concentration, palpitations, breathlessness, ear problems, anxiety, coughing, faints, or dizziness. On top of this, dog owners reported other relevant improvements, such as reduced fear, increased self-esteem, and the feeling of safety, which were not found in the cat-acquiring group or in the controls without pets (Serpell, 1990, 1991).

These results have been validated by other scientists, and they show that a dog brings improved healthiness, better sleep at night, fewer visits to the doctor, reduced needs for medication, as well as less distress, depression, pain, anxiety, loneliness, and aging-related limitations in life (Engelman, 2013; Feng et al., 2014; Friedmann & Son, 2009; Grimm, 2014; Headey & Grabka, 2007; Herzog, 2011; kamioka et al., 2014; Knight & Edwards, 2008; O'Haire, 2009; Oyama & Serpell, 2013; Raina et al., 1999; Wood et al., 2007).

Therapy dogs in hospital settings also increase significantly the quality of care and quality of life, as they may promote both socialization, exercise, verbalization of feelings, relaxation of the mind, and improved mood (Fine, 2010; Bouchard et al., 2004; Caprilli & Messeri, 2006; Gagnon et al., 2004; Penkowa, 2014). As explained later in this book, within recent decades researchers have shown that the health effects are not only psychological but also physical and biochemical.

> Science shows how owning a dog can turn back the aging clock. In fact, living with a dog makes you act ten years younger (Feng et al., 2014).

A population study of 12,297 Norwegians aged between sixty-five and 101 years showed that dog owners are characterized by a significantly better health status than both people who don't own any pets and cat owners (Enmarker et al., 2012). Similar data on the health effects of dogs have been found all over the globe, whether it's European, American, Australian, or Asian populations that are studied (Grimm, 2014; Fine, 2010; Motooka et al., 2006; Oyama & Serpell, 2013; Penkowa, 2014; Serpell, 1996).

A study of elderly's use of physician services show that people increase their visits to the doctor in times of stress and adverse events (Siegel, 1990). However, dog owners are more resilient during adversities as they don't increase their doctor contacts the way other people do, even when burdened by major life pressure and/or bereavement (Siegel, 1990). This finding may have many explanations, but one way or the other, it reflects that a dog mediates resilience and an ability to bounce back.

This finding is corroborated by the German Socio-Economic Panel Survey and the International Social Science Survey Australia, which are longitudinal surveys of two general populations. More than twelve thousand households have participated in the surveys. They have all been interviewed every year since the survey began in 1984 (Headey, 2003; Headey & Grabka, 2007; Headey et al., 2002). Based on the collected data, it became clear how pets, mostly dogs, convey significant health benefits. That is why owners visit their doctor 15 percent less than people without pets. Science also shows how dog owners need less medication like painkillers and are less absent from work or school because of illness when they are compared to the behaviors or needs of matched groups of people who are not dog owners (Headey & Grabka, 2007; Headey et al., 2002; Marcus, 2011; Siegel, 1990). Accordingly, when dogs are allowed in nursing homes, the use of medication for the elderly residents can be significantly reduced, while the institutional expenses for the pharmaceutical treatments may be cut down by 50 percent (Geisler, 2004; Lust et al., 2007; Fine, 2010). Based on such evidence, it was estimated that in the year 2000 alone, pets led to a massive reduction in the national health costs, amounting to 5.59 billion euros for Germany and 3.86 billion dollars for Australia (Headey, 2003; Headey & Grabka, 2007; Headey et al., 2002).

What is perhaps the most interesting part is the reason why dog owners don't need the health-care system's services to the same degree as people without dogs. In particular, attention centers around the finding that dog owners cope better than other population groups when they experience loss and bereavement, during which the dog seems to prevent the need for visiting the doctor (Siegel, 1990). From research interviews it also emerged that owners of dogs have a completely different relationship to their pets than owners of cats or birds have. Consequently dog owners' enjoy a unique pet attachment, bonding, and companionship that were not found in the owners of other pet animals such as cats or birds (Siegel, 1990). This notion is supported by a range of other reports showing that a dog's company can be even more rewarding, soothing, and recuperative than talking to another human (Beck & Katcher, 1983; Becker, 2002; Fine, 2010; Miller, 2010; O'Haire, 2009; Sakson, 2009; Serpell, 1996; Walsh, 2009a,b; Wells, 2007). Dogs make us feel safe, loved, and worthwhile, and they provide us with a purpose in life even when we don't think life has any meaning left.

This is why we consider our dogs full-fledged members of our families, and no less than a third of urban homes include canine family members (Toohey & Rock, 2011). In many Western countries a high level of pet ownership is seen, and so it is not surprising that Australian researchers reported that the most common play activity of girls in primary and secondary school was playing with pets; however, in case of boys in secondary and primary school, pet interactions provide their second and third most common leisure activity (Martin et al., 2014).

In the United States, a third of all Americans and 50 percent of single people report to rely more on their pets than on human relations, and in line with this, there are more households with pets than there are homes with children (Grimm, 2014; Oyama & Serpell, 2013). This trend influences national health statistics since owning a dog makes us less likely to fall victim to stress-related conditions, misery, social isolation, and a range of severe diseases like heart attacks, brain and mental disorders (dementia, depression, and anxiety), cancer, chronic pain, and allergies. As a result these conditions are significantly more prevalent in people without dogs (Becker, 2002; Fine, 2010; Friedmann & Son, 2009; kamioka et al., 2014; Marcus, 2011; Penkowa, 2014; Oyama & Serpell, 2013; Wells, 2011).

Dogs lead to health expenditure savings because their mere presence leads to a substantial decrease in medication usage (Grimm, 2014; Penkowa, 2012). As opposed to those without access to therapy dogs, patients receiving dog therapy cut down their need for psychoactive drugs and painkillers, and all the while the health-care costs go down by 50 percent (Geisler, 2004; Lust et al., 2007).

The observed associations between a dog's presence and improved human health are found after one controls for a range of demographic, medical, psychological, social, behavioral, and/or environmental factors, which in any given study are identified as being relevant contributors to the observations. Hence, all studies include matched control groups without dogs and/or control conditions in which the dog is absent or removed or replaced by another type of pet. These control aspects are a matter of course, as one would otherwise not know whether it's the dog or the lifestyle in general that improves health.

Mind Matters

Dogs are good for us in countless ways, and from scientific efforts in the recent decades, we have gained significant insight into the dog's way of influencing our lives (Barker & Wolen, 2008; Fine, 2010; Friedmann & Son, 2009; Headey, 2003; Knisely et al., 2012; Marcus, 2011; McConnell et al., 2011; McNicholas et al., 2005; O'Haire, 2009; Oyama & Serpell, 2013; Penkowa, 2012; Walsh, 2009a; Wells, 2007,2011).

First of all dogs make us feel empowered, an effect reported in both children, adults, and the elderly, and this is in part due to the dog's ability to distract us from our worries (Beetz et al., 2012a,b; Feldman, 2012; Parish-Plass, 2008; Serpell, 1996). Therefore, dogs alleviate the burden of life's adverse events, such as separation/divorce and bereavement, and promote the owner's resilience and psychosocial functioning (Headey, 2003; Johnson et al., 2002; Siegel, 1990; Walsh, 2009a,b).

It's well-known that an attractive spectacle or stimulus like the sight of a furry dog will distract us, and by the mere distraction we forget our troubles (Serpell, 1996). As such, appropriate distraction can be used as a coping strategy or emotional relief from stressful situations or misery. Hence, doctors often apply distraction techniques for their patients in order to shift the focus away from negative thoughts and engage the mind in a more appropriate way. Thereby, the power of distraction may reduce feelings of stress, anxiety, depression, and various chronic pain symptoms (Engelman, 2013; Marcus, 2011; Osei-Bonsu et al., 2014). The plus side of appropriate distraction became evident in a scientific study that subjected volunteers to experimental pain with or without a simultaneous mental distraction, and the conclusion was that pain sensitivity was reduced and pain endurance was increased in subjects who were mentally distracted (Kumar et al., 2012). This might be why dogs, true masters in distracting us from our surroundings, have such an astonishing ability to reduce pain, stress, and discomfort. This effect is seen in both dog owners, patients who are visited by a friendly dog, and the staff working in clinics using dogs on a regular basis (Becker, 2002; Fine, 2010; Marcus et al., 2012; Penkowa, 2014; Sakson, 2009).

In fact, dogs are continuously reported to significantly relieve some common symptoms, such as aches, stress, anxiety, melancholy, the feeling of loneliness and misery, just to mention some highly prevalent conditions in modern society, all of which take their toll on human health and increase mortality rates (Barker & Wolen, 2008; Engelman, 2013; Ernst, 2013; Friedmann & Son, 2009; Hawkley & Cacioppo, 2003,2010; Marcus, 2013a).

A dog's company can activate our most potent hormones and rewarding molecules (feel-good chemicals), including dopamine, oxytocin, endorphins, beta-phenylethylamine, and prolactin, while at the same time the stress hormones cortisol, epinephrine, and norepinephrine are reduced (Cole et al., 2007; Odendaal, 2000; Odendaal & Meintjes, 2003; Payne et al., 2015). These biochemical changes have a significant impact upon our brains, emotions, and behavior, and this is in part why dogs are able to convey the feeling of harmony, well-being, cohesion, devotion, and bonding, which paves the way for our confidence, good behavior, mental thriving, sociability, and emotional balance (Feldman, 2012; Marcus, 2011; Olmert, 2009; Penkowa, 2012; Serpell, 1996; Walsh, 2009a,b).

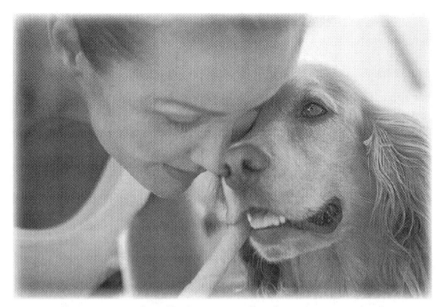

When you pet a friendly dog, your cells release certain molecules and hormones that benefit the brain and mind.

In fact, the more time you let your kids pet friendly dogs, the more their stress hormones drop, as shown by a European research project that studied the effects of social support by a dog (Beetz et al., 2012a).

These hormonal and emotional changes are not only found in us humans. They also apply to dogs (Coppola et al., 2006; Hare & Woods, 2013; Odendaal, 2000; Odendaal & Meintjes, 2003; Romero et al., 2014).

Moreover, memory, learning, and cognitive performance are improved in preschool children when they are tested in the presence of therapy dogs. These results were compared to their performance in the presence of a fake dog (a stuffed toy dog) or a human ally (Gee et al., 2010a,b; Jalongo et al., 2004). Likewise, the kids made fewer errors in a cognitive task in the real dog's presence, and the dog also improved the learning speed and accuracy within the preschool children. At least their scores reflected as much (Gee et al., 2007,2010a,b). Hence, by its mere presence, a friendly dog effectively promoted the children's cognitive capacity, learning, and memory relative to the effects of a fake dog or a human. In general, having a dog in the classroom is shown to be a cost-effective and simple way of improving learning and behavior in children (Kotrschal & Ortbauer, 2003).

Research performed by Andrea Beetz at the University of Rostock in Germany aimed to examine stress reactions in German and Austrian children with learning, emotional, and behavior disorders. The soothing effects of either a friendly dog, a friendly human (female student), or a toy dog were measured with regards to children's stress levels and behaviors, and the study showed what most dog owners would probably guess. A real dog is superior to both controls. Hence, the (real) dog significantly surpassed both the student and the toy in terms of providing comfort and emotional support, relieving the effects of stress, and reducing levels of cortisol (Beetz et al., 2012a). The levels of stress hormone dropped faster and steeper when the kids were together with the dog as compared to the effects of the controls, which explains why many children or adults turn to pets in times of sadness. What's interesting in this regard is the fact that the dog's calming effect was not linked to ownership of the dog. The study used a group of small to medium-sized dogs consisting of a cavalier King Charles spaniel, a Jack Russell terrier, a Norwegian lundehund, and two mongrels.

Among the many interesting findings of this work, the dog's impact was related to the amount of physical touching and stroking of the dog, and this aspect shed light on the molecular mechanisms of action. Touch can increase our hormone levels of oxytocin, which conveys feelings of empathy, confidence, and attachment, while it effectively inhibits cortisol synthesis, leading to calmness and relaxation (Beetz et al., 2012a,b; Olmert, 2009; Onaka et al., 2012). In accordance with this, researchers have shown how anxiety, depression, loneliness, and mental disorders are significantly reduced in dog owners as well as in those who regularly are visited by friendly dogs, and the same effect is found in children and adolescents suffering from behavioral, emotional, or developmental disorders (Fine, 2010; Friedmann & Son, 2009; Le Roux & Kemp, 2009; Marcus, 2011; Martin & Farnum, 2002; McConnell et al., 2011; McNicholas et al., 2005; Wells, 2011).

In fact, the more owners pet, cherish or simply gaze at their dogs, the more oxytocin is released in both the owner and the dog (Nagasawa et al., 2009a,b,2015; Payne et al., 2015). Moreover, dog owners who kiss their dogs release significantly more oxytocin than owners who never kiss their dogs - and the same effect is found in the dogs being kissed (Handlin, 2010). The consequence of this may explain why dogs endow their owners with more confidence and promote social contact and trust in other people (Beetz et al., 2012a,b; Black, 2012; O'Haire, 2009; Wells, 2007). This also reflects that the close bond between dog and man is not just an extension or a replacement of our relationships with other people (Katcher & Beck, 1983; Walsh, 2009b; Zilcha-Mano et al., 2011). In fact, research shows how dog owners enjoy better social support, better family lives, and more friends, and believe it or not, dog owners report better sexual lives too (Irani et al., 2006; Raina et al., 1999). Thereby, the dog is not only a valued pet but also as a loyal, caring comrade who provides emotional and social support, well-being, and numerous health benefits.

Always on My Mind

Another mechanism contributing to the previously mentioned health improvements is the dog's ability to serve as an attachment figure (a significant other with whom an emotional bond is developed), whereby dogs match us humans with yet another skill. Both people and dogs can provide an attachment figure in the dog-owner relationship (Katcher & Beck, 1983; Payne et al., 2015; Zilcha-Mano et al., 2011). An attachment figure helps us feel safe, sound, and loved, whereby we develop self-confidence, self-worth, and a favorable self-image, which are essential feats in terms of emotional development, acceptable psychosocial behavior, and good mental health throughout life. There are four requirements for being an attachment figure, and they include (1) proximity seeking, (2) secure base, (3) separation distress, and (4) safe haven (Katcher & Beck, 1983; Kurdek, 2008,2009; Olmert, 2009; Zilcha-Mano et al., 2011, 2012). These four elements are evoked by both dogs and owners when they are mutual attachment figures because (1) they automatically seek each other's company (proximity seeking); (2) the dog endows his or her owner with increased confidence, which is why the owner is more audacious when accompanied by the dog (secure base); (3) owners bereft of their dogs show separation distress, meaning they are significantly affected by their loss; and finally (4) the dog is often serving as a calming, reassuring, and comforting friend who counters the owner's anxiety, distress, and feelings of weakness, whereby the dog provides a safe haven.

In addition to this, seeking a dog's company and support in times of need might represent a better strategy for stress relief than the one to get from a human relative, even if the latter is unquestionably the most powerful in terms of practical assistance or capacity.

The difference in the bonding towards our dog versus another human being might also explain why most modern people go through divorces and split up relationships, while it is quite rare that we file for divorce from the dog. In fact, modern humans don't seem to mind getting a new spouse or house once in a while, but our dog stays till death us do part.

> "A pet is an island of sanity in what appears to be an insane world. Friendship retains its traditional values and securities in one's relationship with one's pet. Whether a dog, cat, bird, fish, turtle, or what have you, one can rely upon the fact that one's pet will always remain a faithful, intimate, non-competitive friend—regardless of the good or ill fortune life brings us."
> —Dr. Boris Levinson, child psychologist (Levinson, 1962).

This notion finds support in current research showing how pet support may equal human social support with regards to soothing us during distress, sadness, anxiety, and feelings of loneliness, which are not only negative mind-sets but also independent risk factors that make us vulnerable to chronic diseases (Ernst, 2013; Hare & Woods, 2013; McConnell et al., 2011; Sakson, 2009; Serpell, 1996; Shubert, 2012a; Walsh, 2009a; Wood et al., 2007).

When a dog endows us with social support, it also brings great friendship that is always available and easy to reach without the need for making an appointment first. This kind of psychosocial support *ad libitum* has major impact upon our state of mind and resilience (DeCourcey et al., 2010; Walsh, 2009a,b; Wells, 2007,2009,2011). As described in a brilliant book by Dr. James A. Serpell, social support, bonding and reciprocal interactions with others are *per se* key determinants of health and disease resistance, which is due to humans' highly social nature (Serpell, 1996). To this end, it is interesting to know, that scientists have demonstrated that dogs provide a mutual relationship able to meet our psychological, social and emotional needs, as to why the dog-human bond to a large degree mimics an interpersonal bond (Becker, 2002; McConnell, 2007; McConnell et al., 2011; O'Haire, 2009; Wood et al., 2007). Even more so, people who are ostracized or excluded from their usual network can benefit from a dog's company, as science shows it can serve as a satisfactory substitute for human relations (Aydin et al., 2012).

In some research studies, specially trained dogs were brought in at clinical settings, hospitals and nursing homes, and as a result of the dog visits patients showed improved mood, less stress and reduced anxiety (Walsh, 2009a,b). In fact, the overall health benefits are induced by a dog's presence, whether it is our own companion (pet) dog or a professional therapy, activity or service dog (Aoki et al., 2012; Beals, 2009; Cole et al., 2007; Handlin, 2010; Handlin et al., 2011; Nagasawa et al., 2009a; Odendaal, 2000; Odendaal & Meintjes, 2003). Along with the support provided by the pet itself, a dog also leads to other benefits by facilitating our social interactions or talking to others simply due to the dog presence, which makes it easier to talk to strangers (Walsh, 2009a,b; Wells, 2007,2009,2011; Wood et al., 2007).

As explained later in this book, the various dog-mediated effects upon the human brain and mind become even more relevant and needed, when we are succumbing to diseases.

Perhaps you think that lonely, pitiful people compensate for their social insufficiencies by getting a dog, and so, it would make many dog owners look rather pathetic. However, surveys support that dog owners are not seeking their dog as a sort of social replacement therapy, as dog owners generally have very good network of close contacts, friends, and family. Hence, the data indicate that buying a pet is a social supplement, not a surrogate (Hare & Woods, 2013).

Anyhow, these aspects are relevant for elderly people residing in long-term care facilities, as a dog is a most effective way to reduce loneliness, even if the dog only visits once a week (Banks & Banks, 2002). Interestingly, research has also shown that pet attachment as a means for support might sometimes be superior to human social support in terms of reducing negative feelings. Hence, in a study of 159 elderly pet owners, human support was unable to improve the owners' feelings of depression, while dog attachment support altered both feelings of loneliness and depression

(Krause-Parello, 2008,2012). Along with a better mood, the elderly dog owners also showed significantly improved vitality, wellbeing and general health levels, when compared to elderly people with other pets than dogs (Gulick & Krause-Parello, 2012).

Scientific work has also shown that the direct interaction with the dog -not the increased socialization among residents- accounts for the improvements (Banks & Banks, 2002,2005). As such, some of us would likely prefer to be visited by a dog than to join group therapy.

Nevertheless, the dog's impact is highly interesting from a geriatric point of view, since it points toward dog attachment as a coping mechanism that may break highly unfavorable health conditions like loneliness, depression and poor overall health. This specifies how important the human-dog bond is and that its health benefits may go well beyond those of another person's social support. Another take-home message is the importance of letting residents keep their pets rather than imposing a ban upon pet keeping in nursing homes. The latter is often and sadly the case in most institutions, nursing homes and hospices. However, for those who turn to science, the evidence is clear and shows how dogs are able to provide unsurpassed social, emotional and clinical support for their companion people.

From Bodybuilding to Buddy Building

There's no doubt that dogs are good for us in countless ways. The same can be said about physical exercise, which is also an essential part of a healthy lifestyle, and in fact, the best way to get everyone up and going regardless of age and health barriers is to get a dog. Dog owners report how their pets are a key source of motivation to exercise, and on top of this, dog walking facilitates social interactions with other people, the feeling of coherence, and community support. It also increases the bond between the dog and his or her owner (Enmarker et al., 2012; Fine, 2010; Garcia et al., 2015; Grimm, 2014; Knight & Edwards, 2008; Marcus, 2011; Penkowa, 2014; Wood et al., 2007). As a result, dogs can be very powerful motivators of outdoor activity regardless of impediments like rough weather, old age, time of day, minor illness, loneliness, exhaustion, insecurity about walking in the streets, depression, mourning, or other reasons that would otherwise make us cancel a walk without a dog (Abbud et al., 2014; Fine, 2010; Garcia et al., 2015; Knight & Edwards, 2008; Marcus, 2011; Rondeau et al., 2010; Toohey & Rock, 2011). Accordingly, a number of studies indicate that at least some dog owners are more likely to take daily walks and achieve recommended exercise levels than people without dogs (Christian et al., 2013; Coleman et al., 2008; Feng et al., 2014; Johnson et al., 2011; Reeves et al., 2011; Shibata et al., 2012; Toohey et al., 2013). However, many dog owners do not necessarily prefer to walk their dogs, and they still enjoy the health benefits provided by a dog's company and friendship. Dogs go much deeper under our skin than merely serving as exercise promoters as explained later in this section. An interesting observation concerning the owners' eagerness to walk their dogs comes from a Norwegian study conducted at the University of Tromsø, where researchers concluded that owners' engagement in dog walking and the time spent walking are closely related to the owners' degree of attachment to their dogs (Andreassen et al., 2008). The same study also added another interesting association. The more owners loved their dogs, the more they benefitted from dog exposure and vice versa. The dogs also benefit from this walk, and loving dog owners are more willing to take their furry darling out in the fields no matter what as compared to owners who aren't as attached to their pets.

To get to the heart of the matter, Dr. Rebecca Johnson, a professor at the University of Missouri and director of the Research Center for Human-Animal Interaction, performed research studies showing that dogs provide a better walking companion than humans. That's why we'd rather walk dogs than join friends or spouses for walks. Even when the walking companion dog is not our own pet but a loaner dog we are assigned to walk, we are more likely to commit to physical activity. Moreover, walking with a dog instead of a human being results in much better fitness levels and walking speeds, which were increased by 28 percent thanks to the dog, as compared to only 4 percent without the dog (Johnson & Meadows, 2010; Johnson et al., 2011). One of the reasons for this effect might be the dog's need to be taken out for a walk, while human walking companions make various excuses for skipping the walk.

A German study supported this, as it showed how a therapy dog can motivate obese children to become physically active and engage in exercise.

Furthermore, obese kids profit much more from a dog's company than they do from a friend, as the dog's ability to motivate surpasses that of a friendly human (Wohlfarth et al., 2013)

As you would expect, owning a dog makes us even more prone to walk on a daily basis, but when we take a closer look, things become a bit more complex.

First of all, dog owners comprise a very heterogeneous population, and so not all dog owners actually walk their dogs.

A study of 2,533 community-dwelling people found that only 36 percent of dog owners walked their dogs at least three times per week (Thorpe et al., 2006b). Other researchers also reported that no more than 30 percent of dog owners achieved the recommended exercise levels needed for health (Ishikawa-Takata & Tabata, 2007; Penkowa, 2014). Among those who walk the dog regularly, the net increase in walking activity per week is no more than eighteen to nineteen minutes (i.e., less than three minutes per day) (Bauman et al., 2001; Yabroff et al., 2008). In addition, the dog walking performed by elderly owners is described as "nonexercise-related walking" since it is more of a relaxing sauntering than a bout of exercise (Thorpe et al., 2006a).

The dog owner's exercise potential by means of dog walking remains to be realized. Hence, the majority of owners let their dogs run free in the garden, or they hire dog walkers.

Even when we look at those dog owners who take the opportunity to exercise more than people who don't own dogs, the question remains. Is it the dog that truly increases walking activity, or are these owners simply doing more exercise? Perhaps they are more active regardless of their dog ownership. Recent data points to the latter since elderly people who own dogs and are very active physically do report that they were also significantly more active in their youth (Feng et al., 2014). The increased dog walking found in some owners may also replace their usual exercise sessions, and thereby owning a dog does not automatically lead to increased exercise.

However, what can be said is that exercise is healthy for you, and your dog certainly provides you with the perfect incentive to exercise with him or her on a daily basis. However, should you for some reason decide not to walk the dog yourself, you may find comfort in the next section.

You don't necessarily have to walk your furry friend to gain health benefits from your dog. In fact, the health effects from dogs do not rely on whether you walk the dog or not (Arhant-Sudhir et al., 2011; Bauman et al., 2001; Beals, 2009; Fine, 2010; Friedmann & Son, 2009; Serpell, 1996). To be absolutely clear, the human health benefits conveyed by dogs are independent from walking the dog, indicating that dogs are able to change our biology regardless of any potential exercise. Secondly the health benefits conveyed by dogs are found in patients visited by therapy dogs that typically sits next to the patients for ten to thirty minutes, after which the dog leaves. In such cases no physical exercise took place, and yet the dog mediates a range of health benefits. Thirdly research shows that a dog conveys the most health benefits when we are petting him or her calmly inside our home (Motooka et al., 2006).

The latter point is derived from a cleverly designed research study performed in healthy Japanese subjects who were exposed to a study dog, a cavalier King Charles spaniel. The researchers detected changes in the autonomic nervous system by means of electrocardiographic monitoring in the participants as a measure of their overall health (Motooka et al., 2006). This was done while participants were walking with and without the dog, during their routine activities at home, and while they were petting or interacting with the dog at home (Motooka et al., 2006).

Thereby, the experiment could specify how much healthiness we gained from dogs if we (1) walked the dog, (2) walked without the dog, (3) pet the dog or interacted with the dog inside our home, and (4) let the dog into our home while we engaged in routine activities but did not interact with the dog.

The results showed that walking with the dog conveyed greater health benefits than walking the same route without the dog. The researchers also concluded that the dog confers health improvements regardless of walking as a result of the mere presence of the dog in our home. Even if we didn't interact much, the dog's presence brought massive health benefits. Surprisingly the biggest health benefits were obtained when participants were petting or quietly talking to the dog inside their homes (Motooka et al., 2006).

This is of huge interest since it underscores that you don't have to walk the dog to gain its health benefits. You just have to spend some time with your furry friend.

In fact, we may have to revise our very idea of the impact of exercise on certain human conditions since exercise is no panacea for any problem in life (Scheede-Bergdahl et al., 2005). Hence, some of the claims made in relation to exercise have not been thoroughly substantiated, or they were discarded because of lack of evidence. For example, it was proposed that exercise provides a remedy for depression, even though it has still to be verified in larger trials with human participants. In actual fact, some work was done on the subject, and it showed that exercise is not always equally beneficial. In any case, exercise does not always constitute an efficient antidepressant treatment (Krogh et al., 2011, 2012).

While dog owners in general display better health and life quality than people who do not own dogs, it is a bit of a paradox that pet owners in general have increased body mass index and smoke more than controls without pets (Hare & Woods, 2014; Koivusilta and Ojanlatva, 2006; Müllersdorf et al., 2010; Parslow & Jorm, 2003). However, attachment, companionship, and bonding with the dog are more important mechanisms than the traditional risk factor concept (like exercise) as evidenced in dog owners who display significant health gains and reduced rates of various disorder, such as (but not restricted to) diabetes, hypertension, depression, dementia, pain, cancer, and allergies when they are compared to those who do not own dogs (Becker, 2002; Cole et al., 2007; Dimitrijević, 2009; Fine, 2010; Friedmann & Son, 2009; Lentino et al., 2012; Marcus, 2011; Muñoz Lasa & Franchignoni, 2008; Penkowa, 2014; Odendaal, 2000; Oyama & Serpell, 2013; Sakson, 2009; Wells, 2011).

Note, however, that this is not advice against regular exercise, healthy eating habits, and the need to quit smoking. Not at all. The only point here is that scientific data point toward dogs and dog therapy as being superior to many other typical health interventions. And for those who would like to optimize all possible parameters, you shouldn't hesitate to exercise daily or quit smoking, as they are good for you no matter what. Nevertheless, regardless of lifestyles, people aiming at better health would want to spend as much time as possible with their dogs.

> Wise is the one who exercises and eats well. Wisest is the one who keeps a dog close.

I Know You

There're a number of additional reasons why your dog is second to none concerning your reciprocity and attachment, which may explain why dogs provide us with unrivaled stress relief and well-being.

First of all, the dog is always available and is not competitive. The dog has all interest and faith in you ... and you only. Secondly your dog will keep your secrets and abstain from taking advantage of you, and thirdly you can always count on your dog in terms of getting a predictable, supporting, and calming response (Horowitz, 2010; Serpell, 1996; Walsh, 2009a; Zilcha-Mano et al., 2011,2012). The latter should be taken quite literally since dogs share with us the ability to express ourselves nonverbally by means of facial expressions, posture, sounds, and body language. This is one of the reasons why dogs are considered such good friends, as they are able to express sympathy and empathy by miming. Thus, they have a huge advantage over other pets that are much less able or perhaps not able at all to differentially control their facial muscles or body language as part of their emotional expression.

Those who pay close attention can obtain a vast amount of information from their dogs' appearances, as their personality traits and various emotions are expressed by their body language and behavior, including posture, positioning, movements, gaze, tail activity, and vocalizations. Dogs can adeptly communicate their intents and feelings, including their worries, disappointment, sadness, surprise, anger, delight, fear, weariness, jealousy, or trust (Bekoff, 2007; Coren, 2000,2004; Harris & Prouvost, 2014; McConnell, 2002,2007; Mendl et al., 2010; Range et al., 2009; Smith, 2004).

Suggested reading: I highly recommend you read Dr. Marc Bekoff's book *The Emotional Lives of Animals: A Leading Scientist Explores Animal Joy, Sorrow, and Empathy—and Why They Matter* to gain insight into the vast richness of animal emotions or visit his webpage [http://www.literati.net/authors/marc-bekoff/] for more.

In our communication with human friends, we primarily use spoken or written words to describe thoughts, and so humans automatically become very capable of hiding or twisting our true opinion. We can also hurt one another with words. How many times do we tell white lies just to get by or avoid unnecessary conflicts? According to surveys, we all (humans) lie, and telling lies is a very common, frequent, and daily activity in most interpersonal interactions. It contains obvious prosocial benefits, though it also holds an antisocial risk.

Studies show that even some physicians are not always being honest with their patients as up to one-third of medical doctors choose to withhold information from their patients (Iezzoni et al., 2012). In contrast, nonverbal communication, such as that conveyed by our body language, emotions, and facial expressions, is much less deceptive since it is largely controlled by the autonomous (involuntary) nervous system. Therefore, it functions below the level of conscious thought, slyness, and opportunism. This is why we are not in command of the body's emotional signals, and for that same reason most people prefer to use a text message or phone call when they are telling lies. Otherwise, it takes an award-winning actor to do it convincingly, and yet even the best ones fail once in a while.

This is exactly why we trust and rely so much on our dogs. We quickly realize that what we see is what we get, or in other words, dogs don't lie.

In fact, your dog is also most likely to respond in a relevant and timely manner to your outpourings since dogs are true experts when it comes to reading, sensing, and interpreting us (Horowitz, 2010; McConnell, 2002,2007; Serpell, 1996). To this end, the dog's perception of and sensitivity to us are no less than magic, and they outshine the capacity of any human being, most medical doctors, any high-tech medical equipment (Coren, 2000,2004; Fogle, 1990; Horowitz, 2010; Wells, 2012). Just to mention one example, dogs mirror their handlers' cortisol concentration, whereby increased stress hormones in the handler is followed by increased stress hormones in the dogs (Buttner et al., 2015). In other words, a biochemical synchronization of hormonal changes has been demonstrated between the two species. These astonishing abilities deserve an in-depth description because they are utterly enthralling and because they serve as a starting point with regards to explaining the diagnostic and therapeutic potential of dogs within the health-care sector, which is addressed later in this book.

CHAPTER 3

If You're Sick, My Dog Lets You Know

Bring in the Dogs

Dogs are superior to any other species in terms of decoding human behavior, mental states, and emotions (Berns et al., 2014; Horowitz, 2010; McConnell, 2002,2007; Payne et al., 2015; Racca et al., 2012; Siniscalchi et al., 2013b). Also, dogs possess fine-tuned skills to help them communicate with humans, and though there are breed differences in aptitudes, any dog regardless of pedigree is able to exchange complex information with humans. Hence, dogs behave quite differently when they accompany a confident person as opposed to someone who is insecure (Elgier et al., 2009a,b; Faragó et al., 2014; (Hare & Woods, 2013; Jakovcevic et al., 2010; Miklósi, 2007; Silva & de Sousa, 2011; Siniscalchi et al., 2013b).

Accordingly, no other animal is as suitable as the dog for completing missions such as saving people's lives, identifying victims or cadavers after natural disasters, locating bombs or explosives, gas pipeline leaks, invasive species, off-flavors in food, livestock in estrus, or serving as a nonstop guardian of disabled or blind people (Jones, 2011). Truth is that working under such conditions or in such fields is something that necessitates stamina, impetus, and audacity, and who on earth would dare to do it except for heroic dogs?

But how do they do it? Do they have magic senses? Well, nobody knows the full story, but because of the recent decades of canine research, we have gained insight into some important parts of the story, and so this chapter will reveal the scientifically verified information on how the dog senses, perceives, and reacts to the world and us humans. After you have read through this chapter, try to think about its message for a moment, particularly if you own a dog, because the truth is that you are sharing your home with a true genius. Though they never graduated from university, dogs are expert anthropologists and therapists with a natural talent to seemingly apply some of those clinical skills that graduates from universities are often taught.

Canine Anthropologists

From the beginning of our common history humans and canines have converged in terms of behavior, cognition, and emotional states. Hence, combined research in dogs and humans have demonstrated a range of functional similarities, most of which likely emerged as a consequence of comparable environmental selection pressures during our coevolution (Horowitz, 2010; Miklósi, 2007; Reid, 2009; Smith, 2004; Udell et al., 2011).

Though both species lived in proximity and for a long period may have benefitted from reciprocal interactions, the relationship became somewhat uneven when ancestral humans took control of the food rations. This change made canines dependent on human goodwill for food, and as in any other social inequality the subordinate has to adapt to the situation or cut loose. The obvious pick was adaptation with quite a lot of patience and flexibility. So dogs adapted to the new balance by developing a meticulous ability to interpret human behavior and to communicate with their keepers (Gácsi et al., 2004,2009; Hare et al., 2002; McConnell, 2007; Miklósi, 2007; Silva & de Sousa, 2011). By means of a tentative and ongoing approach, dogs found out how and when to loom in order to get what they wanted (food) from their keepers, and to do this without too many misses, they had to develop an acute sensitivity to the behavioral and emotional signals that humans emitted (Call et al., 2003; Lakatos, 2012; Miklósi & Topál, 2013; Udell et al., 2010). So they did, and dogs managed to find out when and how to best behave in order to draw human attention, not to mention when to vanish or express signs of submission.

As a result, dogs have developed a highly attuned communication system based upon their sensory capacity to see, hear, smell, follow, and literally sense humans, and dogs respond by expressing a wide array of visual cues, body language, and sounds. Hence, dogs use postures, actions, looks, nonverbal sound cues, gait, and movements that collectively point to their particular reaction and state of mind (Hare & Woods, 2013; McConnell, 2007; Miklósi, 2007; Miklósi & Topál, 2013; Smith, 2004). In fact, dogs signal their inner states or intentions much like poker players who show their *tells*, and so all you have to do is start looking at him or her. Soon you will become aware of some previously overlooked visible features, such as the dog's activity, gaze, positioning, or physical configuration of the tail, limbs, head, and eyes (Coren, 2000,2004; Horowitz, 2010; McConnell, 2002,2007; Rugaas, 2006). Though dogs are not as verbally eloquent as humans, and despite they don't use words dogs are nevertheless communicating all the time, even if many dog owners often don't notice.

Back in the Ice Age, canines found out how to best read, interact with, and modify human behaviors in a way that secured their survival (i.e., provided continuous food supplies). Indeed, dogs are exceptionally skilled at reading our emotions, intentions, body language, gestures, and behavioral clues, something dogs do much better than any other species. They are even better than our closest primate relatives, the chimpanzees (Call et al., 2003; Hare et al., 2002; Payne et al., 2015; Reid, 2009; Udell et al., 2010). In fact, dogs are so good at adjusting to us that they adapt their physiology by means of hormone concentration according to their owner's mentality and not least the owner's release of hormones (Jones & Josephs, 2006).

A recent study showed that dogs' hormone levels change when their owners' hormone concentrations change, and this synchronization of hormonal changes in owner and dog was independent from the owners' behavior towards their dogs (Buttner et al., 2015). The consequence of this biochemical association is that you can't fool your dog by behavioral expression or by acting, as your furry friend is able to react to your inner biochemistry and the molecular levels of hormones inside your body (Buttner et al., 2015). The synchronization reflects our fine-tuned reciprocity across the species boundary. It's why any dog owner's emotional state is translated into his or her dog's behavior, whether it's negative or positive (Podberscek & Serpell, 1997; McConnell, 2007; Rehn et al., 2014). My point here is to state loud and clear that there are no bad or unbalanced dogs. There are bad, unbalanced owners.

This notion is further supported by other research studies showing how humans and dogs converge on behavioral genetics since our social traits, manners, and bonding abilities emerge to be governed by the same neural, hormonal, and genetic mechanisms (Kis et al., 2014; Parker et al., 2010; Payne et al., 2015). This is yet another indicator of our coevolution and common past.

In contrast to other species, dogs comprehend human communication in ways that other animals do not, as dogs are able to integrate and process various, simultaneous and complex information gathered from humans and their context. Dogs even do this while they perform given tasks like the times when they have to locate hidden items (Gácsi et al., 2004,2009; Kaminski et al., 2012; Kirchhofer et al., 2012; Lakatos et al., 2012; Miklósi et al., 2003; Scheider et al., 2011; Téglás et al., 2012; Topál et al., 2009). Hence, dogs may simultaneously incorporate various expressions, such as our posture, facial mime, movements, hand gestures, involuntary muscle contractions, tone of voice, bodily tension, skin reactions, limpness, gaze, contextual factors, and past experience. They are also able to follow dynamic changes in our expression in order to finally draw the right conclusion (Coren, 2004; Hare & Woods, 2013; McConnell, 2007; Miklósi, 2007; Miklósi & Topál, 2013).

Consequently dogs understand indirect and complex communicative signals even when they are conveyed among other people. Dogs can interpret different behavioral and social clues correctly, and they can grasp contextual clues in order to find meaning (Coren, 2000; Kaminski et al., 2012; Kirchhofer et al., 2012; Kis et al., 2012; Lakatos et al., 2012; McConnell, 2007; Miklósi et al., 2003; Scheider et al., 2011; Téglás et al., 2012).

These abilities of dogs are also manifest because they are rich in mirror neurons, which are essential for their social cognition including the decoding of our emotions, intentions, and states of mind (Grimm, 2014; Hare & Woods, 2013; Reid, 2009; Udell & Wynne, 2011; Udell et al., 2010,2011). As explained later in this book, one of the secrets behind the dog's amazing gifts is the impressive sensory perception allowing the dog to register and react to impending health problems (Coren, 2000,2004; McConnell, 2002,2007; Miklósi, 2007).

> "If a dog will not come to you after having looked you in the face, you should go home and examine your conscience."
> —Woodrow Wilson, twenty-ninth president of the United States

Reveals More Than He Conceals

In delicate ways dogs decode other individuals in order to obtain social, emotional, or practical information that can guide his behavior or reactions toward new or potentially important objects, stimuli, or situations (Coren, 2004; Horowitz, 2010; Merola et al., 2012a,b). To this end, dogs may also differentiate between the emotional states of individuals. Certainly this provides an explanation for why dogs obviously don't trust every human being they encounter. Accordingly, the performance, emotional state, and social behavior of dogs vary depending on their human company. This has been shown in a series of research studies of dogs' performance and reactions to different human emotions. Results clearly varied when the dogs were with their owners, with other familiar persons, or with strangers (Berns et al., 2014; Cook et al., 2014; Gácsi et al., 2013; Kerepesi et al., 2014; Kubinyi et al., 2007). Needless to say, dogs perform better when they are accompanied by their owners or people they trust, in particular when those individuals convey positive emotions. In contrast, negative emotions (expressed by anyone, including the owners) and messages delivered by strangers are not as clear to dogs (McConnell, 2002,2007; Merola et al., 2014; Turcsán et al., 2015).

Consequently you should not use a harsh or negative tone, and you should not let a complete stranger train your dogs if you are not going to participate. Dogs communicate their inner states or intentions to us by using several expression patterns and behaviors. You may learn to "speak dog" if you pay enough attention to the canine way of communicating (Coren, 2000,2004; McConnell, 2002,2007; Miklósi, 2007). Dogs talk to us primarily by using a rich body language and gaze alternation (such as between a desired target/object and the human from whom the dog wants an action) just as they use vocalizations and bodily contact. They also make use of their specific positioning in a room in order to enhance the meaning of their message and intent (Gaunet & Deputte, 2011; Horn et al., 2012; Kirchhofer et al., 2012; Kis et al., 2012; Miklósi, 2007).

What's interesting in this regard is that canines may even learn to communicate by using modern communication equipment in a contextual, relevant fashion, as dogs can use a keyboard in order to request actions from a nearby person (Rossi & Ades, 2008).

Besides, dogs use quite subtle signals to disclose the emotional component of their communication. They can signal whether they find themselves among familiar or unfamiliar individuals. On a very delicate level they express whether they feel concerned or not when they interact with their owner versus a stranger (Bekoff, 2007; Coren, 2000,2004; McConnell, 2002,2007; Miklósi, 2007). As demonstrated by Dr. Miho Nagasawa from the Department of Animal Science at Azabu University in Japan, we ought to pay more attention to our dogs' faces, as they reveal their inner states and emotions. As demonstrated by using high-speed cameras, dogs' facial expressions disclose whether they're happy to see someone and whether they feel safe with this person or not. Hence, only the owner's arrival can make dogs move their left eyebrows, a mime reflecting a positive social emotion evoked by the dog-owner reunion (Nagasawa et al., 2013). The eyebrow did not move due to nonsocial joy like that elicited by attractive toys or when other people (strangers) greeted the dog. When dogs meet strangers, they move their left ears backward, and when they see objects that elicit fear or discomfort, such as a nail clipper or noisy cans, dogs move their right ears instead (Nagasawa et al., 2013).

Similarly dogs will reveal their inner emotional state by using mostly the right or left nostril for smelling. Their right nostrils are used for threatening or alarming scents (such as the sweat from the vet or adrenaline) while the left nostrils are used mainly for nonthreatening or attractive smells like food (Siniscalchi et al., 2011). If you prefer to use the tail movements as an indicator, you need to know that dogs are wagging their tails more to the left side when they are aroused or scared, while they wag more to the right side when they are relaxed and feel safe (Quaranta et al., 2007). These findings reflect that dogs use their right half of the brain for processing threats and alarming stimuli associated with negative emotions, while the left half of the brain is used for more familiar or frequent stimuli associated with positive emotions (Racca et al., 2012; Siniscalchi et al., 2008,2010,2013a). To this end, it should be mentioned that the right brain controls the left side of the body and vice versa. In the case of smell, the right nostril connects mainly to the right brain, while the left nostril connects mainly to the left brain.

While you may think it is difficult to notice such tiny movements, you may wanna take another look next time you're reunited with your wagging dog. We humans—even those who do not own dogs—have a strong and built-in ability to read dogs' facial expressions. Hence, research shows that people in general are able to sense dogs' emotions correctly (at least if they pay attention), and this skill is seen both in those who are experienced and inexperienced when it comes to dogs (Bloom & Friedman, 2013).

Pet Scans

The mentioned abilities of your dog don't leave much to chance. Dogs have a very finely tuned apparatus that allows them to acutely detect our physical, mental, and emotional states, whether in health or disease, and the explanation for this is the dog's sensory nervous system—in other words, the sensory capacity of the dogs brain and mind.

The senses of dogs are so finely adjusted to humans that they can detect even subtle changes in our biochemistry—changes in hormones, signaling molecules and volatile (gas) compounds found in human blood, breath, and urine. Dogs respond to these either spontaneously (without formal training) or because they have been trained to as in the case of dogs used for disease detection (Bjartell, 2011; Horowitz, 2010; Marcus, 2011; Miklósi, 2007; Penkowa, 2012; Smith, 2004; Udell et al., 2011). Dogs' innate sensitivity toward us has grown during our long and common history, and it has reached the point where dogs know more about our internal bodily states than we do ourselves.

In 1989, medical scientists broke the story about a forty-four-year-old woman whose dog reacted so obsessively, relentlessly, and determinedly to a mole on her thigh that she had to go see her doctor. In fact, her dog tried to bite off this particular mole, though it didn't care about her other moles. According to the doctors, the dog saved her life by its prompting her to seek help, as the mole turned out to be a malignant cancer. Luckily her dog's reaction came at such an early point that the cancer could safely be removed, and the woman's life was saved (Williams & Pembroke, 1989).

Since then, scientists have been scratching their heads, as not a soul knew that dogs could detect cancer. Nor did anyone know that malignant cells apparently release some kind of detectable compounds that can be used for cancer detection and early diagnostics.

Though some might dislike the thought of being diagnosed with cancer by a wet nose, we shouldn't underrate the brainpower attached to that nose and its amazing ability to distinguish right from wrong. Hence, while it all started with one woman's mole, dogs are today recognized for their aptness to diagnose various internal cancers, including lung, breast, ovarian, stomach, colorectal, bladder, prostate, and skin cancer (Amundsen et al., 2014; Bjartell, 2011; Boedeker et al., 2012; Campbell et al., 2013; Church & Williams, 2001; Cornu et al., 2011; Ehmann et al., 2012; Le Fanu, 2001; Marcus, 2012a,b; McCulloch et al., 2006; Sonoda et al., 2011; Taverna et al., 2014; Williams & Pembroke, 1989; Willis et al. 2004). In other words, you can't hide from your dog's nose because the nose knows. Their mind-bending capacity to sense what is going on is also illustrated by research into less dramatic behaviors such as studies of dogs' eating habits, which turns out to be deeply influenced by their owners' behavior around the chow. So your dog prefers to eat whatever food you favor, also when you are favouring the smallest (least favorable) snack available. Even if a much bigger snack was also available, dogs tend to follow their owners' indications even if they are obviously unfavorable (pick the smallest snack) (Cook et al., 2014; Prato-Previde et al., 2008). This reflects how much dogs rely on human cues despite that they may lead to a less advantageous result for the dogs (Cook et al., 2014; Prato-Previde et al., 2008). So, next time Fido won't eat the chow you provide, you may wanna reconsider your personal behavior and attitude concerning the specific choice of food. These scientific studies, whether they deal with cancer diagnostics or food selection, point to the dog being a creature strongly influenced by the surrounding humans.

Note that we like to think that we can cheat our dogs by saying we're going to the dog park when in fact we're not but instead going to the vet for an injection. Most likely your dog knows perfectly well what you're up to. Like it or not, most dogs are better mind readers than most humans.

Canine Mind Reader

When dogs developed their exceptional and mind reading skills, they became equipped with the ability called theory of mind (as mentioned earlier). Theory of mind is the ability to understand what others think, want and believe. So in broad terms, theory of mind equals to empathy and mind reading. When humans or dogs make use of this capacity, we are able to perceive, recognize, understand, decode and mimic different emotional states of other individuals (Bekoff, 2007; Hare et al., 2002; Silva & de Sousa, 2011; Udell et al., 2011).

Hence, by means of theory of mind, we are able to predict, explain, and/or anticipate the behaviors, actions, emotions, and desires of other individuals. Notably this is how we can understand one another. We can feel rather than think, research, or analyze.

As for dogs, science supports that they possess theory of mind as part of their social and emotional cognition, especially when they interact with humans (Gaunet and Deputte, 2011; Grimm, 2014; Hare & Tomasello, 2005; Overall, 2011; Reid, 2009; Silva & de Sousa, 2011; Tomasello & Kaminski, 2009; Udell et al., 2010,2011). This is why dogs know who are in need of what and when or why they reckon where or when to beg for food and from whom or which person will pay the most attention to their needs or when to conduct forbidden activities without getting caught in the act. The very same skills also allow dogs to recognize people or other animals that might be in need of help or warmth. Hence, dogs can involve and comfort patients or victims who are strangers to the dog, whether or not the people are used to being with dogs (Grimm, 2014; Marcus, 2011; Sakson, 2009).

Hence, if a stranger is in agony or is crying, most dogs will spontaneously seek the mourning person instead of approaching their owners, for whom they would otherwise always search. As shown by testing, dogs will contact, sniff, lick, nuzzle, and snuffle a stranger instead of their owners if the stranger is showing signs of distress or pain. This behavior reflects empathy and a concern for others, whether they are strangers or familiar persons (Custance & Mayer, 2012; Silva & de Sousa, 2011).

In line with this, dogs also display social anticipation abilities by which they can decode, interpret, and react to their owners' or other peoples' behavior, emotions, and intentions (Coren, 2000; Gaunet and Deputte, 2011; Grimm, 2014; Hare & Woods, 2013; Horowitz, 2010; Kubinyi et al., 2007; McConnell, 2002; Miklósi, 2007; Penkowa, 2014). Accordingly, they are adept at picking out whom to preferably follow or trust and who not to join or rely on.

By their social understanding and mimicry of specific behaviors—for example, contagious yawning—dogs can facilitate bonding and attachment to people (Coren, 2004; McConnell, 2007; Rugaas, 2006; Smith, 2004).

Why Do We Yawn?

Take a big yawn, and you'll see that other people as well as your dog will yawn too. Any vertebrate (from fish to humans) can yawn, but only a very few species, such as humans and dogs, find yawns contagious. In fact, seeing or just hearing the sound of someone yawning makes both man and dogs do it. Taking this trend to a next level, scientists showed that dogs not only catch our yawns but also pay high attention to those from whom they caught it. Hence, in both dog and man yawning from familiar or well-liked subjects is much more contagious than the yawning of strangers. This aspect exposes the fact that contagious yawning reflects an empathy-based, emotional connection between the creatures yawning together, whether they are humans or dogs. This is supported by the fact that autistic children, who lack empathy and social skills, don't catch yawning from others. However, dogs embrace emotional attachment to us in a way that remains unmatched by other animal species (Helt et al., 2010; Joly-Mascheroni et al., 2008; McConnell, 2007; Rugaas, 2006; Senju, 2010; Silva & de Sousa, 2011; Silva et al., 2012; Smith, 2004).

These skills did not emerge at once; however, the dog coevolved with humans, and so dogs had the chance to study us, observe our behavior, recognize our emotions, and capture our scents, sounds, and looks just as they followed us since the beginning of history. And so dogs know us like nobody else.

Their mind-reading proficiency undoubtedly provided dogs with biological advantages that taught them how to behave in order to obtain their own goals (e.g., how to best attract human attention) just as it facilitates dogs' interaction with humans who likely rewarded the most cooperative or receptive or docile dogs with extra food scraps. Selection pressure has enhanced dogs' sensitivity toward us (Miklósi, 2007; Olmert, 2009; Serpell, 1996).

For the very same reason dogs are also fully capable of feeling emotions once thought to be unique to humans. One of these is jealousy, as demonstrated scientifically in dogs that don't like anyone muscling in on their friendships with the owners (Harris & Prouvost, 2014). The study showed that dogs would try different strategies to win back their owners' attention, starting with friendly acts like touching or pushing, and when this doggish diplomacy didn't work, even docile dogs tried barking and whining or getting in between the owner and the intruding object. (In the study, this object was a realistic-looking stuffed dog that able to bark, whine, and wag its tail.) When they realized they couldn't get their owners' attention, even dogs that were described as totally nonaggressive would in fact turn to aggressive measures like biting the stuffed dog in order to get rid of the fake. Moreover, the researchers also tested the dogs' emotional response when owners paid attention to other nonsocial objects like a jack-o'-lantern or read out loud from a book. Interestingly the dogs acted far less jealous when their owners displayed affection for the nonsocial objects. The data indicates that dogs are perfectly able to discriminate between relevant or socially significant rivals (such as other furry rivals) and nonsocial, motionless objects (Harris & Prouvost, 2014).

In fact, the dog's unique sensitivity, reactivity, and readiness in response to humans is a phenomenon that keeps surprising scientists; however, it barely stuns dog owners. In fact, science is merely verifying what most experienced dog lovers intuit. Dogs' emotional lives are no less significant than ours (Bekoff, 2007; Grimm, 2014; McConnell, 2002,2007; Mendl et al., 2010; Serpell, 1996; Smith, 2004).

Meet and Greet the Sweet

How do you behave during reunions with your dog? Do you enter your home and throw yourself on the floor while you pet and sweet-talk to you joyful friend? Or do you follow the horrific advice of those trainers who tell you to act like an alleged alpha leader and ignore your dog for the first five to ten minutes after your return?

Now science supports that acting like the assumed alpha leader is harmful to your dog, as he or she will experience an increase in stress hormones, heart rate, and blood pressure, which are signs of discomfort, anxiety and fear (Rehn et al., 2014).

Remember that in your dog's mind, his or her guardian (the owner) is the primary caretaker and the most important element in securing survival, safety, and welfare. When left alone, most dogs lie down and wait for their attachment figure to return. As soon as the owner returns, dogs react promptly by showing joy and an increase in the hormone oxytocin (which mediates trust, love, bonding, and comfort). Increased oxytocin is followed by a decrease in stress hormones along with contact-seeking behavior and joyful greeting (Nagasawa et al., 2013; Rehn et al., 2014; Romero et al., 2014).

However, if you decide to ignore the dog when you return, two adversities will happen. First of all your dog will be deprived of significant, long-lasting increases in oxytocin and secrete more stress hormones leading to distress, disappointment, and uncertainty. Secondly you will miss one of life's most pleasant, fun, comforting, loving, warm, and hearty moments with your best friend.

In addition to selection pressure based upon dogs' biological advantages, there are further reasons for their proficiency. The course of domestication led to advanced cognition and brainpower in order for the transitional canines to fully exploit their ecological niche at the edge of human campfire (Miklósi, 2007; Reid, 2009; Silva & de Sousa, 2011).

Among all the talents that patients most often request in health-care professionals, empathy or theory of mind is among the highest warranted skills. Many patients feel uncomfortable around doctors and hospital staff. Many associate them with a lack of empathy, compassion, or altruism within the health-care sector.

This is where the dog as a modern therapist might possess a major strength, as dogs embrace inherent empathy, emotional warmth, and social awareness (Bekoff, 2007; Grimm, 2014; Marcus, 2012a,b; Penkowa, 2012). Hence, dogs may comfort not only their owners but also unfamiliar persons like inpatients, who are visited by a therapy dog.

To this end, dogs have an advantage since dogs have always stayed close with humans and been inside our homes, where they have had far more opportunities than any other species to learn how to decode us and respond in the most appropriate manner. That is exactly what has equipped them with theory of mind. Hence, since the beginning of time dogs have attuned themselves to our behaviors, gesticulations, emotional states, energy levels, and physical conditions (McConnell, 2002,2007; Olmert, 2009; Penkowa, 2012; Serpell, 1996; Smith, 2004).

As far as dog owners are concerned, the dog's perception and rapid responses to our condition give rise to some unique benefits, as dog owners likely share their homes with gifted therapists and anthropologists. In other words, who needs Dr. Phil when you have Dr. Fido?

Nature and Nurture

Naturally there are significant differences among dogs and breeds, and in fact, within any given breed and even within one litter, individual dogs will behave and react to their keepers in different ways. These differences basically involve both nature and nurture. Hence, every dog needs training, attachment, friendly company, and multiple interactions with both conspecifics (other canines) and humans in order for them to develop the previously mentioned social skills (Bekoff, 2007; Gácsi et al., 2013; McConnell, 2002,2007; Smith, 2004). To this end, don't be fooled by a dog's physical appearance, as any serious evaluation of canine behaviors indicates how easily we misinterpret canines (McConnell, 2002,

2007). Accordingly, science shows how gundogs like the cocker spaniel and retrievers retain relatively more of the ancestral wolf behavior than their looks (e.g., floppy ears) may indicate, while the opposite is the case for German shepherds, who look quite wolfish on the outer surface, though they haven't retained as much wolf behavior (Goodwin et al., 1997).

Even if an owner buys the best of the best of a given breed from the very best parental lineage, the dog will need plenty of training, environmental stimulation, affectionate company, nurturing, exposure to adventurous situations, social fulfillment, education, cognitive challenges, trust, physical exercise, love, and friendliness in order for the dog's brain to become fully hardwired and well-functioning. These aspects belong to nurture, and in terms of the brain and mind, whether human or canine, nurture is even more important than nature. For this reason the daily environment and the lifestyle that a dog is offered is likely more important for his or her brain than breed, pedigree, or genetic composition are (McConnell, 2007; Miklósi, 2007; Penkowa, 2012; Serpell, 1996). Hence, selective breeding and genetics will not make for a champion. Instead it is the rearing environment, nurturing, daily training, cognitive stimulation, social contact, caretaking, and bonding that shape the brain and mind into a masterpiece.

In other words, don't judge by breed, judge by deed.

Consequently the pedigree of your dog doesn't matter that much as long as you provide him or her with the most enriching conditions. That's why practically any dog of any breed has the potential to become a true champion in terms of performance, problem solving, resilience, social cognition, empathy, and perception (Fogle, 1990; Hare & Woods, 2013; Horowitz, 2010; McConnell, 2002,2007; Miklósi, 2007).

Canine Brainpower

Fortunately recent scientific efforts have explored the dog's perception by means of the senses (sensory nervous system) to shed light upon the still enigmatic achievements performed by dogs (e.g., when they smell their way to a malignant cancer or detect diseases). Consequently our understanding of the canine sensory capacity is mounting. In this regard, dogs are unique among animals, as they may communicate equally well with both conspecifics and heterospecifics (humans). In both cases dogs benefit significantly from a highly developed social nature along with their bilateral communication skills, whereby they make every effort to maintain affiliation, recognize pack members (household members), and reduce antagonism. By doing exactly this, the last decade taught us that dogs not only recognize and bond with us but also may alert their owners to serious health threats, such as sudden drops in blood sugar (hypoglycemia) in diabetics, imminent seizures in epileptic patients, migraine attacks in migraneurs, and even the development of malignant cancers (Chen et al., 2000; Grimm, 2014; Marcus, 2011,2012b; Marcus & Bhowmick, 2013; Penkowa, 2014; Rooney et al., 2013; Wells, 2012).

Doctors still do not precisely know all of the substances or volatile compounds that dogs react to when they alert someone about hypoglycemic fits or seizures, though scientists have begun to explore the different and putative odors involved with these.

In fact, nobody even knew that cancer cells released such chemicals or that dogs were able to pick them up until the world's first cancer-sniffing dog hit the global news in the late 1980s. Not only did the dog astonish mankind, but he also paved the way for a method that has dramatic implications for early diagnosis and the clinical management of some critical diseases. Suddenly calling the dog a most gifted anthropologist may seem like an understatement. Thus, we may not only be dealing with man's best friend. We might be facing mankind's most important friend.

The lesson learned is the fact that dogs may recognize even the most subtle change within the human body, whether it's an emotional, physiological, age-related, behavioral, biochemical, or odorant change. To better understand this, we need to take a closer look at the dog's sensory nervous system, which constitutes the structural foundation (the hardware) of his or her receptivity and perception.

The dog is equipped with multiple sensory modalities that can be divided into the physical senses that we share and know so well (e.g., the visual, auditory, tactile, gustatory or taste, thermal sense) along with the dog's most important sense, the sense of smell (olfaction). However, the dog's sensory system also comprises some less investigated modalities, such as electrostatic, magnetic, and vestibular (position and equilibrium) senses as well as the sense of vibration, atmospheric pressure, and circadian rhythm (body rhythms) (Fogle, 1990; Horowitz, 2010; McConnell, 2007; Miklósi, 2007; Simpson, 1997).

Because of these senses, the body clocks of dogs can be very precise. In fact, many dog owners are woken up by their dogs at the same time every day. In fact, if you know how, you can train your furry friend to react to the clock with an accuracy of within one minute in the twenty-four-hour day/night cycle.

Still the sensory capacity of the dog is not limited to this, as recent data now reveals how dogs register even more delicate signals that are so extremely subtle they may be difficult for us humans to grasp. According to this, science shows that dogs register the earth's magnetic field, and they also possess a sensitivity to ultraviolet light (Douglas & Jeffery, 2014; Hart et al., 2013). Hence, in recent years meticulous research studies have come up with important answers to some of those questions that have always preoccupied many dog owners. For example, in his magnificent book *The Dog's Mind*, which was written by Dr. Bruce Fogle, a doctor of veterinary medicine and head of the London Vet Clinic in England, he suggests that dogs might have a sixth sense, as they seem to be capable of detecting the angle of the sun's rays and may employ electromagnetic navigation in order to steadily steer their ways outside (Fogle, 1990). While Dr. Fogle certainly proved to be ahead of time, recent scientific scrutiny has now closed the gap and explained how some dogs are able to travel through an unknown landscape or cross a continent.

Hence, dogs are amazing creatures. By all accounts they receive also external information through other sensory channels (denoted as extrasensory perception) than by means of the familiar modalities that are well-known to us humans (Fogle, 1990; Horowitz, 2010; McConnell, 2007; Miklósi, 2007; Simpson, 1997).

In the next section aspects of the canine sensory capacity will be detailed, though emphasis is put mainly on those senses that are known to be of primary importance to dogs in the process of decoding of humans and their states of health.

Dog Magnetic

If dogs can use electromagnetic stimuli, they certainly receive some kind of signals that we can only dream of. According to recent scientific scrutiny, dogs are perfectly capable of sensing the earth's magnetic field as shown by a research group led by Dr. Hynek Burda of the University of Duisburg-Essen in Germany and Vlastimil Hart at the Czech University of Life Sciences in Praque.

In 2013, they made a discovery that hit global news headlines as they announced that dogs had a magnetic sense (magnetosensation) by which dogs use the earth's geomagnetic field lines in order to navigate and position their bodies (Hart et al., 2013).

For two years the researchers followed a total of seventy dogs consisting of thirty-seven different breeds, including gundogs (primarily spaniels but also beagles, pointers, and retrievers among others), herding breeds, terriers of various types (fox, West Highland white, Jack Russell, Yorkshire terriers and others), and the dachshund. From their collection of 7,475 observations, it was clear that dogs act in accordance with their geomagnetic super sense, which in fact the scientific community didn't know about until Hynek Burda and Vlastimil Hart published their data in December 2013.

Though it was a novel discovery for scientists, it may not have come as a surprise to many dog owners who have witnessed how brilliant dogs are at navigating their way home or at searching for a specific subject or place. Among the more fascinating examples are the story of Bobbie, a two-year-old mixed Scotch collie/English shepherd that was lost by his family during a trip to Indianapolis in 1923. After their far-reaching search for Bobbie, the heartbroken family decided to return to their home in Oregon, where they never expected to see Bobbie again. However, half of a year later Bobbie suddenly appeared on the family doorstep. The dog all on his own had traveled more than 4,100 kilometers, crossing mountains, plains, and deserts in the dead of winter. He was not surprisingly mangy and scrawny, and his paws were worn to the bone; however, he had found his way home as described in books and the media (Alexander, 1926).

Back then it would be hard to believe how Bobbie did it, but with today's insight regarding dogs' magnificent sensory abilities, we could imagine that Bobbie might not even find it difficult to navigate correctly, though for sure it have been difficult for him, a herding dog, to find enough food to fuel his physical efforts. This is not only a classic tale of dogs' faithfulness and loyalty but also an indicator of the fascinating abilities of our pets.

For the scientific community and society in general, finding the dog's magnetosensation is of tremendous value and offers vast new perspectives that go far beyond the GPS. However, not all dogs are equally adept and one shouldn't forget that most dogs never find their way home, as seen from the many millions of wandering or lost dogs that end up in shelters every year. Consequently not all owners can rely on the dog to find the way home if he or she is lost.

All the recent research data on dogs' sensory abilities, perception, and communication skills may begin to explain how dogs are able to react to cancer, hypoglycemia or epilepsy.

What also has become clear is that dogs communicate by incorporating more than one sensory modality. They communicate by means of multimodal signaling. However, a range of studies of disease-alerting dogs shows that they primarily rely on their most famous sense, namely scent detection, when they diagnose human diseases, including diabetic hypoglycemia, epileptic seizures, and cancers. Dogs can detect diseases simply by smelling the skin or a small sample of urine or exhaled breath (Bjartell, 2011; 2012; Lippi & Cervellin, 2012; Marcus, 2012b).

Accordingly, the most investigated and likely most important senses of the dog will be explained in the next section. As we will see, dogs have abilities that may even fascinate us more than their use of the earth's magnetic field. At least this is the case when we look at the dog's sense of smell, as the dog's nose knows what to look for.

The Sense of Smell (Olfaction)

Smelling occurs by the sensing of chemicals (chemosensation), and in dogs it is the major way of analyzing the world. Dogs detect and discriminate among an enormous series of molecules with different structures and characteristics.

The dog's nose and the brain it connects to are one of nature's most astonishing systems, as they are the foundation for the canine sense of smell (olfaction), which is continuously a source of surprise for scientists. Work in recent years has led to a renaissance of canine brain research and more and more insight into the dog's olfactory achievements and the underlying neurobiology (Lawson et al., 2012; Berns et al., 2014). Dogs' acute sense of smell plays a major role in their extraordinary power to sense human distress, cancer, pain, or disordered homeostasis, and therefore, the biology behind it deserves extra attention.

Because of canine odor detection, dogs can be trained to perform lifesaving tasks, many that we would not be able to accomplish by any other application.

The dog's olfactory capacity is likely the most representative example in terms of why and how the dog completes man. Humans don't rely much on olfaction, as we instead primarily use our vision for experiencing the world (Coren, 2004; Fogle, 1990; Horowitz, 2010).

Because of their unique sense of smell, dogs are employed by police, customs authorities, rescue teams, medical doctors, and the military, where they detect various scents of importance to society or individuals, such as odorants derived from explosives, illegal drugs, firearms, vermin, land mines, booby traps, toxins, money, off-flavors, hidden objects, leaky gas pipelines, invasive plants, pathogens, subjects, or suspects (Coren, 2004; Goodavage, 2012; Hare & Woods, 2013; Jones, 2011; Miklósi, 2007; Quignon et al., 2012). In fact, we have had no allies as valuable as the explosives- or drugs-detecting working dogs, thanks to an unrivaled sensitivity and selectivity of their olfaction.

Another example of dogs' lifesaving scent tracking is search-and-rescue work, where dogs smell their way to find missing persons, runaway children, hostages, or cadavers. More recently the dog's sniffing ability has been applied in the health-care sector. Dogs are able to smell patients' transformed cells or circulating odorant molecules (e.g., hormones, metabolites, and/or volatile organic compounds), whereby dogs provide a tool for early diagnostics (Bjartell, 2011; Penkowa, 2012; Sakson, 2009; Wells, 2012). Cancer cells in particular secrete volatile organic compounds like benzene derivatives and alkanes that dogs can smell, as they are released by means of our breath, urine, sweat, blood, or skin. In fact, we are only beginning to realize where the dog's snout can take us.

Science supports that dogs' sense of smell and their repertoire of scents are at least a million times more sensitive and even more complex than ours, and so it is no surprise that dogs experience the world through their noses (Benbernou et al., 2007,2011; Coren, 2004; Fogle, 1990; Horowitz, 2010; Lippi & Cervellin, 2012). Accordingly, dogs may function well even if they suffer a deficiency in their visual and/or acoustic perception. As long as their olfactory system is working, they are able to stay ahead.

Consequently the dog's nose dominates his or her facial shape, and olfaction dominates his or her brain.

We're Only Humans

Though humans rely on our vision more than any other sense, those of us who own dogs may have picked up some sniffing behavior as demonstrated in a series of interesting tests performed by Dr. Deborah Wells from Queen's University Belfast in Northern Ireland.

In a test of dog owners' sense of smell, the majority or as many as 88.5 percent were able to correctly distinguish the smell of their own dog from an unfamiliar dog when owners were allowed to sniff blankets with either dog fragrance (Wells & Hepper, 2000).

The test did prove that humans can identify their own dogs merely by their individual scents.

Interestingly this effect cannot be extended to other pets or animal species as shown in a similar experiment with cat owners who couldn't identify their pets' odors (Courtney & Wells, 2002).

Consequently the human nose is unequally talented when it comes to recognizing pet animals by means of their odors. Interestingly our ability to identify dogs but not cats by their scents is a natural gift since it did not require any prior training.

Yet there are obvious breed-related differences in the olfactory capacity since breeds with flat noses (brachycephalia), such as pugs, bulldogs, Pekingese, boxers, Boston terriers, and shih tzus, have difficulties with respiration as well as scent detection as compared to the breeds without brachycephalia (Coren, 2004; Fogle, 1990; Miklósi, 2007; Robin et al., 2009). The most proficient scent trackers among canines are not surprisingly the hunting dogs (e.g., cocker spaniels, beagles, retrievers, and bloodhounds). However, a dog's individual capacity reflects not only pedigree or breed-specific neurobiology; since gender, age, nutrition, experience, and history of infections also matter. Male dogs are superior to females for scent tracking, while in general olfactory achievements of dogs are improved by incentives and motivation (Fogle, 1990).

Moreover the environmental stimuli and amount of training you provide are not less important. Whether human or dog, nurture is at least as important as nature if not more important. Hence, the particular enrichment, training, exposure, reinforcement, and challenges that you provide for your dog during his or her development and lifetime in general will in the end determine how proficient your dog becomes (McConnell, 2007; Overall, 2011). This also goes for the dog's sense of smell since the olfactory system is just like any other brain function. It is molded and sharpened by being challenged with stimuli, fun training, and experience (Fogle, 1990; Miklósi, 2007). From my point of view the best way to nurture any dog's nature is to exercise him or her with free running into the fields, forests, grasslands, and wetlands, and from early on you can train the dog while he or she is allowed to enjoy the natural world and the company of other animals. Doing just this on a regular basis will facilitate and consolidate the bond between you to.

At the same time such adventures in nature will keep the dog's mind busy, stimulate the neurons, and benefit the brain.

And there's one more thing for the owner. A little exercise outdoors in sunny daylight will do you good.

Nose Building

The nasal anatomy starts with the moist snout openings (nostrils). In canines these are mobile and able to dilate, whereby the dog can catch the directions of different odors as well as regulate the incoming airflow (Evans & de Lahunta, 2013). From touching a healthy dog's snout, you know it is quite moist, and this is due to the combined secretions of mucus released by different sets of nasal glands (mainly the lateral nasal glands), and the lacrimal glands also contribute through the nasolacrimal duct (Evans & de Lahunta, 2013; Fogle, 1990). There are many points in producing this moisture, but only the most important ones are mentioned here. First the secretions by the dog's lateral nasal glands are in some regards comparable to our sweating, as the nasal fluid allows the dog to dissipate excess body heat during panting (Evans & de Lahunta, 2013). Hence, when room temperature rises by up to 15 degrees Celsius, the lateral nasal glands increase fluid secretion in the order of forty times.

Just as important, the nasal mucus gives the dog the ability to absorb (trap) and dissolve odor molecules from the air, in order for him to capture scents. When odorants reach the dog's nose, they are detected by specialized and highly receptive nerve cells (sensory neurons), which are able to recognize and differentiate billions of different scent molecules. When a given scent is detected, its corresponding sensory neurons transmit a signal to the brain, allowing the dog to process and become aware of that particular odor (Coren, 2004; Jia et al., 2014; Miklósi, 2007).

In other words, for inhaled air to become an awareness in the dog's conscious mind, volatile scent molecules have to be trapped in the mucus of the nasal cavity, where they are caught by dedicated olfactory receptors on the surface of the scent-detecting neurons. Specific receptors are present for different types of odor molecules. Dogs display many more and much more complex scent receptors on their neurons than we do, whereby canines may catch scents even when they occur at exceptionally low concentrations – that is in the range of 1 part per trillion (ppt) or the same as to catch one out of 10^{12} molecules (or one part per 1,000,000,000,000 parts) (Craven et al., 2010; Lippi & Cervellin, 2012). This number (1 ppt) is corresponding to one single drop of water in four hundred Olympic swimming pools.

By means of their diverse and heterogeneous receptor composition, dogs can both detect, track, differentiate, and archive (remember) odors that remain unknown to us simply because they are beyond our nose's capacity (Horowitz, 2010; Evans & de Lahunta, 2013; Jia et al., 2014; Miklósi, 2007). Hence, the canine olfactory cells line a surface area that on average is forty times bigger than the human equivalent, though in some breeds (e.g., hunting dogs) our olfactory capacities may diverge substantially more.

As a scented chemical is bound to an odor receptive cell, a specific signal is sent through the sensory nerve cells connecting the nasal cavity to the brain. For comparison humans are estimated to have five to ten million of these nerves, while dogs are equipped with at least two hundred million and in some breeds up to two billion olfactory nerve cells (Fogle, 1990; Miklósi, 2007; Pinto, 2011; Quignon et al., 2012). In the brain specialized neurons process and integrate the nerve signal so that it results in the conscious experience of a fragrance that governs the dog's behavior, emotions, cognition, memories, instincts, and conditioned responses.

The dog's scent detection is both in relative and absolute terms superior to ours, which is reflected by the fact that one third of the dog's brain is involved in olfaction (Jia et al., 2014). Perhaps even more important than relative size is the dog's nasal features and the molecular configuration of the olfactory system, which surpasses what has been found in any other animal (Robin et al., 2009; Salazar et al., 2013).

Chemosensation

In fact, the dog's sense of smell does not rely only on one default olfactory pathway, as dogs use a number of different anatomical systems, each of which have specific and overlapping functions in olfaction (Miklósi, 2007; Quignon et al., 2012).

The main olfactory pathway is analogous in humans and dogs and consists of the olfactory region. But only in dogs does this region contain hundreds of millions of olfactory nerve cells (the neuroepithelium). These cells form a cellular layer that coats the convoluted nasal structures (turbinates) found in the rear of the dog's nasal cavity. The neuroepithelium have olfactory receptors on the surface that detect odorant molecules, and they are concentrated in the nasal mucus (Craven et al., 2010; Fogle, 1990; Pinc et al., 2011). Once they catch a scent molecule, olfactory signals are generated and transmitted to the olfactory bulb, a brain structure serving as a filter that discriminates among odors, removes background noise (by filtering out insignificant odors), and augments the transmission of significant scents. From the olfactory bulb information is disseminated to several areas in the brain, leading to the conscious experience of a given smell (Berns et al., 2014; Horowitz, 2014; Jia et al., 2014).

However, the neuroepithelium's chemosensation is far from being fully characterized, and so scientists engaged in olfaction research won't be jobless in the near future. This is reflected by the fragmented knowledge of some apparently unconventional neurons found to express nonolfactory, trace amine-associated receptors (TAARs) within the neuroepithelium of the main olfactory region. The TAARs are sensitive to hormones like phenylethylamine and pheromones like isoamylamine and trimethylamine, which are natural components of urine. Their concentration reflects an individual's gender, social status, and stress levels (Tirindelli et al., 2009; Zhang et al., 2013). Hence, by subtle chemical changes, a vast array of information is available for the one who can sniff.

Our lack of knowledge about olfaction may explain why the human race hasn't been able to create an apparatus or machine that can match the dog's sense of smell, and so our furry friends still remain the very best, most sensitive, and reliable method when it comes to diagnostic scent detection like in case of sniffing out cancer, alerting us to diabetic hypoglycemia, migraine attacks, or epileptic seizures, and tracing criminals, fugitives, illegal drugs, toxins, bed bugs, vermin, etc. They can also detect explosives, firearms, land mines, booby traps, and the like. You can bet on this: If it has a smell, Fido will find it (Grimm, 2014; Hügler, 2012; Jones, 2011; Marcus, 2011,2012b; Marcus & Bhowmick, 2013; Penkowa, 2014; Rooney et al., 2013; Wells, 2012; Wells et al., 2008).

The olfactory ability of the dog lies at the far boundaries of what we are able to fathom. Dogs may recognize an individual's odor on a steel tube that the person touched for only five seconds. Moreover, dogs can detect a specific human scent from lightly fingerprinted glass slides that are kept outdoors for weeks. That's just to mention some of the amazing skills of our furry friends (Coren, 2000,2004; Fogle, 1991; Le Fanu, 2001).

Ebola Screening

Early detection of potentially deadly infections such as Ebola, Clostridium difficile or Methicillin-resistant Staphylococcus aureus (MRSA) is of paramount importance as a strategy to prevent a pandemic. Right now our best strategy might be the canine way since dogs can recognize infectious microorganisms, even though they are too small for us to visualize and can only be seen in a microscope (Bomers et al., 2012; Coren, 2000,2004; Desikan, 2013; Grimm, 2014). Hence, dogs can be trained to detect potentially deadly bacteria such as Clostridium difficile, which may pose serious threats to society because of its wide-ranging resistance to antibiotics and a tendency to cause very serious and fatal infectious disorders (Bomers et al., 2012). In fact, a dog can identify bacteria with an extremely high level of sensitivity and specificity, both in stool or tissue samples and in the patients (Bomers et al., 2012). According to this, dogs are of great value to society when health-care services are scarce or when emergencies occur.

In addition to the main olfactory region found in the nasal cavity's rear end, a separate cluster of olfactory neurons exists in a lower part of the nasal cavity, an area named the septal organ of Masera (Tirindelli et al., 2009). This organ, which has been described mainly in rodents, contains cells that in structure and function remind one of the neuroepithelium, though there are subtle differences. Because of its location (in the airstream of relaxed respiration), the septal organ of Masera possibly functions as a first filter to notice any potentially harmful or interesting odors passing by, and when one is noticed, it may activate. One will sniff in order to get the odors transported to the main neuroepithelium. However, the septal organ of Masera is yet to be elucidated in dogs. Likewise, the Grueneberg ganglion is a nasal structure containing sensory receptors involved in olfaction, although it's possible role in the dog remains elusive (Quignon et al., 2012; Tirindelli et al., 2009).

A different and highly specialized olfactory region within the dog's nose is the vomeronasal organ (or the Jacobson's organ), which is a blind-ended pouch of specialized sensory cells located close to the floor of the nasal cavity and just behind the upper incisors. The vomeronasal organ is connected to both the nasal and oral cavity whereby volatile chemicals entering either nose or mouth can reach the organ's specialized sensory cells. When a signal is received in the vomeronasal organ, cells within a special region of the olfactory bulb are activated (Salazar et al., 2013). The vomeronasal organ is specialized for detecting volatile substances like pheromones and sex hormones carrying information relating to species-specific emotional, social, and behavioral states, and so it guides the dog's social interactions, mating behavior, and self-confidence (Coren, 2004; Fogle, 1990; Horowitz, 2010). However, the dog also has pheromone receptors in the neuroepithelium of the main olfactory region (Quignon et al., 2012; Tirindelli et al., 2009). Besides, there most likely also exist some additional scent receivers or pathways within the dog's nose, though they have yet to be characterized.

In both dogs and humans pheromones are involved in diverse behaviors relating to reproduction. For example, dogs produce trace pheromones that urge others to follow, and they also produce alarm pheromones that put conspecifics on alert or may induce aggressive attacks (Coren, 2000,2004; Fogle, 1990; Horowitz, 2010; Miklósi, 2007). Interestingly, some of the pheromones of dogs and humans are shared, and this could explain why man and his best friend may seem to exchange information on a rather subconscious level (Horowitz, 2014; Tirindelli et al., 2009).

Yet another separate sensor contributes to scent transmission in dogs, as the trigeminal nerve, a major cranial sensory nerve, is also used for detection of larger odiferous molecules (Miklósi, 2007). Besides, the trigeminal nerve is part of the airway's first line of defense system, as it is mainly involved in the detection of inhaled irritants, toxins, or noxious substances. Hence, the receptors of the trigeminal nerves react to specific chemicals classified as pollutants, ammonia, ethanol, irritants, alcohols, carbon dioxide, acetic acid, menthol, capsaicin, and various others. In addition, the nervous system of the nose also contains some autonomous nerves that control a range of normal functions, such as the blood flow to the nose, secretion from the glands, and reflexes like sneezing (Evans & de Lahunta, 2013).

The Sniff

When the dog normally inhales air, it will flow from the nose to the lungs, and then it is exhaled. However, as any dog owner knows dogs also have the sniff. The sniff is easily recognized, as it consists of consecutive trains of sniffing accompanied by characteristic nostril movements, and at the same time the dog's normal breathing pattern is disrupted.

The sniff is a highly advanced mechanism by which dogs draw in air containing particularly important odors that are then kept inside the nasal champer instead of being inhaled to the lungs and then exhaled. Thus, the dog is able to accumulate and store important odors for later use.

During the sniff the dog creates an odorant whirlwind that won't block incoming or outgoing airstreams, as the whirlwind instead creates an optimized scent transport to the olfactory part of the nose (Craven et al., 2010). The dynamic air flow keeps renewing the volatile scent molecules, which thereby do not fade, and so the dog is allowed to register and differentiate even the smallest components of an odor of interest. That's why dogs will sniff anything that they find attractive or important (Fogle, 1990; Horowitz, 2010). Hence, dogs hold a complex air flow system inside their noses, and the sniffed scents can be saved for later use, recognition, or comparisons.

Take a Whiff

For a human being it is quite impossible to really fathom what it feels like to experience life through the snout, mainly because our own olfactory sense is in a rather sad plight as compared to that of our furry friends (Coren, 2004; Fogle, 1990; Howard, 2006; Penkowa, 2012; Serpell, 1996).

Accordingly, we rapidly adapt to an odor—that is, if we can catch it. Hence, our experience of scents (e.g., perfume, a cup of tea, a flower, etc.) lasts only for a brief moment, after which it seems gone with the wind because we're no longer aware of it. Even if we wanted to sense the world by olfaction, it would be difficult. Modern human life is filled with "olfactory noise" because of all those artificially added scents found in most of today's consumer products. Hence, our clothes, cars, food, beverages, personal care products, tissues, accessories, and household items have all been coated with some industrial additives that hold fragrances, aromas, perfumes, or other olfactory inputs.

Dogs remain true to their roots, as they certainly prefer natural body odors over artificial additives. Consequently they meet and greet by sniffing one another, and in particular they may start with the head region and mouth in order to smell body fluids like saliva or nasal mucus. However, when dogs meet one another, they only spend a short while on the nose. They rapidly turn to focus on the rear end (or the crotch of people) since this is where they find many pheromone-releasing glands, apocrine sweat glands, anal glands, and informative odors released from feces, urine, and mating activity (Coren, 2004; Fogle, 1990). As a result, this is where dogs may find out about the physical, mental, and emotional state of other living beings. They can retrieve and differentiate olfactory information regarding age, social rank, sex, mood, energy, confidence, behavior, and various health issues by odors relating to diseases, injuries, metabolism, recent surgeries, and/or drugs (Coren, 2000,2004; Fogle, 1990; Horowitz, 2010; Jezierski et al., 2012; Miklósi, 2007).

This kind of information is the canine equivalent to our newspapers, health records, and most kinds of text messages or communication relating to other people. Because of their olfactory capacity, a tendency to prefer natural body odors over deodorant, and their attuned way of bonding with us, man's best friend has emerged as a prime diagnostic method with regards to human health conditions and diseases.

In terms of smelling, this sense has a huge advantage over the other major senses because both sounds and sights may vanish while scents hang around in the air, on surfaces, or as a track on the ground. Consequently the sense of smell is a window to the past, while the other senses are only useful then and there (Coren, 2004; Fogle, 1990; Horowitz, 2010). Human skin is constantly shedding, even when you can't see it, and the constant flaking of our skin leaves an invisible trail behind us that most dogs' noses can without difficulty track. The same goes for other species. For instance, hunting dogs will easily lead you to the quarry to find prey. Dogs can also determine who and how many people were present in an area, whether they were male or female, when they left, and in which direction they traveled, just as your dog does so when he applies his 'pee mail' on your walk as he sniffs and makes urine marks (Coren, 2000,2004; Fogle, 1990; Horowitz, 2010; Jezierski et al., 2012; Miklósi, 2007).

This kind of scent tracking has been studied for decades, while the odors detected by dogs as they register human diseases have only in recent time been the subject of scientific scrutiny.

The Gustatory Sense: A Matter of Taste

A dog's sense of taste (gustatory sense) is one of the few senses that is functioning as soon as life begins, yet science doesn't pay much attention to it despite its extensive mentioning and branding in commercial ads for modern dog chow. One reason for the divergent focus of attention paid by the academic world versus producers of dog food commercials might be that nobody really knows what is going on when dogs enjoy their dinner.

Hence, compared to the ever-increasing scrutiny of canine scent detection, research is lacking with regards to the mechanisms of taste sensations. Nevertheless, because a taste can signal either delight or disgust, the gustatory sense provides both man and dog an essential survival tool.

What we do know is that the experience of taste starts with detecting a gustatory molecule from ingested particles. The chemosensory detection occurs by means of different sets of receptors located on the taste buds (papillae), most of which are on the tongue and in the oral cavity, though abundant taste buds are also distributed in the canine throat (Evans & de Lahunta, 2013; Fogle, 1990).

To experience its taste, a gustatory chemical must be dissolved in the dog's saliva in order to reach the receptors, which have evolved to detect sweet, salt, bitter, sour, and savory components in foods (Coren, 2004; Horowitz, 2010). Accordingly, dogs are not true carnivores. They are omnivres just like us. While these five taste sensations are familiar to us humans, we can only guess as to what it may taste like when dogs drink water since they are most likely experiencing something different than we do. Hence, dogs have a special set of receptors that are tuned to detect water molecules, and logically they are located at the tip of the tongue, exactly where dogs curl their tongues backward when they are lapping water (Coren, 2004; Crompton & Musinsky, 2011; Fogle, 1990).

> **Let's Drink to It**
>
> In contrast to humans trying to spoon in water with the tongue, dogs do it differently, as they curl their tongues backward before they let the curled tip slip into the surface of the water. Then they plunge the body of the tongue forward and much deeper into the liquid in order to form a pouch filled with water. However, instead of scooping the water back in the mouth, they make use of adhesion, whereby a column of water adheres to the tongue's surface, as to why most of it moves against gravity and ends up inside the mouth (Crompton & Musinsky, 2011). The lower part of the adhered column of water will drop as soon as the dog closes the jaws around the retrieved part, and as any dog owner knows, the lower part will move perfectly - on the floor.

So dogs are neither overly sensitive nor snobbish if they act a bit fussy about drinking water as many dogs do, and the reason is that they do so because they can actually tell a real difference between different sources of water (Coren, 2004; Fogle, 1990). This is interesting since in terms of quantities humans have more than five times as many taste buds than dogs do. However, we must admit to be behind canines in terms of taste qualities, as they in some regards are the true connoisseurs that are able to experience flavors that we don't (Coren, 2000,2004; Evans & de Lahunta, 2013; Fogle, 1990). Perhaps the water taste is responsible for the fact that dogs prefer foods that are moist, mushy, warm, and thereby more palatable. It is a bit of a modern paradox that most dogs are fed hard kibble and pellets dry as a bone.

Dogs are considered to use primarily their sense of smell, then the texture of the food and only lastly, they pay attention to the food's taste (Fogle, 1990). This illustrates how closely the chemosensations of taste and smell are interconnected. Anyone with the flu or a stuffed up nose knows this, as we can't taste much without the ability to smell it.

This bridging of the chemosensory systems has implications for working dogs that are required to find important items, such as narcotics, missing humans, or game on a hunt. Hence, dogs will become even better at tracing down the scents of their targets if they have previously tasted them (Fogle, 1990; Horowitz, 2010). Thus, even the best of best gundogs used for the successful hunting of woodcocks will be able to complete their mission faster or more precisely if you feed them a morsel of woodcock. Eating it leads to the absorption of its molecules into the dog's circulating blood stream, and this will make it easier for the dog to recognize and track down more woodcocks. The same applies to police or law enforcement dogs searching for illegal drugs, and for that reason they may receive a tiny amount of the target compound. That way they can take full advantage of the canine detection system. When seizure alert dogs, as described later in this book, snuffle and start licking their owners, it may represent the way these dogs notice that an epileptic attack is about to follow.

In that regard, dogs use their mouths and tasting when they need to examine something up close. At a distance their other senses work perfectly, but up close right before their faces, they rely much on their mouth and tongue, which thereby come to serve as the tool for having "a closer look" (Horowitz, 2010). By adding a few licks to their sniffing of someone or something, dogs may rapidly analyze all the incoming data not least in their vomeronasal organ. Accordingly, this highly specialized organ is located in between the oral and nasal cavity, as it collects information from the nose and mouth in order for the dog to make a conclusion based upon a combination of olfactory and gustatory scrutiny (Evans & de Lahunta, 2013; Salazar et al., 2013).

By means of this ability, dogs can serve as sentinels regarding materials and substances. This is the case when dogs serve to differentiate between water from different sources or with different levels of purity. Besides, taste sensation may add to the dog's capacity for detecting potential problems with contamination, environment violations, infestation with microorganisms, gases or heavy metals, pollutants, pests, or any other type of aberrant elements (Coren, 2004; Grimm, 2014; Fogle, 1990). To this can be added that dogs perhaps perceive gustatory information from airborne molecules. In their respiratory system, such as inside the larynx and on the vocal cords, dogs display an assortment of taste buds (Koizumi, 1953; Yamamoto et al., 1997). However, whether they are true taste buds or have other functions in chemosensitivity, has yet to be fully explored (Horowitz, 2010; Yamamoto et al., 1997).

Vision: The Sense of Sight

As explained in chapter 1, the hominins carefully watched the savanna's mighty wolves, and at some point they returned the gaze and began keeping a watchful eye on us (Olmert, 2009; Smith, 2004). Dogs' untiring watching of humans has been inherited and fine-tuned through vast numbers of generations. That's why it is a predominant trait of today's dogs.

Hence, dogs are observing our comings and goings, our habits, our friends and spouses, and in general the habits and behaviors connected to our circadian rhythm just as they witness how we emotionally react to any possible situation. In fact, dogs are watching us like nobody else.

This is facilitated because we invite our dogs into our most private lives and our homes (including in most cases our bedrooms), and consequently we share with them all those secrets that are never disclosed to other humans. The great thing is that dogs enjoy this privilege like nobody else, and if they could talk, they would likely express their appreciation of this accessibility, and it is even more likely that they would also ask to join us when we leave for work, reflecting just how very social their nature is.

Despite the fact that we also share our homes with other critters like insects, microbes, vermin, bugs, houseflies, dust mites, lice, and mice, there is one major difference between these creepy-crawlies and the dog. Only the dog cares.

Canines are spectators with a visual capacity that evolved primarily in response to particular survival skills—hunting for food. Many million years ago canid food tended to run away, masked by its herd, which often migrated on the savanna in particular around sunset (twilight) and sunrise. Hence, canines developed an acute ability to see and track movements, panoramic flickers, and subtle or masked changes in motion, all of which they do best in dim light or at night (Coren, 2000; Fogle, 1990; Horowitz, 2010; Miklósi, 2007). In other words, they are visually primed for hunting down prey at dusk. This makes canines proficient predators, stalkers, guardians, shepherds, or at the core, observers.

Though most modern dogs will never have to stalk or kill their food, it does not mean they have stopped looking.

In fact, dogs pay huge visual attendance to us. They gaze at us. They see us out of the corner of their eyes, and they never seem to get tired by looking at us (Coren, 2004; Horowitz, 2010; Serpell, 1996). Dogs perceive our daily activities, even the slightest movements and changes in behavior and tempo, carefully monitoring the surrounding field of view.

This superiority does not come free, as the dog performs poorer than us in terms of resolution up close and the range of colors (Coren, 2000; Fogle, 1990; Horowitz, 2010; Miller & Murphy, 1995). Hence, while humans evolved trichromacy (i.e., the ability to detect three primary colors, namely blue, green, and red), dogs have dichromatic vision, meaning they mainly perceive the world in two primary colors (blue and green).

However, the assumptions made on behalf of dogs with regards to their use of chromaticity, luminous efficiency function, and spectral sensitivity levels are not always based on sufficient scientific scrutiny. Hence, many sources claim to know what is actually processed or experienced by the dog's senses and visual brain. Times might be changing. Recent science indicates that dogs use color cues much more than we previously thought (Kasparson et al., 2013). So regardless of the number of cone pigments detected in the canine retina, nobody really knows what or how much color the dog's brain actually is able to experience or how sensory color inputs are processed. At least we shouldn't underestimate canine color vision, and in particular this is supported by recent research showing that dogs rely predominantly on different color information during visual testing in daylight (Kasparson et al., 2013). Researchers at the Russian Academy of Sciences in Moscow tested eight different dog breeds in terms of visual recognition capacity, and the researchers concluded that during natural photopic light, colors are more informative for canines than the levels of brightness are (Kasparson et al., 2013). Hence, these data dispel the myth that dogs mainly see black-and-white objects, and besides, the scientists proved that dogs register yellow colors, which indicates that dogs may also see some reddish color in addition to their detection of blue and green. At least one thing is certain, we humans have a long way to go before we can state for sure, what dogs can or cannot detect with regards to color nuances.

Regardless of color sensitivity, the dog's visual system certainly surpasses human vision with regards to distant and very delicate motion.

They can register a hand signal up to a kilometer away or a subliminal contraction of a muscle in another living being (Fogle, 1990; Miklósi, 2007; Miller & Murphy, 1995).

A dog detects not only our intentional movements but also involuntary ones and reflexes, such as tiny twitches, tensions, tics, and pent-up bodily energy (Coren, 2000; Horowitz, 2010). Hence, your dog registers even the most subtle changes in you, including those that would remain unrecognized by people. This goes also in the dark, where dogs' vision surpasses ours. This is due to the canine anatomy since dogs' retina contains a reflective layer called *tapetum lucidum*, which is able to reflect incoming light within the eyeball, thereby increasing the available light to the retina and allowing for dog's superior night vision (Coren, 2004; Evans & de Lahunta, 2013; Fogle, 1990).

Whether in bright or dim light, dogs not only recognize us. They also do quite a lot of visual differentiation too. Hence, dogs discriminate between different human faces and their different emotions, such as a happy smile or a straight face. This ability has been demonstrated in dogs even when they are only presented with photographs of their owners along with strangers, by which dogs also could discriminate between males and females (Adachi et al. 2007; Nagasawa et al., 2011). Like humans, dogs prefer the face of a smiling person over a blank facial expression which reflects that dogs process emotional expressions much like we do. We look, we feel, we think, we recognize, and then we decide (Bekoff, 2007; Grimm, 2014; McConnell, 2007; Miklósi, 2007). This is not to say the dog uses vision as his or her primary sense since that's not the case, but dogs developed their aptitude for reading human clues most likely because it provided a major advantage in terms of their coexistence with human beings.

What we call *visible light* is the light waves visible to us humans, but as we will see in the next section, dogs can see much more than us. Light consists of waves defined by their wavelengths, which are measured in nanometers (nm). Humans' visible light consists of waves within the range of 400 to 700 nm, which we perceive as the three primary colors—red, green, and blue.

Light with a wavelength of around 700 nm is seen as red, while light waves around 500 nm are green. And those around 400 nm are blue.

Humans don't see wave bands longer than 700 nm, which would reach infrared light. Nor do we see light waves shorter than 400 nm, which reaches the ultraviolet spectrum.

Secret Superpower Sight

Dogs not only see the world around them by means of the visible light waves that are familiar to us humans. Novel research has revealed that dogs perceive a broader spectrum of wavelengths, and so they see light outside the visible range of humans. This is due to dogs' lenses being UV transparent. That's why their retinas receive wavelengths of the UV spectrum (Douglas & Jeffery, 2014). In other words, your furry friend has UV vision, allowing him or her to perceive UV colorations and luminescence. Hence, dogs see everything from UV glowing urine trails from other animals, psychedelic stripes on flowers, and flamboyant feathers on birds, all the while we humans remain oblivious to this. It is hard to imagine what a dog's world looks like because UV waves normally are invisible to us as a result of our UV blocking lenses. Accordingly, not only can dogs hear sounds or detect scents that are outside the range of humans, but they also see things that we totally miss.

Until the publication by the two London-based professors Ronald Douglas and Glen Jeffery came out in 2014, the general notion was that UV vision is rare in most mammals. That is why the recently published work is nothing but outstanding. In the publication thirty-eight different mammalians ranging from small rodents to carnivores (including dogs, cats, ferrets, and suricates) to primates, ungulates, and cloven-footed animals are examined, and a large number of these are demonstrated to receive UV light (Douglas & Jeffery, 2014). Interestingly among the thirty-eight animal species investigated, dogs are in the top (together with small rodents and the hedgehog) when it comes to how much UV light the lens transmits to the retina.

The retina is the eye's light-sensitive layer lining the back of the eyeball. It converts light waves into nerve signals sent to the brain. All of this translates into meaningful visual scenes (Wunderlich et al., 2010). What is fascinating from a developmental point of view is that dogs surpass the whole plethora of examined primates, carnivores, ungulates, and cloven-footed animals with regards to UV transparency of the lens (Douglas & Jeffery, 2014). What is just as fascinating is the potential of being able to discriminate both visible light plus the UV spectrum of light, though one shouldn't be surprised if science one day reveals that dogs also perceive yet unexplored signals. Concerning the point of having UV vision, it is most likely used for specific functions, such as prey detection, navigation, trailing of various targets, improved vision in darkness, and ultimately for survival and mate selection. In addition, UV waves in the natural world are used for communication because animals have UV-reflecting markings (UV coloration) on their faces and bodies, and these serve as important social signals and reveal the emotional states of animals (Lim & Li, 2006; Pérez i de Lanuza & Font, 2014). This kind of UV-induced communication most likely also applies to dogs, and it only adds to the mounting pile of information that we humans are missing.

> Truth is that nobody can say for sure just how much our dogs can grasp, but next time your dog is seemingly barking at "nothing at all" in the dark, you are almost certainly wrong.

While the findings published by Ronald Douglas and Glen Jeffery are novel, the subject is also in the making, and subsequently much remains to be further investigated with regards to the dog's sensory capacity. As an example of how much further the most recent data can take us, we will shortly look into some scientific facts derived from birds because their navigation properties have been subject of scrutiny for decades. Hence, studies of the orientation of migratory birds reveal that very complex interactions occur between the visual system's detection of light waves and the magnetosensation (Wiltschko et al., 2013). Hence, it turns out that birds' magnetic compass information is dependent on the rays of light both in terms of the light's intensity and wavelength (color). Most likely such complex integration and interconnection of the different sensory modalities will also apply to our furry friends. Even if many new questions arise, we may one day be able to find out just how dogs are able to navigate across huge and to them unknown landscapes or continents, be it in daylight or darkness.

To encapsulate the latest advances within the canine sciences, it looks as if we are heading toward an era of new answers to old questions.

The Sense of Sound

Our sense of hearing never sleeps, and it doesn't rest in dogs either. In fact, dogs have a more sensitive hearing capacity than we do (Coren, 2004; Miklósi, 2007).

First of all the dog's ears are mobile, whereby they can scan an area for sounds and collect the auditory input by which its location, possible source, intensity, and the frequency of the sound waves (pitch) can be determined (Evans & de Lahunta, 2013; Fogle, 1990; Horowitz, 2010; Leeds & Wagner, 2008; Molnár et al., 2009). Because of the mobile ears, dogs elevate, turn, or rotate their outer ears, which thereby work like a sound radar, allowing them to identify direction and distance of the acoustic source before the sound waves are differentiated, and processed in the brain (Horowitz, 2010; Siniscalchi et al., 2008).

With such a fine-tuned and broad-ranging sense of hearing, dogs can hear numerous notes and noises that remain perfectly quiet to us. For example, they may listen night and day to the household bugs like ants, earwigs, spiders, termites, beetles, cockroaches, vermin, lice, and mice. Their ears also detect all the clocks, alarms, ringtones, fluorescent lamps, computer buzzing, noise from the street, radio, TV, etc.

Suddenly I Couldn't Hear You

Almost every dog owner has experienced what might be called "selective hearing," which describes a situation where we're experiencing a sudden case of acute canine deafness. It seems as if someone ignores what they don't want to hear.

To some of us, it might even take place on a weekly basis, or at least every time the dog has better business to do instead of coming when called. It is not a physiological condition or a disorder, as your dog certainly can hear the words, though his or her conscious mind does not appear to receive the information. After you have called the dog's name all over the park, you will realize why this feat is named selective hearing, a euphemism describing our disappointment as the dog's owner and trainer.

You will find it in human beings as well. For example, when the wife asks her husbond if he wants to join her for the opera, he may seemingly ignore her. However, when she mentions something of interest to him, such as formula-one, beer, or football, he instantly responds as if he has been listening all the time. This kind of selective hearing or selective attention may be done consciously or subconsciously.

These cases may seem mundane to most, and so they are since they happen on a daily basis during our interactions with either people or dogs.

The dog's hearing is in many ways superior to human auditory perception. Dogs receive sounds from four times more remote sources than us, and yet they may even locate its precise direction or the source of origin in hundredths of a second (Coren, 2004; Leeds & Wagner, 2008). When we are comparing the human and canine sense of hearing, we find the biggest difference in the high-frequency range. Dogs detect the sounds we humans can perceive, and they also have the sense of hearing ultrasonic vibrations (i.e., sound waves with frequencies far above the human range) (Coren, 2004; Miklósi, 2007). In terms of frequency, dogs can register tones up to 55,000 Hz, while we humans are able to detect sounds up to 20,000 Hz (Fogle, 1990; Horowitz, 2010). However, we are not very receptive in the range above 12,000 Hz, and even in the range of 3,000 to 12,000 Hz, dogs' acoustic sensitivity is much finer than ours. In fact, when considering higher-pitched sounds, dogs are so much better than us that comparisons don't make much sense.

The reason for canines to be so adeptly attuned to higher-pitched sounds has to do with their evolutionary origin. Wild predators benefitted from being able to detect high-pitched sounds like the squeaks that are made by smaller prey. As a result, being able to quickly track sudden shrieks would equal a successful hunt, at least in those days when deer, antelope, or wild sheep were out of reach (Coren, 2004; Fogle, 1990; Miklósi, 2007). This is also why many modern toys for dogs have high-pitched squeakers since their intense shrieks will naturally attract a dog's interest.

I'm Listening

Dogs' ears are in particular finely attuned to sounds that are socially meaningful, such as the human voice, which obviously carries significance to dogs, as we are the source of their food and housing. The dog's mind is in general highly attuned to us humans, but a recent discovery drives the point home since it reveals that the brains of dogs and men are in fact quite alike in terms of processing human voices and their emotional meaning (Andics et al., 2014). In other words, not only humans but also dogs have brain regions that work to find meaning and make sense of human vocalizations, and so these specialized brain areas are highly sensitive to the emotional content of vocal sounds. While most dog owners already know that our furry friends seem to understand perfectly our outpourings, it is the first time that these brain similarities have been scientifically proven, and they certainly offer an intriguing neurobiological glimpse into the richness of the dog's brain and mind (Andics et al., 2014).

Consequently dogs are able to detect even the most subtle changes in vocal signals, such as a subliminal variation in rhythm, loudness, tempo, frequency, attitude, pitch, style, regularity, sharpness, repetitions, quantities, accent, weakness, stanza, nasal twang, and emotional valence (Fogle, 1990; Horowitz, 2010; Leeds & Wagner, 2008). As a result, dogs can engage in very sophisticated communication with other individuals, be they conspecifics or humans. In particular, the language of dogs builds upon four cornerstones, (1) pitch, (2) duration, (3) repetition, and (4) intensity (volume), which altogether make it possible for your furry friend to decode your intention, emotion, and most likely behavior. In other words, it doesn't matter much *what* you utter. It all comes down to *how* you say it (McConnell, 2002). First of all dogs are incredibly sensitive to the pitch of your voice. In fact, they can tell apart sounds that only differ by one eighth of a tone (Coren, 2000,2004).

In general, high-pitched sounds mean "I pose no danger," "I want something," or "I'm sad or in pain," while low-pitched growls basically mean "Stop it," "I warn you," or "Piss off." The more dangerous an animal is, the more low-pitched sounds it emits. Looking at the duration of a sound, a short duration translates into higher intensity of the dog's emotional state, and long duration reflects that cognition and conscious decision-making are involved. If the dog makes many repetitions of a sound expressed at rapid rates, it reflects excitement and urgency. The sound's volume reflects importance. These elements altogether result in emotional expression and social communication, which are both used and decoded cleverly by dogs (Coren, 2000,2004; McConnell, 2007; Scheider et al., 2011; Smith, 2004). So it is easier to train a dog to sit or stay (remain inactive) when your voice is low and calm and when you are using long-lasting sounds. A raised pitch of exciting, short, repetitive outbursts will facilitate any active, moving, or lively reaction such as a prompt return or the rapid fetching of items (McConnell, 2002; Smith, 2004).

To this end, beware that dogs associate your higher-pitched vocalization with reward, while harsh, low-pitched sounds have the opposite effect. Don't be surprised if your dog displays selective hearing while you call his or her name with a voice filled with disappointment and dissatisfaction. The dog hears you perfectly well, and by his or her inattentive behavior, the dog is conveying a message to the frantic person yelling his or her name. It is not complicated. The dog is simply trying to tell you that right here and now you're the most boring option and that the dog has found something more rewarding than you.

Canine Concert

Dogs' sensitivity to the emotional content of sounds is reflected by their interpretation of music, as dogs react in a distinct manner whether they listen to classical music, operas, mainstream pop music, background noise, human voices, or hard-core heavy metal played by Metallica (Leeds & Wagner, 2008; Wells et al., 2002). Like us, dogs relax deeply and settle down quietly in response to classical compositions like Vivaldi's "Four Seasons", Grieg's "Morning", or Beethoven's "Ode to Joy". To unwind and yet feel uplifted, dogs and people prefer Schubert's "Serenade", Debussy's "Arabesque", or Dvorak's "New World Theme". If instead the aim is to wake up, get aroused, and get going, there's no better way than playing Metallica (Leeds & Wagner, 2008; Wells et al., 2002).

In fact, the German composer Richard Wilhelm Wagner, best known for the four operas constituting *The Ring Cycle*, strongly appreciated the musical preferences of his cavalier King Charles spaniel named Pep (Coren, 2004). Pep could tell apart passages in E-flat major and E major, to which he either wagged his tail calmly (E-flat major) or got up all aroused (E major). Consequently the dog's reactions to different musical phrases directed the composer in creating his concept of musical motif as well as the famous opera *Tannhäuser*. After Pep died, Wagner was supervised by an operatic expert named Fips, who also happened to be a cavalier King Charles spaniel (Coren, 2004).

Most importantly, the context in which a sound is expressed along with our body language and behaviors naturally also matters a great deal to dogs' decoding of sounds and how they will respond to a message (Molnár et al., 2009). This is reflected also in dogs' own use of vocalizations, such as barking, which is all but a shower of meaningless or boisterous noise (McConnell, 2007; Miklósi, 2007). Dogs vary their barking depending on situation, target, and context, as their barks reflect the signaler's emotion, motivation, and intent (Coren, 2000, 2004; Fogle, 1990; Yin & McCowan, 2004). Hence, human listeners who are familiar with the nuances, grades, pattern, and variations found in a dog's barking will be readily able to interpret the meaning (Coren, 2000; McConnell, 2002). Moreover, dogs can quite easily be identified individually by means of their specific (personal) bark spectrograms (Yin & McCowan, 2004). Accordingly, dogs discriminate between barking sounds made by different dogs or a single dog in different situations and contexts. Just by listening to conspecifics, a dog can also tell apart individual dogs as a result of vocalization in specific circumstances or contexts (Molnár et al., 2009). The point is that dogs not only hear sounds, they listen to them.

By being very good at listening, often much better than any human, dogs extract a great deal of information from acoustic tonality, rhythmicity, intensity, speed, and frequency, and that's why most dogs can instantly tell just by merely listening to our voices how we are doing or how much we are trying to cover.

> Any dog's vocalization varies with context and intent, as barking reflects the signaler's inner state and target. Hence, barking is a complex and sophisticated way to communicate.

Add to their vocalization all the details dogs get from their other senses as they interpret us, their human companions, and then one may start to fathom just *how much* these critters grasp when it comes to knowing humans.

This is part of the reason why your furry friend seems to know what is happening to whom, where, and when as well as how rewarding or punishing it may be and what to expect.

Dogs also use the sounds made by other individuals to make a judgment about their physique, gender, and energy (Coren, 2000; McConnell, 2002,2007; Molnár et al., 2009). For example, dogs use the acoustic information to form a visual representation that includes a body size assessment of the one who is making the sound (Faragó et al., 2010). In other words, your dog is able to predict the body size of an individual by means of listening to the acoustic features of his or her vocalizations. This was shown in a scientific experiment where dogs sat listening to a tape recording of different growls made by ten unfamiliar dogs of different breeds, ages, and sex (Taylor et al., 2011). When hearing a given growl, the dogs were able to extract information about the size of the growling dog. This means that another individual's voice is conveying its sound waves to the dog's brain (Taylor et al., 2011). This finding has also been shown in humans, as we are ourselves capable of extracting size information by means of hearing a dog growl. We know that with bigger size, the sound of voice gets more and more low-pitched (Coren, 2004; Taylor et al., 2008). We are also able to tell the difference between dogs' barking at nothing versus barking at something of importance (Coren, 2000; McConnell, 2002,2007). Any dog owner will excel at that without much effort.

However, dogs not only integrate sound and size in order to obtain socially relevant information in real life. They do it just as well when they are listening to a tape recorder (Taylor et al., 2011). By listening to recordings of different unfamiliar human voices, dogs are able to impulsively foretell the gender of each person (Ratcliffe et al., 2014). In other words, when your dog listens to the household's utterings, he or she might know much more about each of you than you would guess.

The conclusion from this and other auditory studies of dogs is that one should never underestimate the ability of dogs to perceive, appraise, and react to vocalizations, whether they are emitted from a human or another dog.

The data also reveal that dogs hold high levels of perceptual and cognitive abilities, as they can integrate multimodal sensory information across sounds and sights in order to gain valid information of social relevance. Accordingly, we might not be surprised to find that dogs are able to tell people apart and let us know when somebody is in need of help or have become sick.

Snooping Around

Dogs' social cognition has been taken to a next level by research showing that our furry friends are quite adept at eavesdropping on us (Freidin et al., 2013; Kundey et al., 2011; Marshall-Pescini et al., 2011). Hence, the dog secretly acquires information from third parties, such as a group of interacting humans, even though these people don't address the dog at all. Hence, when a family is having a discussion, the household dog is not only waiting passively for the quarrel to finish. Instead the furry member of the family is most likely following, perceiving, and analyzing the scene. Information based upon human social interactions is then used by the dog to decide who to rely on or trust. This is the case when dogs make use of eavesdropping on third-party humans who engage in a conversation, gesticulatory communication, emotional interaction, and/or generous versus selfish food-sharing behavior (Freidin et al., 2013; Marshall-Pescini et al., 2011). A series of experiments show that eavesdropping dogs extract information by using various simultaneous cues like the tone of voice, gesticulation, and emotional outbreaks. That's why dogs' performance decreased if the investigators masked some of these cues. Interestingly listening to human voices (talking) seemed to be the more important to eavesdropping dogs' performance than the sight of visual cues (human gesticulation), though dogs performed best when they could integrate both auditory and visual cues (Marshall-Pescini et al., 2011). However, the most interesting conclusion from these experiments is how dogs indeed analyze social and emotional reciprocity of a group rather than the individual behavior executed by each participant (Freidin et al., 2013).

Accordingly, dogs have developed a sensitive talent for understanding and bonding with us human beings, whereby they effortlessly distinguish between our positive or negative behaviors and emotions. That's why dogs have a natural talent for decoding people's personality, inner state and emotions (Miklósi, 2007; Turcsán et al., 2015).

These are rather complex abilities, and they may in fact shed light on how dogs—even without any formal training—are able to tell apart potential hazards or adverse health in their owners.

In fact, we humans are expectedly the most important in our dogs' lives, and therefore, it makes sense that they are so delicately attuned to us. Exactly *how* attuned is illustrated by the subtle fact that hormones released into the blood stream of dogs are significantly influenced by their owners' hormone levels (Jones & Josephs, 2006; Penkowa, 2012). This kind of biological reciprocity is seen in many situations, one of them being the reunion of owner and dog even after a short separation (Rehn et al., 2014). As shown in an elegant Swedish study performed by Kerstin Uvnäs-Moberg and collaborators, it makes a huge difference to your dog's emotional state and his or her hormone levels whether you choose to (1) talk to, touch, and pet your dog, (2) only talk to your dog, or (3) neither talk to nor pet your dog when you return home even after a twenty-five-minute separation (Rehn et al., 2014). Moreover, this emotional and hormonal contagion occurs not only when the dog sees you coming home but also for a while after your return. So if you talk to, touch, and pet your dog as part of a merry, cheerful contact-seeking "welcome home" greeting, your pet will experience a significant and long-lasting sense of pleasure because of the release of heartwarming hormones and reduced stress hormones. Consequently, if you return home without engaging in any greeting, interaction, petting, or talking, you will prevent the dog from enjoying the soothing and relaxing molecules, and his or her stress hormones will spiral up too (Rehn et al., 2014).

Hence, on a very physiological and biochemical level, it appears that dogs absorb and imitate our multifarious mental states, gestures, and behaviors, as dogs carefully watch, listen to, and interact with us.

This also indicates why being a dog owner calls for a certain amount of thoughtfulness, concern, empathy, and love.

Sounds for Hounds

Another indicator of the dog's delicate and context-dependent sense of hearing and its impact upon the canine mind is the fact that playing certain kinds of music promotes specific behaviors or emotions in dogs. Hence, clinical tests support that certain compositions of classical music can relax dogs that are aroused, be it inside their homes, when they are driven in cars, or when they are housed in shelters (Leeds & Wagner, 2008; Wells et al., 2002). Science also indicates that the dog's brain cells respond to music in a way that is comparable to humans. That's why dogs register a melody, beat, or rhythm pattern and detect resonance. Accordingly, dogs react quite like humans when they listen to different types of music (Leeds & Wagner, 2008). In short, classical compositions (like Bach's "Air on a G String" or Beethoven's "Moonlight Sonata") significantly relaxes and unwinds dogs, while Metallica's heavy metal generally arouses dogs just like it does with people (Kogan et al., 2012; Wells et al., 2002).

Studies show how dogs react both physiologically and psychologically to the different types of music, and they also show that dogs mimic the response found in human music listeners. Hence, both dogs and humans display music-induced changes in their breathing, respiratory rate, heart rate, brain waves, vigilance, sleeping, vocalization, and body movements (Kogan et al., 2012; Leeds & Wagner, 2008; Wells et al., 2002).

The dog's humanlike reactions to different music genres are highly interesting in light of our evolutionary convergence and the bond between a dog and his or her keeper. Hence, dogs are not only highly attuned to the sound of us and even more so to the individual voice of their owner. They are also sensitive to the acustic landscape of humans and the music genres often preferred by us.

The dog's brain associates and processes simultaneously sensory inputs like hearing and vision in order to generate a meaningful mental representation and act in response to a task or emotionally charged situation (Miklósi, 2007; Siniscalchi et al., 2008). For example, dogs are able to identify their owners' faces from a photograph when they hear the owners' voices (Adachi et al. 2007). Likewise, the research showed that dogs did not react normally to their owners' photographs if they were preceded by a stranger's voice calling the dog's name. Hence, the dog brain apparently integrates sound, sight, and emotional perception with their working memory and cognition when they interact with us (Siniscalchi et al., 2008).

These findings are supported by research showing that dogs (just like us humans) use the right half of their brains for processing threats and alarming stimuli, while the left part of the brain is used for more familiar or frequent stimuli (Siniscalchi et al., 2008,2010,2011).

This supports that the dog's processing of sensory inputs, contextual integration of the received data, perceptual complexity, and cognition is likely not that different from ours (Coren, 2000,2004; Fogle, 1990; Howard, 2014; McConnell, 2002,2007; Miklósi, 2007; Siniscalchi et al., 2008). Accordingly, despite the fact that your pet does not apply linguistics, the dog might be the (only) one who always listen to your sayings and the one who always senses your state of mind.

The dog is even more likely to be the only one who unconditionally and patiently offers all the time you need, the one who will show heartfelt interest and careful listening both when you talk seriously, when you chat, when pour your heart out, or when you simply babble.

While it may seem as if the dog has no clue as to what you are talking about, Fido will in a split second have gathered all the information needed in order to know how you are doing. The dog knows your tone and tune, and he or she can catch layers in your voice that reveals whether you are happy, angry or sad, worried or cocky, resilient or weak. He or she likely also knows a few things that are still unknown to you (Coren, 2000,2004; Fine, 2010; Grimm, 2014; Horowitz, 2010; McConnell, 2002,2007; Miklósi, 2007; Penkowa, 2014; Smith, 2004).

According to the amazing sensory capacity of dogs along with their impact upon our healthiness, the rise of pet therapy and in particular the launch of therapy dogs within hospitals should come as no surprise. Actually owners of furry companions sometimes take for granted the fact that dogs can sooth and comfort us.

CHAPTER 4

The Rise of Dog Therapy
and Therapy Dogs

Because of their remarkable ability to decode us humans, dogs know when and where to intervene, as they possess a natural ability to spot those among us who need to be soothed, comforted, and cheered up (Becker, 2002; Miller, 2010). This is exactly why dogs have been applied by therapists or as therapists for a very long time, dating back to at least in the ancient Greek civilization and likely also before that (Serpell, 1996). While humans have also interacted with other animals, nothing compares to the dog, as we most notably have always valued the deep bond and emotional connection with dogs (Shipman, 2010; Walsh, 2009a).

Since ancient times dogs have been acknowledged for their beneficial impact upon various critical or painful situations encountered by humans. In our time a plethora of research has proven the dog's value and health benefits for a vast number of human physiological and psychological conditions (Fine, 2010). This started in the 1960s when efforts grew toward evidence-based and scientifically controlled research to be published in medical journals. Particularly within the last three decades, the proofs of the canine concept have been rising, and they include scientific demonstration of the dog's major effects with regards to health benefits, improved recovery, and survival following diseases (Fine, 2010; Penkowa, 2012; Friedmann & Son, 2009; Wells, 2011; Wisdom et al., 2009). The rising number of scientific publications based upon dog therapy and/or therapy dogs and the seriousness with which the research is carried out are altogether indicators of the scientific community's acceptance and inclusion.

Find Your Fit

As described in this book, the dog's major mechanism of action involves the human brain and mind, which serve as the control tower over the major bodily systems (the immune system, cardiovascular system, and hormone system). Dogs influence a very broad range of human health conditions. Consequently dogs are now recognized for their impact upon specific diseases, treatment regimens, and rehabilitation. They provide better quality of life for those in hospitals, psychiatric institutions, nursing homes, private homes, and society in general (Becker, 2002; Fine, 2010; Marcus, 2011; Miller, 2010; Penkowa, 2014; Vormbrock & Grossberg, 1988; Wells, 2011; Wisdom et al., 2009).

In fact, both pet dogs and professionally trained or certified dogs like service, assistance, or therapy dogs are now applied in diverse and manifold programs that all have the benefit of humans as primary goal. These programs involve therapy or interventions for patients, diagnostic detection of cancer or other conditions, disease prevention, and rehabilitation programs. The types of dogs involved in such tasks are divided into categories—therapy dogs, psychiatric service dogs, autism dogs, diabetes alert dogs, activity or mobility dogs, cancer-sniffer dogs, guide dogs for the blind, service dogs for the disabled or for rehabilitation programs, seizure- or migraine-alerting dogs, antistress support dogs for postcombat soldiers and disaster-hit victims, grief dogs for the bereaved, hearing alert dogs, emotional support dogs, educational dogs for reading, and prison dogs for better inmate behavior (Chen et al., 2000; Jalongo et al., 2004; Grimm, 2014; Hügler, 2012; Marcus, 2011; Marcus & Bhowmick, 2013; Morris & Esnayra, 2011; Muñoz Lasa et al., 2011; Penkowa, 2012,2014; Walsh, 2009a,b; Wells, 2012; Wells et al., 2008).

Hence, we may at some point begin to classify dogs according to their lifesaving roles or medical specialties rather than their breed, genetic strain, or pedigree, which doesn't really provide that much information about the individual dog.

In fact, science supports that genetics and pedigree are not as important for your dog's behavior, state of mind, or aptitude as are his or her environment, training history, exposure to adventures and challenges, physical exercise, and social interactions (DeGreeff et al., 2012; Gácsi et al., 2013; Marshall-Pescini et al., 2009; Smith, 2004). This is why any breed or individual dog can become a therapy and/or service dog. It is simply a matter of the human on the other end of the leash because what really shapes your dog's brain are the daily inputs, education, care, and lifestyle that you provide for him (McConnell, 2002,2007; Miklósi, 2007; Serpell, 1996). This is supported by science, which by the way has never been able to provide solid evidence of a more or less intelligent breeds (Hare & Woods, 2013; Miklósi, 2007). For that reason today's very popular idea of breeds that are particularly clever or the opposite is nothing but gossip and folktales. There are no dumb dogs, only dumb owners.

Choosing & Using

However, not all nations exploit the dog's health-promoting and therapeutic effects. The United States, Australia, Japan, and Germany have put dogs into clinical practice within their health-care system, and as reported, implementation of dog therapy produces specific goals as measured by the medical health-care staff (Fine, 2010; Hare & Woods, 2013; Headey and Grabka, 2007; Knisely et al., 2012; Nagasawa et al., 2009b). Dogs in hospital settings are not only fighting diseases. They also provide an advantage in terms of reduced health-care costs, higher satisfaction, and quality of life of both patients, their relatives, and the health-care staff (Bouchard et al., 2004; Caprilli & Messeri, 2006; Fine, 2010; Gagnon et al., 2004; Headey et al., 2002; Marcus, 2011; O'Haire, 2009).

Looking ahead, therapy dogs offer the perfect growth opportunity for hospitals and health-care facilities, which often struggle with financing and patient entitlement. In addition, the global population is aging, and with greater age comes an increased request for health-care services and in particular, the growing concept of "aging in place" (ie. staying in one's own home despite old age) will put forward other needs for supportive care delivered at home. Yet in the near future fewer younger people will be available to take care of the elderly. On top of this, multiple and intersecting pressures are expected to drive the transformation of health-care delivery and financing from volume- to value-based systems. That's why the health-care system is facing an unparalleled need to change. To this end, a suitable solution is applying canines such as therapy dogs and dog therapy for patients, assistance or service dogs for rehabilitation or assisted-living programs, and cancer-sniffer dogs for screening and diagnostic purposes. Dogs can be trained to perform various services that go beyond those mentioned previously, and so dogs are ultimately allowing more and more people to live better lives.

Today various organizations, such as the Delaware Assistive Technology Initiative, which is located at the Center for Disabilities Studies at the University of Delaware, educates highly specialized dogs that aid fragile or disabled individuals so that they can live independently in their own homes (http://www.dati.org/newsletter/issues/1999n1/dogs.html). These dogs are taught to open doors, pull up a person, assist walking up and down stairs, support transfer from/to chairs, cars, beds, or wheelchairs, etc. The dogs also turn the light switches on and off and press elevator buttons. These dogs are taught to identify and carry objects like telephones, packages, books, or clothes. In other words, dogs may provide a much-needed tool for the "aging in place" concept.

Let's Get Serious

At present scientific studies have supported the use of therapy dogs and dog therapy for patients suffering from a vast range of conditions that include cardiovascular diseases, brain disorders (neurological, psychiatric, developmental, and behavioral disturbances), and diseases of the immune system (including allergies), and a range of malignant tumors (Becker, 2002; Knisely et al., 2012; Marcus, 2012a,b,2013b; Miller, 2010; Penkowa, 2012,2014). Moreover, today's therapy dogs ameliorate the feeling of pain, loneliness, anxiety, stress, social isolation, and hypertension. Dog therapy also reduces anger and violent behavior, while it improves mood, social behavior, confidence, cohesion, and life quality (Beetz et al., 2012a,b; Ernst, 2012; Marcus et al., 2012; Miller, 2010; Serpell, 1996; Wells, 2011).

The value of dog therapy is reflected by the fact that the US National Institutes of Health (NIH) in 1987 released a recommendation of the use of pet therapy (The health benefits of pets. Workshop summary; 1987 Sep 10-11. Bethesda (MD): National Institutes of Health, Office of Medical Applications of Research. 1987). The NIH recommendation declared, "Future studies of human health should consider the presence or absence of a pet in the home and the nature of this relationship with the pet as a significant variable."

The message is that no study of human health can be considered comprehensive if the animals with which they share their lives are not included.

The seriousness and validity of dogs' roles in medicine and science are reflected by the amount and quality of published research, case studies, textbooks, and other academic publications on the subject as well as the introduction of university courses on the topic (Fine, 2010; Marcus, 2011; Muñoz Lasa et al., 2011; Palley et al., 2010; Penkowa, 2012,2014; Wells, 2011,2012). There are also reports of surveys showing that almost 50 percent of psychiatrists, psychotherapists, and psychologists have used or have prescribed a therapy animal in order to help their patients (Ernst, 2012).

Hence, students may join university-based programs in order to obtain academic credentials with regards to the field of dog therapy and human-animal interactions as used clinically for treating human patients. Such courses are offered in the United States by the University of Denver's Graduate School of Social Work, the Oakland University's School of Nursing, and Harcum College (Palley et al., 2010). Furthermore, academic institutions, including Virginia Commonwealth University's Medical Center and the University of Pennsylvania's School of Veterinary Medicine, have integrated human-animal interactions and therapy animals into their scientific strategies.

As part of the scientific acceptance of dogs' potential roles in medicine, the American Heart Association has summoned experts in the field in order to make an official statement on the matter (Levine et al., 2013).

The scientific statement by the American Heart Association is certainly comforting to dog owners, as it supports that dogs are indeed a pleasant shortcut to improved cardiovascular health. The scientific statement is endorsed by the American Association of Cardiovascular and Pulmonary Rehabilitation, the American Society of Hypertension, the American Society for Preventive Cardiology, the National Heart Foundation of Australia, the Preventive Cardiovascular Nurses Association, and the World Heart Federation, and it was published in the journal *Circulation* (Levine et al., 2013), which is the prime journal for cardiologists, cardiovascular surgeons, and cardiac experts.

Dr. Fido

Dog therapy is an ancient medical aid used for the first time in a period without laboratory tests, technology, placebo-controlled studies, or scientific publications (Serpell, 1996). Yet dog therapy has survived for thousands of years, and today the method is a soaring element of modern, evidence-based, clinically controlled research programs (Becker, 2002; Fine, 2010; Marcus, 2011; Miller, 2010; Penkowa, 2014).

By integrating current knowledge into this concept, the health-care system may be endowed with an intervention that can treat conditions for which pharmaceuticals or surgeries are ineffective or potentially hazardous.

In the most recent decades a growing trend of global green movement and environmental sustainability has emerged along with increased global awareness that medications are not always safe or effective in treating every single patient with identical diagnoses. This new age-integrative medicine has promoted more individually and patient-focused practices that seek to accommodate both ancient and modern methods.

Hence, we have seen an increasing trend of merging complementary or alternative therapies with the established Western-style conventional technologies of the health-care business. That's why clinics all over the globe offer acupuncture, meditation, music therapy, herbal compounds, among other treatments along with the traditional pharmaceuticals and surgery.

As part of today's trend, animal-assisted interventions (AAI) have been established as a therapeutic modality in the clinic and have become a burgeoning research field.

Benefitting from AAI depends to some extent on personal values and preferences, and so it's not for everyone to receive dog therapy. However, for those people who don't have a problem with dogs, there are many health benefits to be derived from the human-dog bond, whether they own dogs or spend time with other people's dogs, which may be the case with AAIs (Becker, 2002; Fine, 2010; Miller, 2010; Penkowa, 2014).

To dig deeper into AAIs, it is necessary first to define what it specifically involves or not. AAIs are typically classified into either animal-assisted therapy (AAT), animal-assisted activity (AAA), and service dog programs (Fine, 2010; Marcus, 2011; Penkowa, 2012).

Animal-Assisted Therapy (AAT)

By definition, AAT (which in this book covers canine-assisted therapy or dog therapy) is a goal-directed intervention in which a specially skilled dog is an integral part of a patient or recipient's treatment. AAT is delivered by the dog and his or her human handler or service partner, who is either a health professional or a certified, professional dog handler. Typically the dog visits the patient in the ward for ten to thirty minutes per session, after which the dog leaves the patient until their next session.

AAT is designed to promote specific improvements in human physiological, mental, social, or emotional health, for which specified goals and objectives are defined for each session, patient, or medical condition. AAT is applied in various clinics, care facilities, or therapeutic settings and can be performed either as a group or individual therapy.

According to the specified goals and specific objectives, AAT has to be documented and evaluated in order to measure the recipient's progress.

For example, AAT can be applied for a patient with a brain injury who is on the road to recovery from an accident or trauma. The patient would often suffer from limited mobility, walking problems, and a lack of strength and balance. By its presence the therapy dog motivates the patient to touch, stroke, brush, and/or move around with the dog. To increase mobility, muscle strength, coordination, or motor balance, the patient may also walk the dog, while the handler would assist by walking alongside them. The distance or speed of walking, muscular volume, endurance, coordination skills, and/or other parameters of mobility progress are recorded, documented, and evaluated as part of the patient's functional recovery (Fine, 2010; Marcus, 2011; Penkowa, 2014; Snipelisky & Burton, 2014). As such, the therapy dog should not be seen as a placebo intervention but a medical option that not only treats disorders but also fosters harmonic, social, biophilic interactions between man and nature, promoting health and mental balance. In the sections describing stroke and patients with brain injuries, more details with regards to AAT are provided.

A subgroup of therapy dogs used for AAT include those owned by the doctor or therapist. The dog is closely working with these individuals as he or she serves as a co-therapist (Fine, 2010; Marcus, 2011; Penkowa, 2014). Consequently such a canine co-therapist has a regular seat in the doctor's consulting office just as he or she will join in on ward rounds and/or on a doctor's call. These canine co-therapists are in some countries designated intervention dogs, doctor dogs, or rehabilitation dogs. Nonetheless, they are complying with a therapy dog providing AAT within a clinical setting.

Animal-Assisted Activities (AAA)

By definition, AAA (which in this book is similar to canine-assisted activity or dog visits) is a casual session that isn't goal-directed, where a friendly, calm pet dog meets and greets people, either individuals or groups. The session can be repeated with many different recipients since AAA is not specifically targeted for a particular patient or goal and is not meant to treat a specific medical condition. Basically it is a pet dog visiting people who engage in activities with the dog or simply pet the dog. The recipients will typically obtain motivational, educational, psychosocial, recreational, and/or therapeutic benefits that enhance their quality of life.

AAA is delivered by the pet and a volunteer (often the owner) who meet some basic criteria. Unlike AAT, the content of an AAA session is spontaneous, and it does not involve documentation or evaluation (Fine, 2010; Penkowa, 2014).

An example of AAA is when a volunteer dog owner takes his or her pet to visit the elderly residents of a nursing home. Informal petting or playing will occur, and aside from signing in and out, no measurements or medical records are kept. The recipients will typically experience better moods, less anxiety, pain, or loneliness, increased appetite, a sense of cohesion, and life quality after the dog's visit.

Service Dogs

Service dogs are in some countries designated as assistance dogs, and they may be subgrouped according to their main functions, such as mobility/walker dogs, guide dogs for the blind, hearing dogs for deaf people, and likewise (Abbud et al., 2014; Duncan, 2000; Fine, 2010; Marcus, 2011; Penkowa, 2014; Rondeau et al., 2010). Service dogs are profoundly different as compared to dogs performing AAT or AAA, as service dogs are living with and owned by an individual patient for whom only the dog provides its services and so it goes around the clock (Marcus, 2011; Miller, 2010; Vincent et al., 2015). Consequently service dogs are highly and individually trained or specialized to provide assistance and perform a range of tasks for the benefit of people with disabilities. In general, service dogs increase the autonomy of the owners such as in the case of guide dogs for blind people, hearing dogs for deaf people, dogs that assist or pull wheelchairs, walking dogs for people with mobility or balance impairments, etc.

A service dog lives together with the disabled person, yet he or she is not a pet animal. A service dog is always on duty and will accompany the owner in any public place, including those areas where animals are normally prohibited. This reflects how service dogs are legally defined and protected by law (Duncan, 2000). However, to be considered an official service dog, the training has to be directly related to the specific disability in order to act in accordance with the personal needs.

In the case of deaf people who cannot hear doorbells, smoke alarms, phone calls, among other things, a service dog will be the one who alerts the deaf person to certain sounds. However, if a deaf person owns a dog that opens doors and picks up items from the floor but is unable to alert his or her owner to sounds, this is not officially or legally a service dog since he's not performing tasks that are directly related to the disability. Medical alert dogs that are trained and certified to warn their owners well before imminent seizures, migraine attacks, or episodes of diabetic hypoglycemia are usually also classified as service dogs.

Any Dog

However, whether you enjoy the company of a dog as part of an AAI program or as a dog owner or trainer, the mechanisms of action upon our health are most likely identical. In that regard, the purpose of making a distinction between AAT and AAA or for that matter other kinds of human-dog interactions is merely for research purposes and statistics. Hence, separating the effects of receiving AAT or AAA or being a dog owner does not make much sense if you are a human being who simply wants to know what a dog can do for your health. Evidently nothing compares to owning your own furry companion, though the point here is that a dog causes specific effects within us, whether we are his or her happy owner or not.

In fact, few studies have compared the outcome of AAI with dog ownership, and in general it is to be expected that anyone would get more from owning a pet dog as compared to having AAI since the latter only spends little time with the critter. As mentioned in the coming chapters, the difference between being a dog owner or recipient of AAI is only a matter of the magnitude of the effect or the time it takes before the benefits set in (Penkowa, 2012). In some cases of human cancer, the dog's anticancer effect increases with increased exposure to dogs, and in that regard, dog ownership naturally surpasses AAI in terms of the outcome (Tranah et al., 2008).

However, for most parts of this book, the dog's effect upon human health is described regardless of ownership status.

Milena Penkowa, M.D., Ph.D., DMSc

Let's Get Honest

Living in an era of digital technology and virtual realities, it is easy to overlook the significance of unconditional love and devotion. The more we live life on the Internet, the easier we tend to forget the importance of being touched, how rewarding unselfish goodwill is, or the secure feeling of having a best friend nearby, all of which boost life quality and health (Olmert, 2009; Serpell, 1996). The clinical use of therapy dogs or dog therapy as a medical treatment within the health-care system is to some degree still met with reluctance or skepticism rather than open-minded curiosity. Regardless of those who subjectively feel it's irrational to consider animals as medicine prescribed for improved health, the concept is soaring, and so we may face a future where dogs might be a rather conventional approach. This practice extends at least with regards to human diseases of both the brain, mind, cardiovascular and immune system as well as cancer, since these conditions have been the center for most research.

This reflects how the dog has moved from being an outdoor worker in the past to becoming an integral part of academic business, from herding to healing. Though the list of health-related conditions that can be improved by a dog is long, the list is anticipated to expand as our medical insight grows. Along with this, for today's patients dogs remain the only clinical approach that doesn't depend on digital technologies and clinical utensils, whereby they provide the patients' with a much-needed link to the outer world. Dogs are perhaps the only icon of certainty and stability that you are left with as soon as you enter a hospital bed. This view is supported by numerous testimonies of how dogs have changed the lives of people ranging from children to the elderly in hospitals, nursing homes, and like institutions.

The dog's major mechanism of action involves the human brain, which serve as the control tower over the bodily systems. That's why dogs have such a broad range of use in terms of human health.

As a result, the dog has proven to be not only man's best friend but also our healthiest friend.

CHAPTER 5

Dogs Benefit the Brain and Mind

The brain remains the most complex, enigmatic, and uncharted part of human life, and so it is the only organ in the human body that has yet to be mapped and fully understood. In the last decades our knowledge of the brain's biochemistry, emotions, processing of thoughts, mental flexibility, and functional behavior control has been revolutionized, but still our understanding is incomplete as many aspects remain to be explained (Howard, 2014; Kandel et al., 2013; Penkowa, 2010).

For instance, no one can explain exactly how or why a specific thought or emotion emerges inside your head at a given point or in any given situation, and in the same situation other individuals may think about something completely different. Those are quite fundamental parts of human life, and yet nobody knows how they got there. The same goes for our individual emotions or outbreaks, abstract thinking, temperament, intelligence, and/or reflections on life. Again, these are quite ordinary features of a human being, but they are not explained in any academic textbook. Our incomplete knowledge of the normal brain is logically an obstacle to scientific development, but an even bigger problem is that we are lacking knowledge of the disordered brain.

Milena Penkowa, M.D., Ph.D., DMSc

The Brain Disease Challenge

Because of the incomplete understanding we have, we cannot cure any brain or mental disease, neurological or psychiatric diseases, including developmental, personality, and/or behavioral disorders, addictions, strokes, pain syndromes, and headaches (Greenberg et al., 2012; Howard, 2014). However, by using medications, assistive devices, physiotherapy, disability aids, and to some degree surgery, symptoms can be decreased and the progression of disease delayed, so the burden upon the patient is considerably lessened and quality of life improved.

Neurological and psychiatric disorders are in fact one of the biggest threats to human health because they are chronic and incurable. Their severely disabling effects often continue for many years or decades (Greenberg et al., 2012; Penkowa, 2010,2012). Moreover, their occurrence is rapidly increasing because of many factors like the global aging of populations, lifestyle aspects like obesity, and the increasing capacity of modern medicine to prevent death and/or keep patients alive despite their conditions.

Consequently the overall burden from neurological and psychiatric diseases and disorders is much greater than the number of deaths would suggest.

According to the WHO (World Health Organization), the burden from neurological and psychiatric diseases will become even more serious and unmanageable on a global scale in the near future. Accordingly, a major challenge is to improve on parameters that restore and create a life of acceptable quality for the patients and their families.

Even if we still cannot explain how the brain creates individual thoughts or emotions, mounting research have approached how the human brain processes information and stores it as memory (Howard, 2014; Kandel et al., 2013).

What is also clear is that no two brains are alike, not even in identical twins. When it comes to our personalities, mind-sets, and/or attitudes, human diversity is far more pronounced than physical appearance. Hence, the very idea of using medications in a "one size fits all" fashion is most likely not the most appropriate. On the other hand, it is a rather unattainable goal to medicate every patient individually since every standard treatment regimen has to be developed and tested in a certain number of individuals before the drug can be approved for the market. Hence, we are not about to see pharmaceutical industries developing drugs on a single-patient basis.

Accordingly, to be able to manage patients with respect to their personal conditions or preferences, something else is needed. This is exactly where the dogs come in.

Dogs and Brains

The beneficial effect of dogs upon patients with neurological or psychiatric diseases is the result of several mechanisms. First of all science shows that the dog's major mechanism of action involves specific changes in the human brain (Handlin et al., 2011; Marcus, 2013a; Penkowa, 2012). These changes in the brain include physiological, cellular, and molecular benefits, and they relate to behavioral, emotional, and psychological effects (Aoki et al., 2012; Fine, 2010; Mormann et al., 2011; Olmert, 2009; Penkowa, 2014). At the end of this chapter we will go deeper into the cellular and molecular mechanisms behind the dog's effects.

On another level dogs can be trained to serve as assistive aids that can physically help paralyzed or deranged patients live better and become more mobile and independent (Marcus, 2011; Muñoz Lasa et al., 2013; Vincent et al., 2015). Another advantage of dogs relates to psychiatric diseases, which make a person unable to recognize his or her state of mind or distort the individual's personality. For the same reason patients are insecure about themselves and their surroundings, and most often they don't trust other people either. They trust psychiatrists or medical doctors even less.

Quite the opposite is true in the case of dogs since even the most confused, insane, paranoid, or psychotic patients don't seem to argue with or blame friendly animals. For these various reasons dogs are able to improve the life of those who suffer from neurological and psychiatric diseases (Penkowa, 2014; Wisdom et al., 2009). As explained later in this chapter, there are a range of cellular and molecular mechanisms of action that explain the effects of dog therapy with regards to the human brain and mind. However, to bridge the field of neurobiology, therapy, and cerebral recovery with therapy dogs and the basic features of being human, let's first look at some relevant features of our fascinating brains.

This Is Your Brain Wired on Neural Networks

The human brain weighs around 1.4 kilograms and contains an overwhelming number of cells, which consist of neurons and glial cells (Herculano-Houzel, 2012; Howard, 2014).

The brain, its brain stem, and the spinal cord form the central nervous system (CNS), which is the part of the nervous system embedded in skeletal bones (i.e., the skull and backbone). All the nerves outside your CNS form the peripheral nervous system, which connects the CNS with your body. This reflects the brain's position as a complex, integrated, information-processing, and executive boss that controls and monitors all bodily parts and functions (Howard, 2006). Sensory neurons carry information from the body's sensory receptors to the brain, allowing us to detect vision, sounds, smells, touch, temperature, etc. Motor neurons transmit signals from the brain to the body's muscles, allowing us to move and take action.

Inside the brain the neurons form the basic cellular entities and building blocks. Neurons are highly specialized cells that stick out their nerve processes or branches that are finger-like projections extending from the cells. These branches make up the brain's neural networks, trillions of cables that conduct and transmit signals to and from other neurons.

A neuron will convey signals to thousands of other neurons by means of a high-speed electrical signal that is transmitted through the neural networks.

When the signal gets to the end of a cable (a nerve process), it will be handed over to the receiving neuron's process by means of a small chemical messenger molecule (a neurotransmitter), which flows through the tiny gap (the synapse) separating one neuron from another with the goal of reaching a receptor on its target cell. As soon as the neurotransmitter finds its receptor, a new electrical impulse is initiated in the recipient neuron, which will then let the information flow to other neurons. On average each neuron communicates with thousands of other neurons, and so most of the time trillions of synapses are being used by your brain as it releases hundreds of different neurotransmitters, each conveying specific messages or emotions that can vary depending on the site of their release within the CNS.

For instance, the neurotransmitter dopamine is signaling reward and pleasure in some areas of the brain. It will enable us to enjoy life's rewards and also motivate us to pursue the source of such rewards. In the brain stem, dopamine is involved in voluntary movements and motor control. That's why a loss of dopamine-producing neurons in this particular area will lead to Parkinson's disease. Likewise, there are other important neurotransmitters like serotonin, oxytocin, endorphins, and prolactin, each of which is involved in particular states of mind, brain, or bodily functions in both man and his best friend (Howard, 2014; Meyer-Lindenberg et al., 2011; Mitsui et al., 2011; Penkowa, 2014; Yoshida et al., 2009). Basically the synaptic flow of chemicals is responsible for the brain's activity (i.e., our thoughts, personalities, behaviors, emotions, and habits) (Kandel et al., 2013).

Brain Building

Neurons are anatomically organized within the central nervous system (CNS) according to their major functions. That's why different brain regions are each responsible for particular tasks, such as memory, language, smell, hearing, vision, conscious thought, reward, and various emotional responses.

The density of neural networks or the number of synapses in your brain is continuously changing due to a high level of plasticity. Hence, the brain reinforces and prunes active connections leading to outgrowth of neural processes (more neural networks) and formation of new synapses. The opposite happens to connections or capacities that are left unused. In other words, when we engage in mindful activities like playing a musical instrument or learning a foreign language, our neural networks will grow along with our skills. In case we decide to stop playing music or don't speak the foreign language, our brain will remove those synapses that were shaped for those activities. This is the brain speaking since neurons are demanding and energy-consuming to keep, and so if you don't use them anyway, why keep them? In other words, use it or lose it.

This is important in case you want to get the most out of life since the major determinant of the brain's performance and capacity is the density of the neural networks and the number of active synapses. Hence, the total weight of the human brain is not the foundation of brainpower (Bamidis et al., 2014; Howard, 2006). Our brain structures and functions are formed primarily by the inputs we get in life (McConnell, 2007).

If you want to train your brain, don't worry too much about genetics. Instead take a closer look on your surroundings, experiences, habits, and daily lifestyle. Bodybuilding is not enough. You need brain building too if you want to become the best version of yourself (Bamidis et al., 2014).

Exercise, the right nutrition, and a good lifestyle are just as important for the brain as they are for your body. That's why eating habits, sports/physical activity, and your amount of cognitive work, sleep patterns, stress management, social relations, task-solving experience, and other environmental enrichment influence your intellectual performance and mental resilience (Bamidis et al., 2014; Dresler et al., 2013; Howard, 2014).

However, there is more to keeping a healthy brain, as we humans are social by nature. That's why we need to belong to somebody, interact with others, exchange support, get attached, and be touched. So a healthy mind is the one enjoying positive and rewarding company, friendships, family, and other social support, which may well include the company of a dog (Hawkley & Cacioppo, 2010; Kamioka et al., 2014; Penkowa, 2012; Serpell, 1996; Zilcha-Mano et al., 2011,2012).

Frayed Ends of Sanity

Although the normal human brain and mind have yet to be fully understood, the situation looks a bit more complex when the nervous system is hit by disease. As the global population is getting older, the frequency of neurological and psychiatric diseases is increasing. Unfortunately they are disabling, chronic, and incurable. That's why the patients and their families most often lose the right of self-determination and control, as they cannot decide much for themselves in terms of pharmaceutical or surgical strategies, medical options, and hospitalization. Many patients live for decades while they suffer from brain or mental disorders, and so there is a solid need for supplementing strategies and therapy in order to not only ameliorate further the disease symptoms but also in order to improve the patients' mood, quality of life, and cheerfulness.

Though neurological and psychiatric diseases and/or injuries pose a major challenge to the health-care sector, no cure exists for these conditions. Yet much knowledge has been obtained regarding the prognosis of some diseases, but exactly why and when some people develop Alzheimer's disease (AD), schizophrenia, panic disorders, depression, or Parkinson's disease (PD) remain to be elucidated.

When someone has to live many years with this kind of chronic disease, there is a huge need for supportive and assistant approaches that may facilitate patients' quality of life, energy, resilience, vitality, motivation, social activity, sense of belonging, and safety. In this regard, dogs have been shown to provide great benefits as an accompanying or supplemental strategy that ameliorates the burden of the brain's incurable diseases (Beetz et al., 2012b; Bernabei et al., 2013; Burton, 2013; Fine, 2010; Friedmann & Son, 2009; Kamioka et al., 2014; Knisely et al., 2012; Muñoz Lasa et al., 2011,2013; Penkowa, 2014; Püllen et al., 2013; Wisdom et al., 2009).

Canis Honorabilis

If people wanted to honor a special dog in the past, they would either erect a statue such as in the case of the world famous dog named Greyfriar's Bobby, of whom a statue sits in Edinburgh, Scotland. He became known for his extreme loyalty and devotion expressed in the graveyard surrounding Greyfriar's Church, where Bobby is said to have spend fourteen years lying on the grave of his beloved owner until the dog finally died (http://greyfriarsbobby.co.uk/story.html).

Nowadays we are not into statues. Instead we head for digital media where today's hero worship takes place. If anything is brilliant, it gets to be published in the most prestigious scientific journals, and if it is second to none, it might be published in *The Lancet Neurology* (http://www.thelancet.com). This is exactly where Dr. Fido made headlines in September 2013

(Burton, 2013), and as far as science is concerned, nothing beats that in terms of respect and status. So this is the modern equivalence to a statue. In the publication, which can be found in volume 12 of 2013 in the September issue of *The Lancet Neurology*, Dr. Adrian Burton addresses the benefits derived from therapy animals, be they real dogs, fake robot seals, or dolphins (Burton, 2013).

Obviously the practical benefits of using a dog rather than a large ocean pool with dolphins are evident in terms of application, implementation, safety, and feasibility. This is particularly relevant when patients are suffering from neurological and psychiatric diseases, which cause physical disabilities, paralysis, fear of going into water, and various other symptoms that are not always well-matched with a huge swimming pool of dolphins. Hence, most patients prefer to stay in a safer place and get a visit by a friendly, soft-furred, pettable pooch.

Dementia and Alzheimer's Disease

Many people were never taught the difference between dementia and Alzheimer's disease, or perhaps they don't know there is a difference. The difference is quite simple though since dementia describes a symptom, as dementia is not a diagnosis in itself, and this symptom consists of memory loss, learning difficulties, and blurred thinking. So dementia symptoms are found in many different diseases or diagnoses, such as stroke or intoxication and Alzheimer's disease (Greenberg et al., 2012; Howard, 2006).

Alzheimer's disease is a complete diagnosis that comprises a pattern of characteristic symptoms among which the most prominent or early symptom is dementia. The changes are often tiny in the beginning, but for most patients they have already grown severe enough to disturb daily functions and life in general. However, there are also other symptoms than dementia in those diagnosed with Alzheimer's disease, as the patients may experience depression, insomnia, restlessness, and personality changes (Greenberg et al., 2012).

While the distinction between a diagnostic entity (disease) and a single symptom of a given disease is important to doctors, it doesn't make much difference to patients or to their dogs.

Whether a patient is burdened by Alzheimer's disease or a condition leading to dementia, a loss of mental and cognitive functions will take place. This is due to the shrinkage of the brain caused by a loss of its neurons, which degenerate and wither throughout the brain (Hidalgo et al, 2006). While the brain tissue eventually decays, the mind loses nearly all its functions, and though research has pointed to some targets for future treatment strategies, we still cannot cure the disease (Howard, 2014; Penkowa, 2006,2010).

Dementia and Alzheimer's disease are widespread, fast-growing, and much-dreaded conditions not only affecting the elderly but the whole family. The disease progresses with ongoing brain cell damage and loss of cognitive and socioemotional functions.

Clinical research in Alzheimer's disease and various types of dementia have shown that dogs, both pet dogs and those working in AAT and AAA programs, can ameliorate the symptoms and improve behavior, communication, social responses, emotions, and cognition in both in- and out-patients as shown in various settings, such as nursing homes and hospitals and geriatric departments (Filan & Llewellyn-Jones, 2006; Friedmann et al., 2014; Kamioka et al., 2014; Knisely et al., 2012; Marcus, 2011,2013a; Snipelisky & Burton, 2014).

In these patients the normal verbal use of language is often lost, but when they are visited by a dog, patients often verbalize how they like being with the dog, how friendly the dog is, and how they can identify themselves with it (Fine, 2010; Tribet et al, 2008).

In a study performed in Frankfurt (Germany), 105 demented, elderly patients with cognitive, mental, and functional impairments took part in dog-assisted group therapy lasting for thirty minutes every fourteen days for a total period of fourteen months (Püllen et al., 2013). The dog-assisted group therapy resulted in significant improvements of the patients who showed better mood, became more active, improved their attention levels, social behavior, and communication, while at night they slept better because of the experiences with the dog. On the same day as the dog visited and again on the next day, a very frequent topic of the conversation with patients was the dog. At the same time no side effects or adverse events occurred.

The researchers could also conclude that in terms of the hospital and the patients, it was safe to bring in the dog, a labrador retriever who was subject to veterinary control.

This is in general the case, as no adverse or harmful effects or allergies have been reported in relation to AAT and AAA in hospitals, institutions, and clinics (Fine, 2010; Johnson et al., 2002; Kamioka et al., 2014; Marcus, 2012a; Snipelisky & Burton, 2014).

In addition, it was demonstrated how a therapy dog's company leads to improvements of patients' prosocial contact seeking, emotional states, communication and friendly interactions with other people, as measured by the number a patient smiles, seeks eye contact, touches other individuals, talks and expresses joy (Bernabei et al., 2013; Filan & Llewellyn-Jones, 2006; LaFrance et al., 2007; Perkins et al., 2008; O'Haire, 2010; Richeson, 2003; Tribet et al., 2008). At the same time the company of a dog leads to reduced agitation and less aggressive behaviors, which otherwise can become a significant problem in patients with Alzheimer's disease (Barker & Wolen, 2008; Marx et al., 2010). Hence, the number of aggressive and noisy outbursts was reduced, and the general level of noise in the department was diminished during a dog's visit. After the dog left, the situation reverted to its previous state (Walsh et al., 1995).

Likewise, a study compared a dog's impact on aggressive behavior in institutionalized patients with Alzheimer's disease (Churchill et al., 1999). These patients were prone to become agitated in the evening, a dementia-related behavior known as the sundown syndrome. The sundown syndrome makes patients confused and agitated while the sun goes down and/or perhaps throughout night. Hence, sundowning patients are likely to wander, and therefore, the syndrome puts quite a lot of stress on caregivers or family. When these patients were exposed to either a dog with its handler or the handler alone, it soon became clear that the dog—and only the dog—improved their behavior as agitation, including sundowning, diminished while prosocial interactions, contact with others, and mood improved (Churchill et al., 1999).

These behavioral changes are part of the dog's ability to promote a general relaxation of the patients, and in conjunction with this, language and verbal skills of the patients are improved, leading to better self-esteem and a sense of cohesion (Bernabei et al., 2013; Penkowa, 2012; Tribet et al., 2008; Walsh, 2009a).

At this point one may consider if a toy dog (plush dog) or a pet robot, such as the AIBO made by the Sony Corp., could be used instead of a real dog for demented patients. While patients do react to AIBO as well as they react to a toy by looking at it or talking to it, they are in fact fully aware that AIBO is nothing but a robot (Tamura et al., 2004). In a study performed in the lab of Dr. Ádám Miklósi at the Hungarian Academy of Sciences in Budapest (Hungary), researchers compared how much people liked to interact with either the AIBO or a real puppy (Kerepesi et al., 2006). They found that both children and adults stopped playing with the AIBO quicker than they did with the real puppy. Researchers judge the AIBO to have a limited capacity to keep us engaged. Hence, we tend to show an initial curiosity toward such a living robot; however, that soon ends, and we lose interest in the robot, which in spite of everything is nothing but a piece of dead metal. Interestingly dogs are also drawing a line between a robotic experimenter and a living human being, and even when the robot displays a sort of social, interactive behavior, the dog is still differentiating it from humans (Lakatos et al., 2014).

Not surprisingly, research confirms that clear benefits are obtained when humans are together with a real dog instead of an artificial dog, such as playing with a toy or robotic dog, watching a video with puppies, or reminiscing about dogs. For instance, patients' communication levels and verbal abilities are improved the most by the real dog as compared to the group of artificial dog-related stimuli (Beetz et al., 2012a; Friedmann et al., 2014; Marx et al., 2010). For comparisons, on average demented people talked about twenty-three things/subjects when they were with a real dog, while a fake dog (toy) made them talk about three things/subjects (Marx et al., 2010).

Hence, research concludes that live, social stimuli and interactions with a real dog rather than a robotic or plush dog are superior with regards to the cognitive and mental benefits for the elderly with dementia (Cohen-Mansfield et al., 2011).

These effects are also described in a book by Dr. Aubrey H. Fine, a book that explains how the dog's presence is associated with less confusion and agitation among demented patients (Fine, 2010). The tendency of demented patients to wander and get lost both in unfamiliar and familiar places can also be dealt with (Fine, 2010). Hence, by letting a trained dog join patients out for a walk, the dog can be called back, and the patient will follow him and return. Some dogs may even join patients for longer walks during which the dog by himself decides to return and makes the patient follow.

What might be more surprising is that as little as two weekly visits from a therapy dog may improve demented patients' sense of time by increasing their orientation to the days of the week when the dog visits (Katsinas, 2001). This effect is in itself quite sensational since losing track of time is very salient in dementia. However, it does not mean we are going to cure Alzheimer's disease by means of a dog visit, but it shows that dogs can influence the course of disease to a degree that surpasses the effects of medications. Hence, strategic implementation of dog therapy in nursing homes, clinics, hospitals, and geriatric institutions may indeed result in better quality of life for these patients.

The benefits of a dog's visit is primarily evident when the dog is present since demented patients' behavior would return to a baseline after the dog has left. However, other studies have shown that the dog's effect lasts on a long-term basis since the benefits continued after the dog session was over (Fine, 2010; Marx et al., 2010; Kanamori et al., 2001; Walsh et al., 1995). To this end, a study of elderly residents living in long-term care facilities in southern Mississippi showed that receiving dog visits significantly reduced the feeling of loneliness and that a dog's visit once per week was just as effective in reducing loneliness as receiving three dog visits per week (Banks & Banks, 2002). Most likely the explanation for this is that a therapy dog may convey an enduring change that will keep the feeling of being lonely at bay in between visits. The impact of reducing loneliness in itself has a huge effect on human health since social isolation leads to increased disease frequency (morbidity), increased rates of cancer and cardiovascular disease, not to mention increased mortality (Hawkley & Cacioppo, 2003,2010; Serpell, 1996).

For anyone burdened by Alzheimer's disease and/or dementia, the most devastating consequence is the loss of remembrance. In that regard, the most dramatic effect is that a dog may to some degree improve patients' memory and in particular their fond memories of the past, including those relating to their own pets (Bank & Banks, 2002; Marcus, 2011). In a study lasting three months a therapy dog visited patients every fortnight for a total number of six visits. The recipients of the therapy dog were patients with Alzheimer's disease or vascular dementia (dementia caused by reduced blood flow to the brain, usually because of a stroke or series of strokes). After these six visits researchers could measure a memory improvement of 8 percent, whereas the control group (not receiving dog visits) showed a memory deterioration of 7 percent after the three study months (Kanamori et al., 2001). Furthermore, anxieties and phobias were cut down to half of their usual occurrence by means of the therapy dog, while in control subjects (not visited by the dog), anxiety and phobia tended to increase.

Another example of unexpected effects as a result of a dog's presence comes from a study of elderly residents who suddenly would recollect and verbally explain a series of personal memories from the past, and so they told the dog about it spontaneously during the AAT session (Banks & Banks, 2002).

If you'd like to watch such an encounter for yourself, I recommend that you go to this link: http://laughingsquid.com/daughter-posts-video-catching-an-incredible-moment-between-non-verbal-father-with-alzheimers-and-loving-dog, which shows an amazing moment where a dog seeks contact with a nonverbal patient with Alzheimer's disease.

By measuring the concentration in saliva of the protein chromogranin A, researchers can determine how negatively affected patients are, as chromogranin A serves as a disease marker that increases because of an arousal of the nervous system and/or an agitated mind. Interestingly in patients with dementia, chromogranin A levels drop to less than half as a response to the dog's sixth visit, while it went up in those who did not get any visits by the dog (Kanamori et al., 2001).

As the most important effect relates to the patients, therapy dogs are also able to positively influence the caregivers and families (Barker & Wolen, 2008). The dog may also build a bridge between patients and their families or caregivers (Marcus et al., 2012; Oyama & Serpell, 2013). This is a hugely important aspect of AAT since dementia most often will isolate patients from the outside world, including even the closest relatives (Marcus, 2011).

Obviously a dog cannot provide a cure for Alzheimer's disease, but neither can any doctor. Yet there are so many aspects to life that a dog can improve for these patients, and these go far beyond the capacity of the human doctors.

Unfortunately no cure exists for Alzheimer's disease or dementia, though some pharmaceuticals may slightly delay some of the patients' progressively developing symptoms. In unison, unwanted side effects from the drugs are following as to why the care and management of these patients are facing serious challenges. Conversely dog therapy is not invasive and causes no adverse reactions, yet it is inexpensive and universally available. In fact, using dogs as part of an overall therapeutic strategy is a rather safe, uncomplicated, and limitless approach (Javelot et al., 2012).

Parkinson's Disease

Parkinson's disease is a chronic brain disease that causes severe movement problems and affects how the patient moves, speaks, thinks, and behaves. It arises because of the destruction of some specific neurons in a small area known as substantia nigra (the black substance) situated in the upper part of the brain stem. Normally these cells produce and secrete the neurotransmitter dopamine, as to why parkinsonism is caused by the lack of dopamine (Greenberg et al., 2012; Howard, 2006; Kandel et al., 2013).

Like in the case of dementia, Parkinson's disease is a progressive disease, which means it will gradually get worse. It often starts with subtle hand tremors and later on develops into stiffness of the limbs, whereby patients can't move their bodies just as easy and rapid as before. Later patients lose the control over their muscles, and their physical control, coordination, and balance are lost. Sleep problems, dementia, and depression will also accompany the disease (Wagle et al., 2014).

According to the MNT Knowledge Center (http://www.medicalnewstoday.com/info/parkinsons-disease), just about one million Americans live with Parkinson's disease, which sixty thousand people are diagnosed with in the United States annually. In the United Kingdom, approximately 127,000 persons suffer from Parkinson's disease, and on a global scale approximately ten million people suffer from this disease.

As stated by the Parkinson's Disease Foundation (http://www.pdf.
org/en/index), the economic toll of the disease is huge (around $25 billion
annually in the United States), and for each patient the average yearly
medication costs are in the range of $2,500 to $10,000. For unknown
reasons men have a 50 percent higher risk of getting Parkinson's disease
than women. Although no available cure exists, a range of symptomatic or
supportive interventions can improve patients' functioning, independence,
and the quality of life. This is where the dogs come in.

Researchers have examined the effects of AAT upon elderly people
suffering from different age-related disorders like Parkinson's disease, as a
therapy dog visited the elderly in their long-term care facilities in southern
Mississippi (Banks & Banks, 2002). The dog came either once or three
times a week for a period of six weeks, and the same dog was used for each
participant throughout the study period. Whether the dog was applied
once or three times a week, it caused the same degree of beneficial effects—
significantly reduced loneliness and a tendency to increase social behavior,
even including talking to the dog (Banks & Banks, 2002).

While the study also included persons with other disorders, such as
stroke, diabetes, cardiovascular diseases, pulmonary disease, hip fractures,
and osteoporosis, the effects of the dog are likely to be extraordinarily
valuable for the patients with Parkinson's disease since they often drift
away from the world and people around them as a result of their lack of
voluntary control over their bodies including also the ability to speak,
process sounds and control the voice (Tsanas et al., 2012). Most often this
leaves Parkinson's patients with a fixed, inexpressive face, and they do not
talk to others then. When a dog approaches and nuzzles these patients,
they are brought out of their shells and get reconnected to those around
them (Becker, 2002; Fine, 2010; Olmert, 2009; Salmon & Salmon, 1982;
Serpell, 1996).

This is of great importance since we won't be able to cure Parkinson's
disease in the near future, and so being able to increase quality of life and
the feeling of belonging can make quite a difference to the patients and
their surroundings.

This was demonstrated by deploying a dog in a nursing home where
residents were burdened by various disorders, including also Parkinson's
(Salmon & Salmon, 1982). The dog went to accompany the residents in a

specific department within the nursing home for a period of six months, while residents in another department served as the controls and did not get a dog. The aim was to investigate how such a residential dog in a nursing home could affect the elderly, and the conclusions were quite positive since the dog led to happier, more vigilant, more social, more obliging, and more responsive patients (Salmon & Salmon, 1982). In the control department residents were not showing these positive changes. On the contrary, they deteriorated, becoming more bedridden and withdrawn. This is supported also by other data indicating that institutionalized patients may benefit profoundly from a dog as they improve on a range of emotional, psychosocial, and physical parameters (Fine, 2010; Serpell, 1996; Wells, 2007,2011).

Research has shown how Parkinson's patients benefit significantly from having dogs. Since they will have to take the dogs out, they get some balanced exercise many times a day with the dogs, which will assist the patients with several daily routines, perform specific tasks, and protect the patients against falling or becoming injured in falls. Parkinson's service dog can make sure that patients remain independent for longer, feel more personal freedom, and stay physically active despite their disease (Marcus, 2011; Penkowa, 2014; Serpell, 1996).

Because of their amazing and reliable abilities, of which numerous anecdotes are published in just about any media, a number of organizations train and/or provide these custom-trained service dogs, which in some regions are recognized either as Parkinson's walker dogs or assistance dogs.

The Parkinson's Association created a division called *Paws for Parkinson's* (http://www.parkinsonsassociation.org/resources/paws-for-parkinsons), which is a program that aims to pair patients with service dogs specialized for Parkinsonian problems, as described in the magazine *San Diego Pets* in April 2014 (http://www.sandiegopetsmagazine.com/view/full_story/17680504/article-Paws-for-Parkinson%E2%80%99s?instance=petpress).

Furthermore, the organization Paws with a Cause (https://www.pawswithacause.org/what-we-do/service-dogs) breeds, raises, and trains service dogs at no cost to eligible, approved recipients. In the United Kingdom, the organization Canine Partners (http://www.caninepartners.co.uk) trains their carefully selected dogs for the individual needs of an eligible and certified recipient who will be educated, thoroughly assessed, and continuously supported in order to take best care of both the dog and the recipient. In fact, Canine Partners make use of a rigorous assessment procedure in order to spot appropriate applicants for their highly specialized dogs, whereby they make every effort to ensure a happy and healthy human-animal relationship.

A nationwide listing of worldwide organizations that are engaged in training and service dog programs for individual purposes can be found by visiting the Land of PureGold Foundation's website (http://landofpuregold.com/service-groups.htm) or the website of the Assistance Dogs International (http://www.assistancedogsinternational.org).

Anyone interested in service/assistance/walker dog programs may contact these or any of the other organizations to get information on how to best obtain a dog educated to help a person with Parkinson's disease.

A Parkinson's dog is trained to help with practical things like turning on or off the light switches, picking up difficult-to-reach objects (like keys or credit card), opening and closing doors, helping to get dressed and undressed, assisting during walking by providing balance, and supporting a person, or helping one get up. The dog may also help you to overcome Parkinson's freezing and immobility, or he may clear your way in crowded spaces by placing a gentle physical pressure on the surrounding people's legs or instead guide your way out of a crowded area that would otherwise aggravate freezing of gait. A Parkinson's dog can also fetch medications from customary places and remind patients to take their scheduled medicine. Likewise, the dog conveys antidepressant effects, increases physical exercise by walking with the patient, and establishes social interactions with other people, which are all highly relevant quality-of-life aspects relating to Parkinson's disease. They can also load and unload the washing machine, collect the post (instead of attacking the mailman), and press buttons on various devices. Besides, the dog will make just as good a friend and calming companion to a Parkinson's patient as he will for any other person.

In most cases Parkinson's disease is believed to be caused by a combination of genetic and environmental risk factors. Hence, many studies have explored various risk factors in relation to the occurrence of the disease, and it has been shown that pet ownership reduces the risk of getting Parkinson's disease. In fact, the risk seems to decrease more and more with longer exposure to pets, and so owners who were exposed to their pets for more than ten years have a twofold reduced risk of becoming Parkinson's patients (Behari et al., 2001). However, living with a dog for shorter periods or less than five years in total may likely be too short to bring about the preventive effect (Tanner et al., 1989).

> Having a dog for at least ten years halves the risk of Parkinson's disease (Behari et al., 2001).

However, no large-scale, clinically controlled publications or reviews have been published with regards to AAT for Parkinson's. This is a bit unexpected since studies published more than a decade ago have shown how the company of a pet or therapy dog increases levels of dopamine in humans (Odendaal, 2000; Odendaal & Meintjes, 2003). This ought to incite huge interest in the application of dog therapy for Parkinson's since the disease develops as a result of dopamine depletion as a result of the death of dopamine-producing neurons localized in the aforementioned substantia nigra (Greenberg et al., 2012; Howard, 2014; Kandel et al., 2013).

However, one study performed by Nekisa Zakeri and Dr. Peter G. Bain at the Department of Clinical Neuroscience, Imperial College London, Charing Cross Hospital Campus in London examined the effect of a pet dog in a case of Parkinson's disease, and for the first time they showed how a dog conveys a range of advantages to Parkinson's patients (Zakeri & Bain, 2010). The applied dog significantly changed the patient's life for the better, as he gave rise to major improvements in clinical symptoms as well as a reduction in the need for pharmaceutical treatment. Hence, this very important study has taken a huge step forward with regards to dog therapy for Parkinson's management, as it showed how a dog—in this case a highland terrier—may convey much more benefit for the patient than being merely a walking aid (Zakeri & Bain, 2010).

Though a walker dog will certainly make his or her owner's life easier and more independent, there are many more benefits that may follow in addition to the patient's mobility. The study by Zakeri and Bain (2010) revealed that a dog also may reduce the neurological deficits, slow down disease progression, and decrease the need for pharmaceuticals. Thus, from the case report published by Nekisa Zakeri and Peter G. Bain, something novel emerged. They revealed how a pet dog without any formal training conveyed a range of neurological, physiological, and medical improvements for someone with Parkinson's disease.

Motor functions like walking as well as nonmotor functions, such as bowel function, appetite, and sleep patterns, were remarkably improved after the pet dog arrived in the patient's home (Zakeri & Bain, 2010). Psychosocial functions were also improved, and by the following year after the dog's arrival, the patient's anti-parkinsonian medication could be reduced. Six years later the effects attributed to the dog still persisted, and the patient's medication had not undergone any ensuing adjustments. The latter is in itself quite remarkable since Parkinson's disease management almost always requires significant modifications of the dosage, administration routes, and/or drugs of choice because of an eventual lack of desired effects and/or intolerable side effects (Greenberg et al., 2012; Howard, 2006).

Since this is a case report (a single patient's case), one cannot deduce anything in general, but it is nevertheless out of the ordinary to find out about the dog's lasting effect on Parkinson's. Considering the dog's extraordinary influence as reported in the paper by Zakeri and Bain (2010), time has come for a needed change in the way medical doctors and society approach Parkinson's disease. Immense pharmaceutical research is conducted, and along with it enormous resources follow. This is not bad though, but the point is we might be missing out on nonpharmaceutical interventions, such as those involving therapy, service, or pet dogs. In fact, by May 2014 there are more than seventy-three thousand published scientific papers dealing with Parkinson's disease according to a simple search in Pubmed (www.Pubmed. org), which is a major database of scientific papers. However, only one of the seventy-three thousand publications deals with the dog's effects on the disease.

All the existing drugs on the market have serious side effects, are quite expensive, and require careful planning to hit the correct concentration at the right time. Thus, the absence of scientific publications focusing in the dog's possible impact upon the disorder is baffling.

The explanation for this is multifaceted and are beyond this book's focus, but we all should ask ourselves whether the time has come for a showdown with the past and our ongoing and often uncritical expectations for the pharmaceutical industry?

And there is one more thing. Being with a dog elevates significantly the levels of dopamine, which is depleted and consequently missing in Parkinson's disease. Excellent work performed by the late professor Johannes S. J. Odendaal and his senior colleague Roy Alec Meintjes, a professor at the University of Pretoria in South Africa, first showed that a dog's company made our human cells release significant amounts of dopamine (Odendaal, 2000; Odendaal & Meintjes, 2003). It only takes fifteen to thirty minutes together with a dog who may or may not be your own pet before dopamine flows in the blood stream.

As a consequence, dogs hold an untapped potential with regards to Parkinson's disease, and our four-legged therapists cause no side effects or unnecessary expenditures.

Epilepsy

Around 3 percent in the United Kingdom and 4 percent in the United States develop epilepsy at some point in life, which means they suffer seizures or epileptic attacks suddenly without much premonition. There are several different types of attacks that may last from a few seconds to many minutes, and symptoms may range from minor or partial seizures to severe convulsions where patients are rendered unconscious (Greenberg et al., 2012). The symptoms arise because of a burst of abnormal activity in the brain, which suddenly transmits electrical impulses that are uncoordinated, uncontrolled, and unhealthy.

In the long run epilepsy not only affects the muscles because of the convulsions but may also disturb sensory functions, emotional states, cognition, and behavior (Howard, 2006). This is due to the nature of the disorder, side effects to the antiepileptic medication, and the pressure from society's often unfriendly attitude toward disabilities like epilepsy.

> - Sixty-five million people on the globe have epilepsy.
> - More than two million in United States have epilepsy.
> - Every year in the United States, 150,000 new cases of epilepsy are diagnosed.
> - Around 33 percent have uncontrollable seizures because of a lack of effective treatment.
> - In around 60 percent of cases, the cause is unknown.
>
> This information comes from the Epilepsy Foundation
> (https://www.epilepsy.com).

Patients with epilepsy have repeated attacks that will come and go throughout their lifetimes. Thus, epilepsy should not be confused with the condition of having one single, nonepileptic seizure, which close to 5 percent of people experience or witness. For instance, high fever in children may cause an episode of febrile convulsions just as lack of oxygen, low blood sugar, toxins, or drugs may provoke a sort of reactive seizure, and such a single episode does not classify for epilepsy (Greenberg et al., 2012; Howard, 2006).

Among the many lifesaving jobs dogs do, one of the most amazing achievements is their ability to sense an imminent epileptic attack. Dogs are able to warn the patient or those around the patient in due time (typically fifteen to forty-five minutes) before the convulsions and/or unconsciousness begin (Brown & Strong, 2001; Di Vito et al., 2010; Fine, 2010; Kirton et al., 2008). Thanks to such seizure alert dogs, the patient get the needed time to move away from dangerous places like traffic, take antiepileptic medication, find a safe, quiet place to lie down, or call for help (Brown & Goldstein, 2011; Dalziel et al., 2003; Kirton et al., 2004; Strong et al., 1999).

Scientific attention to this ability in dogs was particularly drawn two decades ago because of some sporadic anecdotes suggesting how family pet dogs were able to sense their owners' onsets of seizures (Edney, 1991,1993). Since then, neither the scientific nor public attention has decreased.

Logically speaking, dogs alerting their owners to imminent seizures is beyond what any doctor or researcher would ever dare to fancy, and still today nobody knows exactly what it is these dogs can sense. In fact, before the first anecdotes nobody knew that some minutes to hours before an attack epileptic patients actually showed or emitted or secreted *something*, and whatever that was, their pet dogs not only seemed to know but would also let them know. Such news naturally shook the scientific community and fascinated even more people. That's why the mechanism behind it has been the subject of debate and research ever since, and so it will likely remain the same for at least a couple of decades more. However, researchers seem to converge on a set of mechanisms that include the sense of smell (like scent detection of pheromones, hormones, transmitters, sweat, or other biochemicals), subtle behavioral clues (observation of microscopic gestures, tensions, or altered positioning), and/or physiological parameters like heart rate and respiration (the sound of heartbeats or changes in breathing patterns or otherwise) (Brown & Goldstein, 2011; Brown & Strong, 2001; Dalziel et al., 2003; Miklósi, 2007).

Anyway, there are two types of canine seizure specialists, the seizure alert dogs and the seizure response dogs (Fine, 2010; Kirton et al., 2004,2008). Seizure alert dogs react prior to the looming epileptic attack, and accordingly, they respond when nobody else has any clue. And they do so with great precision and reliability (Brown & Goldstein, 2011; Dalziel et al., 2003; Kirton et al., 2004; Strong et al., 1999). The dogs convey the message to the owners or other people by behavioral changes or sounds, as they typically starts to contact and lick the owners and even become restless, jump up, bark, and/or whine (Brown & Strong, 2001; Di Vito et al., 2010; Kirton et al., 2004; Miklósi, 2007). In fact, the contact seeking and in particular the licking might reflect how the dog can use chemosensation in order to find out what is about to happen.

In contrast, the seizure response dogs react during or immediately after the seizure, as they typically protect the convulsing subjects by guarding against other people, starting emergency response systems, or positioning themselves to physically support the patient during the attack (Di Vito et al., 2010; Kirton et al., 2004,2008). Another mechanism used by both types of seizure dogs is licking the patient, a simple gesture that is known to break off the seizure, an effect that comes as a result of its sensory modality, which activates certain neural and hormonal mechanisms (Di Vito et al., 2010; Edney, 1995; Kirton et al., 2004). In other words, the result of the dog's licking behavior reflects what was described earlier in this book, namely the power of touch.

Because of these amazing skills of our four-legged friends, there are today various professional organizations working with seizure alert dogs or seizure response dogs (Brown & Goldstein, 2011; Brown & Strong, 2001; Dalziel et al., 2003; Fine, 2010; Strong et al., 2002). The dogs are specifically trained for months or even years before they are certified to assist epileptic patients, while in some cases it may be the patient's own pet dog that is properly trained.

There's something more to it though. Scientific studies keep showing that the frequency of seizure attacks is reduced significantly when patients receive seizure dogs (Brown & Goldstein, 2011; Brown & Strong, 2001; Fine, 2010; Strong et al., 1999,2002). Hence, the dog gets to perform his or her task fewer and fewer times after arrival, which is a phenomenon ascribed to the calming effect of the dog.

The dog's calming effect is in this case an extended version since a major handicapping factor in epilepsy is the loss of control that goes along with an epileptic seizure, and so the risk of having a seizure, including the risk of getting injured, rather than the seizure itself may be the biggest problem and source of anxiety for the patient. They also fear having seizures in public, since other people often react with fear, disgust, or embarrassment toward the patient, who often gets stigmatized because of the manifest loss of control during seizures. The patient cannot control the reaction from others, and so many epileptics choose isolation over social interactions (Räty & Wilde-Larsson, 2011).

What only makes things worse is the fact that modern society has idealized the image of being in control and living an independent life, whereby the mere unpredictability of having a seizure and its evident loss of control profoundly conflict with the glorified image of our time. Subsequently patients with epilepsy are stigmatized, which in itself promotes negative feelings, distress, and anxiety.

Hence, when these patients get seizure alert dogs, they not only get four-legged companions and devoted friends. They are also given a feeling of safety and control, thanks to the dogs letting them know when seizures are looming (Strong et al 1999). The dog's calming and reassuring effect should not be underestimated because a strong link exists between seizure frequency and psychological distress (Sahar, 2012). As a result, the frequency of epileptic seizures is significantly reduced in those patients who receive seizure alert dogs as shown by studying their condition before and after the dog's arrival (Brown & Goldstein, 2011; Strong et al., 1999). In fact, no less than a 43 percent reduction of the seizure frequency rates was demonstrated after patients got dogs, and the effect kept growing throughout the study over a period of six months (Strong et al., 2002).

Other researchers found that 69 percent of epileptic patients experienced improvements in their seizure frequency after receiving seizure alert dogs, while 43 percent of those patients who received instead a seizure response dog saw improvements in frequency and severity (Kirton et al., 2008).

Among the tasks performed by the seizure response dogs were emergency notifications, such as fetching a phone, rolling the patient on his or her side to reach a recovery position, and switching off electrical devices to avoid accidents that otherwise used to occur (Kirton et al., 2008). As shown in the same study, various breeds are suitable, although the main priority was breeds belonging to hunting dogs, such as the cocker spaniel (English) and labrador retriever, whereas also some poodles (toy and standard poodles) plus a border terrier participated.

The prophylaxis of seizures by the seizure response dogs is somewhat baffling, as this type of dog wasn't trained to warn before an attack. However, it turned out that the majority of the dogs trained as seizure response dogs did in fact spontaneously develop alerting behavior after their deployment in the patients' homes, and most reported no missed incidents (Kirton et al., 2008).

This phenomenon is in general also found in pet dogs that may turn into seizure alert dogs without any formal training (Dalziel et al., 2003; Di Vito et al., 2010). Hence, 40 percent of pet dogs spontaneously become seizure-sensitive when they live in a family with epileptic children (Kirton et al., 2004).

What's no less interesting is the fact that patients with seizure dogs also reported improvements in the intensity of their epileptic convulsions plus shorter duration of each seizure attack, which along with the reduced frequency of seizures could only be ascribed to the dog's arrival (Kirton et al., 2008).

Another contributing factor to dogs' antiepileptic actions is likely their natural ability to attract attention and engage our minds since mental occupation in itself is shown to reduce seizure attacks. As shown by science, epileptic propagation is countered if many neurons are occupied by an activity. This leaves fewer brain cells susceptible to an abnormal (epileptic) recruitment, whereby the spreading of epileptic discharge can be blocked (Wolf, 2002). These aspects are relevant in terms of strategic management of epilepsy since treatments primarily target the single seizure rather than the overall disease. One should also take into account that millions continue to suffer from uncontrollable seizures despite the latest introduction of novel pharmaceuticals, and in contrast to dog therapy, all drugs cause numerous and/or intolerable side effects.

Stroke

Stroke is a major cause of death and disability in the Western world. It is a condition when brain cells abruptly die because of a lack in blood supply and therefore a lack in oxygen. There are two types of stroke. One is caused by an obstruction of the blood flow typically because of a blood clot that hinders the supply of oxygen to certain parts of the brain (ischemia). That's why this type of stroke is called an ischemic stroke. The other type of stroke is the result of a rupture of an artery leading to a bleeding inside the brain, namely a hemorrhagic stroke (Greenberg et al., 2012; Howard, 2014; Kandell et al., 2013).

Though the two types of stroke may sound like two very different or even opposite conditions, they are in fact quite similar, at least in terms of their consequences—disruption of the normal blood flow to the brain. Whether patients are hit by ischemic or hemorrhagic strokes, their brain cells will suddenly die, leaving behind an area of dead brain tissue that is called an infarct (Greenberg et al., 2012; Nordqvist, 2014).

Stroke patients typically experience sudden symptoms that often include aphasia (loss of speech), paralysis in one side of the body or in a limb, vision loss, severe headache, dizziness, confusion, lack of balance, and other disabilities. Consequently having a stroke is always a medical emergency. Those patients who survive strokes likely also experience some cognitive problems, loss of memory, and mood changes (depression). As a result, stroke survivors usually face long-term, rigorous rehabilitation with speech-language therapy in order to regain the ability to communicate. This is exactly where dogs come in since they are true masters in terms of communication without words (Becker, 2002; Coren, 2004; Fine, 2010). In addition, nobody can reach out and motivate us as much as dogs, and there can be no doubt that persistent motivation is an essential part of the physical training needed in order to get back on track after a stroke. Studies show that dogs motivate us to overcome various physical, mental, and environmental impediments to rehabilitation and training programs (Abbud et al., 2014; Fine, 2010; Knight & Edwards, 2008; Muñoz Lasa et al., 2011,2013; Rondeau et al., 2010; Toohey & Rock, 2011).

In a study performed at the University of Alabama, post-stroke patients with aphasia were offered dog-assisted speech-language therapy with a male Newfoundland in addition to the traditional (without dog) speech-language therapy (Macauley, 2006). Only patients with severe post-stroke aphasia accompanied by evident frustration (as judged by their grimaces, intonations, and refusals to talk) were enrolled, and the idea was to compare the effects of speech-language therapy with or without a dog's presence. This experimental design allows researchers to compare the outcome of traditional speech-language therapy (without a dog) with the outcome of having a dog present during speech-language therapy.

The research setup is interesting since speech-language therapy focuses on a skill (verbalization) that dogs are devoid of. Hence, the dog's odds are unfavorable as compared to using dogs in other kinds of therapies, namely those involving physical exercise or body language, both of which are part of a dog's natural repertoire. Nevertheless, in terms of the formal linguistic skills of the patients, dog-assisted speech-language therapy was at least as efficient as the traditional speech-language therapy. However, the dog-assisted therapy was significantly better in terms of the participants' self-reported outcomes, as all patients stated that their language skills improved most when the dog was present (Macauley, 2006). When the researchers compared other outcomes, it became clear that the dog had a huge impact upon the rehabilitation since patients showed significantly increased motivation, enjoyment, engagement, satisfaction, and happiness because the dog was part of the therapy program (Macauley, 2006). In fact, patients even rated their clinicians as more competent, dedicated, comprehensible, courteous, and well-prepared when the dog was present despite the fact that clinicians would strive to act unaffected by the dog's presence. The latter is very interesting, and it's something that therapists should never play down. Besides, it also reflects the fact that the patients showed emotional and social improvements during their rehabilitation programs, which likely are just as important measures as the linguistic goals.

The fact that the dog was able to reduce participants' difficulties and made them speak more spontaneously and emotionally engaged was not only reported by the patients but also by their family members, caregivers, and the clinicians (Macauley, 2006). For decades similar results have been described by other researchers, and they support that AAT is an exceptional catalyst for motivating stroke patients to improve their functioning and communication (Adams, 1997; Fine, 2010; Muñoz Lasa et al., 2013).

In a Canadian study of a male stroke patient with very severe aphasia and mental deficits who was admitted to the Rehabilitation Center of the Ottawa Hospital, researchers investigated the effects of adding a therapy dog to the speech-language inpatient program (LaFrance et al., 2007). The dog joined the patient for his one-hour therapy sessions held once a week for a period of five weeks. Moreover, after the speech-language training conducted in a therapy room, the dog and its handler would accompany the wheelchaired patient on his way back to the ward, whereby the dog took part in both verbal (speech-language) and nonverbal (walking) activities. During the walk the patient got to hold the dog by the leash, which would both increase his well-being, feelings of confidence, and his chances of talking or interacting with bystanders who would automatically pause to greet the dog (LaFrance et al., 2007). For a period of four weeks before plus two weeks after the five weeks of AAT, the patient followed a similar program—only the therapy dog was missing. When the researchers compared the patient's outcome in the different periods (with or without the dog), significant improvements were found only when the dog was present (LaFrance et al., 2007). Only in the presence of the dog the patient showed remarkable improvements in both verbal and nonverbal abilities, and he also became more socially active and contact-seeking, showed interest in others, smiled, and laughed more. His attempts at verbalization, the use of spontaneous speech, sentence production, and general language skills were significantly improved when the dog was present. However, as soon as the dog left after the scheduled five weeks of AAT, the patient's condition deteriorated. His verbal, nonverbal, and social skills regressed to their deficient level, which were present before the dog's arrival (LaFrance et al., 2007). From this study performed in Ottawa, Canada, you would only have to drive a few hours to arrive at another Canadian stroke rehabilitation unit where similar results were obtained by means of dogs. Hence, researchers in Québec showed how therapy dogs as part of AAT as well as service assistance dogs could promote the patients' mobility skills, leading to higher walking speed and better gait function in stroke patients (Rondeau et al., 2010).

As traditional neurological and neurosurgical treatment strategies tend to focus on stroke patients' medical emergencies in the acute phase, they don't allocate as many efforts to the prolonged phase of rehabilitation nor to preventive interventions. In view of that, for any surviving post-stroke patient, and not least from a community point of view, prevention of stroke by means of lifestyle interventions and post-stroke convalescence leading to recuperation of survivors cannot be overemphasized. In that regard, therapy dogs may impact the burden of stroke as much as medicine. Dogs not only convey rehabilitation as described previously. They are also the key to lowering risk factors of stroke, as a friendly dog's company lowers blood pressure, heart rate, fat contents in the blood, and stress hormones (Aiba et al., 2012; Becker, 2002; Grimm, 2014; Marcus, 2011; Penkowa, 2014).

Hence, not only certified therapy dogs but also family pet dogs can change the risk, course, and outcome of a stroke. Nevertheless, don't forget that anyone suspected of having a stroke should always be taken immediately to hospital in order to ensure correct emergency handling.

Traumatic Injury to the Brain or Spinal Cord

Traumatic injury refers to tissue damage caused by an unexpected physical impact from the outside, whereby injuries (trauma) are distinct from a disease that gradually develops from the inside. Blows, crushes, or stabs to the head or spine, such as those seen in violent attacks, gunshots, motor vehicle accidents, falls, or high-risk sports (where athletes are heading a ball or receiving repetitive punches) are the most frequent contributors to neurotraumatic injury, which is a major worldwide cause of death and disability in all age groups (Greenberg et al., 2012; Penkowa, 2010).

> Now about one in five people worldwide are living with at least one disability, and most of us will be burdened by some kind of disability during our lifetime, according to Centers for Disease Control and Prevention (http://www.cdc.gov).

What's tricky about a traumatic brain injury is that it causes both a primary and secondary injury to the brain. The primary injury is the immediate cell death resulting from the initial causal accident. The secondary injury is an aftereffect of the trauma and it results from indirect complications within the brain tissue. The secondary damage can affect large areas of tissue that were not initially injured and it typically progresses for weeks or months after the primary injury. In the end the secondary delayed injury may lead to more cell death than the accident did (Penkowa, 2006; Penkowa et al., 1999).

Symptoms remain more or less chronic, and their severity reflects the degree and size of the injury. Consequently, if victims stay alive after severe traumatic incidents, the majority will suffer from a chronic loss of mobility, as their motor control is either partially gone (paresis) or it may be completely lost (paralysis). Survivors become disabled and may have to use wheelchairs for the rest of their lives (Greenberg et al., 2012). Other frequent symptoms include the loss of sensation, impaired cognition, emotional dysfunctioning, personality, and/or mood changes. Neurotraumatic injuries not only change the life of the individual patient. They also come down hard on the entire household.

Injured or otherwise disabled individuals will need assistive devices, such as mobility aids, reaching aids, alarm systems, adaptive tools, and nursing or supportive care, in order to live more independently. However, whether patients are young or old, they generally become more and more socially isolated, and so it is no surprise that their quality of life goes down (Howard, 2006; van Koppenhagen et al., 2008).

In order to ameliorate patients' condition and promote independency, a special group of mobility-service dogs have successfully been trained in order to help disabled citizens achieve autonomy and independence, which are key determinants of life satisfaction in the years following the accident (Muñoz Lasa et al., 2011,2013; van Leeuwen et al., 2012; Winkle et al., 2012).

Hence, several worldwide organizations such as Canine Partners in the United Kingdom (http://www.caninepartners.co.uk) make such mobility-service dogs to the recipients' individual needs, as the dogs may perform a multitude of different tasks. Some are listed in the text box following.

Service dogs can be trained to open/close doors, turn on/off lights, pull you up from a chair or the floor, call 911 on rescue phones, help you in/out of the tub, alert you at specific time points (medication time), put on/off clothings, find and fetch various objects and medicine, drag a wheelchair, help with shopping and carrying packages, draw a person into safety in case of fire or emergency, drag laundry to the washing machine, load/unload washing machine, fetch food and beverages from the refrigerator or cupboard, pick up items from the floor, and/or organize the household or yard by carrying and depositing designated items.

Service dogs empower injured or disabled patients to function independently, prevent injuries, and summon help in case of emergency, and they are aware of their surroundings. In total, service dogs can perform more than a hundred possible tasks in order to assist the patient (Allen & Blascovich, 1996; Blanchet et al., 2013; Muñoz Lasa et al., 2011; Rintala et al., 2008; Vincent et al., 2013; Winkle et al., 2012).

For practical information, you can visit www.assistancedogsinternational.org, http://www.tdi-dog.org, http://www.servicedogsforamerica.org, http://www.servicedogseurope.com/mobility-service-dogs, http://www.caninepartners.co.uk, http://www.mira.ca/en, https://www.pawswithacause.org/what-we-do/service-dogs, http://www.petpartners.org, http://4pawsforability.org/mobility-assistance-dog, http://www.littleangelsservicedogs.org, or http://www.dati.org/newsletter/issues/1999n1/dogs.html.

More than 1.2 million citizens in the United Kingdom are wheelchair users, and the majority will benefit from having a mobility-service dog. The dog conveys a range of psychological, emotional, and social benefits along with its physical and practical way of transforming life of the patient (Allen & Blascovich, 1996; Camp, 2001; Muñoz Lasa et al., 2011,2013; Rintala et al., 2008; Shintani et al., 2010). Disabled Europeans may also find mobility-service dogs by visiting Service Dogs Europe (http://www.servicedogseurope.com). In the United States, there are a number of different organizations to turn to, as mentioned in the previous text box. Beware that mobility-service dogs are in some areas designated mobility-assistance dogs, as seen in the following organizations: Service Dogs for America (http://www.servicedogsforamerica.org), 4 Paws for Ability (http://4pawsforability.org/mobility-assistance-dog), or Little Angels Service Dogs (http://www.littleangelsservicedogs.org), just to mention a few. However, depending on your location, you may instead have to search for dogs under the name of intervention or rehabilitation dogs, as therapy dogs are called in some countries, while service dogs might be designated assistance dogs (Abbud et al., 2014; Rondeau et al., 2010). For example, if based in Canada, you will encounter intervention or rehabilitation dogs that are equivalent to therapy dogs used by health professionals in their clinical setting, while an assistance dog is the Canadian version of a service dog that is living with and owned by the patient. Such dogs are found by contacting the MIRA Foundation in Canada (http://www.mira.ca/en), which also has an affiliation in North Carolina (http://www.mirausa.org), and in France (http://www.miraeurope.org).

A range of clinical, scientific studies have demonstrated how recipients with mobility loss benefit from getting a service dog/assistance dog in their homes (Allen & Blascovich, 1996; Camp, 2001; Hubert et al., 2013; Muñoz Lasa et al., 2011; Rintala et al., 2008; Shintani et al., 2010; Winkle et al., 2012). One study compared people with mobility impairments six months before and after they received a service dog trained for their specific needs, and in addition, the recipients were also compared with a control group consisting of future service dog recipients who by the time of the study were applicants placed on a waiting list (Rintala et al., 2008). Whether they were service dog recipients or nonrecipients (applicants), most of the study participants (60 to 66 percent) suffered from both upper and lower body impairments, while 33 to 40 percent had lower body impairments. Generally the recipients stated they were highly satisfied after they got the dogs. The dogs made them significantly less dependent on other people or caretakers. After the service dog's arrival, the need for paid assistance in the home of the patient was significantly reduced, while there were no changes in the homes of the nonrecipient control group (Rintala et al., 2008).

In fact, the beneficial effects of service dogs on people with disabilities have been known for decades, and so has the economical savings resulting from getting a service dog, as published almost two decades ago by Dr. Karen Allen at the State University of New York at Buffalo and Jim Blascovich at the University of California, Santa Barbara (Allen & Blascovich, 1996). In addition to the physical and psychological health improvements, the recipients of service dogs also obtained financial benefits, as they could cut down drastically (by 68 percent) their weekly expenses for personal assistance services, including health-care workers, household assistants, cleaning services, and help from family members (Allen & Blascovich, 1996). After the dogs' arrivals recipients also notably increased their attendance rate at school and employed working hours. The service dog owners also experienced better integration into the community, more social interaction within the neighborhood, and increased use of public transportation as compared to the controls who were on a waiting list for service dogs (Allen & Blascovich, 1996).

Among the daily benefits most often provided by a service dog are retrieval of various items, activating emergency call devices in case of emergencies, emotional support, turning on/off lights, opening doors, carrying of things, barking to alert family members to let the participant into the house, picking items off the supermarket's shelves, companionship, and help to stand, walk, and balance the body. Moreover, family members became less worried about the patient's situation thanks to the dog.

Overall, studies support that service dogs provide their recipient households with a range of positive benefits relating to mental and physical health, social activity, societal status, and economy, whereby a service dog substantially increases quality of life (Allen & Blascovich, 1996; Camp, 2001; Hubert et al., 2013; Muñoz Lasa et al., 2011; Rintala et al., 2008; Winkle et al., 2012).

Because trauma patients often depend on wheelchairs and manual walking aids, the influence of a service dog was specifically investigated in manual wheelchair users with spinal cord injuries who were examined before the dog's arrival, during training with the dog, and up to seven months after the service dog's arrival (Hubert et al., 2013). The study showed that the traction and assistance provided by the dog conveyed physical benefits for manual wheelchair users, as they could operate the wheelchair with less effort and for longer distances. Hence, patients suffered less shoulder pain, which may in the long run prevent shoulder degeneration and improve shoulder health. The latter is important since significant shoulder pain and degeneration are very common in wheelchair users, and in particular these increase with time because of the repetitive, strenuous forces of wheeling. The wheelchaired recipients of a service dog also showed improvement in their general mobility, prosocial behavior, and activity of daily life, as they got to move around more competently in different settings and conditions thanks to the dog (Hubert et al., 2013). In fact, the overall impact of having a service dog might be even bigger than we imagine, as shown in a Japanese study comparing disabled patients living with a service dog with a matched control group that had comparable disabilities but no service dog, though they were deemed eligible for receiving one (Shintani et al., 2010). Overall, the service dog owners showed significant improvements in physical functioning, vitality, mental health, emotional states, and psychosocial functioning when compared to the controls without a dog. What's even more astonishing is how much the disabled dog owners' mental health and life quality surpassed not only those of disabled control subjects but also the levels found in the general background population in Japan. Hence, an overall mental health score was computed from various parameters such as emotions, balance, psychosocial well-being, harmony, calmness, mood, sociability, and mental quality of life, and surprisingly it turned out that disabled owners of a service dog did not only score better than the disabled controls without a dog but in fact scored higher than the average Japanese citizen without any disability (Shintani et al., 2010). This is despite the fact that the studied dog owners were physically disabled and therefore typically burdened by poorer mental health, social isolation, lack of self-esteem, low quality of life, depression, and stigmatisation when compared to the background population without disabilities (van

Koppenhagen et al., 2008; Winkle et al., 2012). Yet the disabled dog owners turned out to be experiencing better lives with fewer problems or sorrows. Such findings likely indicate a very high level of synergy derived from the many different ways that dogs may enrich people's lives (Abbud et al., 2014; Allen & Blascovich, 1996; Counsell et al., 1997; Hubert et al., 2013; Muñoz Lasa et al., 2011,2013; Shintani et al., 2010; Walsh, 2009a; Winkle et al., 2012). Details of these mechanisms of canine actions will be explained later in this chapter.

Psychiatry: Disorders of the Mind

The human psyche is perhaps what dogs influence the most, as dogs more than anything seem to possess forces shaping our very thoughts, behaviors, and moods. Hence, dogs may not only improve our mental well-being, emotions, and mood but specifically counter a vast range of conditions, such as depression, anxiety, PTSD (post-traumatic stress disorder), autism, schizophrenia, psychosis, violent attacks, substance abuse/addiction, eating disorders, imprisonment, bereavement, sexual abuse issues, and a range of developmental, conduct, and personality disorders (Bardill & Hutchinson, 1997; Bernabei et al., 2013; Cirulli et al., 2011; Dietz et al., 2012; Dimitrijević, 2009; Fine, 2010; Friedmann & Son, 2009; Grimm, 2014; Marcus, 2011; McConnell, 2007; O'Haire, 2010,2013; Oyama & Serpell, 2013; Parish-Plass, 2008; Penkowa, 2014; Serpell, 1996; Walsh, 2009a,b; Wells, 2007; Wood et al., 2007).

Although other animals may alleviate certain mental problems, the dog is most often preferred because of his or her superior skills with people, trainability, availability, and a matchless prosocial empathy (Marcus, 2011; Miller, 2010). As explained in chapter 2, the dog's fluffy fur also facilitates sensory inputs by means of touching and petting. They, too, have a natural ability to distract us, unwind our thoughts, provide empathy, and make us laugh. That's why dogs provide the optimum source of pet therapy.

These effects upon the human mind are not only the results of AAT/AAA research. They also become obvious when one is studying the mental health of the dog-owning populations, as dog owners are characterized by improved psychosocial health and less psychiatric problems than the background population (people without dogs) (Knisely et al., 2012; McConnell, 2007; Raina et al., 1999; Siegel, 1990; Serpell, 1990,1991,1996; Wells, 2009,2011; Wood et al., 2007).

The dog's effect on the brain and mind are supported by research studies that have identified how interacting with a dog affects a variety of electrophysiological, neurobiological, metabolic, and neurochemical mechanisms in the human brain. Hence, a dog's company changes significantly the activity and cognition in the frontal lobes of the brain, the impulse firing rates in specific subsets of neurons, and the brain's release of specific chemicals, such as neurotransmitters, signaling molecules, and hormones (Aoki et al., 2012; Beals, 2009; Cole et al., 2007; Handlin, 2010; Handlin et al., 2011; kamioka et al., 2014; Nagasawa et al., 2009a; Odendaal, 2000; Odendaal & Meintjes, 2003; Marcus, 2013a; Penkowa, 2014). These changes are found as a result of our interactions with dogs, including the times when we pet, touch, play together, or talk softly to our furry friend, and the changes observed are found regardless of ownership—that is, whether it's our own pet or a professional therapy dog. The specific changes and their mechanisms of action inside the human brain are described in a section of its own later in this chapter.

When you think about it, it is noteworthy that a dog can alter the human brain's processing, activity, and functioning in the normal background population. And if a dog can improve the health of people in general, it is not surprising that canines convey even bigger health benefits for those beset with psychological, social, emotional, and/or mental problems (Grimm, 2014; Bernabei et al., 2013; Cirulli et al., 2011; Dietz et al., 2012; Dimitrijević, 2009; Fine, 2010; kamioka et al., 2014; O'Haire, 2010,2013).

No cure exists for any psychiatric disease, which at its best can be only calmed down a little bit. Unfortunately the psychiatric drugs used today induce a number of hazardous side effects that the scientific community rarely call attention to. In fact, antidepressant drugs may lead to suicide, and likewise these drugs and a range of other psychoactive medications may also cause chronic brain impairment as revealed by one of the most influential medical doctors, Dr. Peter R. Breggin (Breggin, 1993,1999,2011,2013). Dr. Breggin is a psychiatrist based in New York who left his position at Harvard Medical School and John Hopkins University in order to run his private clinic and author several scientific articles and books on the subject of psychiatric drug facts (Breggin, 1993,1999,2011,2013). From the works of Dr. Breggin, who by many is considered to be the "conscience of psychiatry," most psychoactive medications lead to severe, life-threatening emotional and physical withdrawal reactions. Accordingly, it is not only dangerous to start popping psychiatric pills but may also be very unsafe when you want to withdraw. Hence, there has to be another way, and indeed there is. To put it in short, until there's a cure, there's a dog.

Anxiety

Dog owners have long been known to report being less worried and frightened, while their feeling of safety is increased in the company of their furry friends (Serpell, 1990,1991). From a variety of clinical studies applying therapy dogs, this trend has been supported. Data reveal how AAT reduces the level of anxiety and phobias in hospitalized patients with psychiatric diseases (Barker & Dawson, 1998; Barker & Wolen, 2008; Dimitrijević, 2009). It only takes a single thirty-minute session with a therapy dog to minimize anxiety responses in patients suffering from psychoses, schizophrenia, mood disorders, and other mental illnesses (Barker & Dawson, 1998; Barker et al., 2003; Dimitrijević, 2009; kamioka et al., 2014; Penkowa, 2014).

This might be the result of various biochemical mechanisms, as dog exposure increases our levels of relaxing molecules and decreases transmitters igniting arousal and nervousness (Cole et al., 2007; Handlin et al., 2011; Nagasawa et al., 2009a; Odendaal, 2000).

In particular the dog's ability to increase our oxytocin levels and reduce the stress hormones epinephrine, norepinephrine, and cortisol might explain why most people unwind and calm down in response to the company of furry, wagging friends (Cole et al., 2007; Fine, 2010; Odendaal & Meintjes, 2003; Yoshida et al., 2009).

In fact, sessions with a therapy dog are twice as effective in reducing anxiety in patients with psychotic disorders as compared to the control (comparison) therapy (Barker & Dawson, 1998). In the study the control sessions consisted of recreational activities that contained educational presentations, music, and/or art classes. Therefore dogs are also second to none in reducing anxiety in other types of patients, such as those suffering from chronic heart conditions. In these individuals clinical symptoms and the amount of anxiety-promoting chemicals in the blood were reduced relative to those who did not receive AAT (Cole et al., 2007).

Another option in the case of anxiety disorders is to get a psychiatric service dog that can alert one to an imminent attack of panic or uncontrollable anxiety by means of sensing the body's physiological changes preceding an attack just like dogs alerting people to epileptic seizures (Fine, 2010; Marcus, 2011).

Another feat of such dogs is their grounding of the panicking person, a task also denoted as "deep pressure therapy" in which a medium-sized dog place his or her body atop the owner's abdomen and/or chest or in some cases in the owner's lap, as the pressure of the dog's body in a physical and then psychological way will alleviate anxiety and evoke a calm feeling (Miller, 2010). Witnessing dogs performing such grounding during a panic attack is nothing less than impressive, in particular since it works in a few minutes, though just a minute before the patient was madly terrorized, sweating, trembling, choking and overwhelmed by fear. However, the mere presence of a service dog at your side 24-7 is the most important element in the emotional support provided, as a friendly dog wagging his or her tail provides a sense of ease and calm to anyone nearby.

Likewise, dogs may function as a psychiatric and medical therapy for patients undergoing procedures that are innately frightening or conjure frightening images, such as in the case of electroconvulsive therapy, sometimes also known as electroshock therapy. Hence, before their scheduled electroconvulsive therapy sessions, patients were either exposed to fifteen minutes of a therapy dog's company or (with the control intervention) fifteen minutes of reading magazines (Barker et al., 2003). As shown in this study, the dog could substantially reduce patients' fear relating to electroconvulsive therapy, as compared to the control intervention.

Moreover, there are further benefits since applying a therapy dog also seems to improve the relationship between the health professional (the therapist) and the patient (O'Haire, 2010). This is a very important and relevant issue to consider in psychiatry, which is most often characterized by patients' distrust and disbelief in the system, concept, and its staff (O'Haire, 2010). A general effect of having the therapy dog in the ward is that its mere presence will change the way patients regard the staff, who are perceived as being more sympathetic when they appear with the dog as compared to the same staff without the dog (Beck & Katcher, 1983; Fine, 2010; Grimm, 2014; Serpell, 1996; Schneider & Harley, 2006; Walsh, 2009a).

Depression

Depression has become the health-care sector's biggest challenge, and according to recent data, at least 350 million people worldwide live with depression, which today is humanity's leading cause of disability (D'Souza & Jago, 2014).

The medical management of depression poses a number of serious challenges. First psychosocial treatment strategies are the preferred first-line option ahead of pharmaceuticals, and while psychosocial therapy remains more successful than taking antidepressant drugs, it is also vastly more time-consuming, at least in the short run. That's why many patients aren't part of such interventions (Alladin, 2013; D'Souza & Jago, 2014). When we turn to the antidepressant drugs, of which abundant generic options are available, we can see that they are not very efficient. According to Irving Kirsch, a professor of psychology at the University of Plymouth (UK), the therapeutic efficacy of antidepressants is entirely due to a placebo effect, as described in Kirsch's book *The Emperor's New Drugs: Exploding the Antidepressant Myth* (Kirsch, 2009). Hence, other scientists support the notion of Dr. Peter R. Breggin as mentioned previously.

Irving Kirsch reached his conclusion after he methodically reviewed most clinical trials of antidepressant drugs published since the 1960s, including those trials that were kept hidden from the public. Another problem with the modern medicalization of depression is that antidepressant drugs carry a huge range of very serious or fatal side effects, which paradoxically include an increased risk of suicide (Alladin, 2013; D'Souza & Jago, 2014; Kirsch & Low, 2013). However, the pharmaceutical business keeps marketing their ever-increasing drugs, and so those diagnosed with depression will have to take charge of their treatment even if they feel totally disempowered, as the patient is the one who should decide whether to pop pills or start proper therapeutic interventions (Alladin, 2013; Kirsch, 2009).

From a medical point of view one of the most appealing methods demonstrated to counter depression and stave off disempowerment is obtaining a dog (Bernabei et al., 2013; Fine, 2010; Friedmann & Son, 2009; Le Roux & Kemp, 2009; Walsh, 2009a,b; Wisdom et al., 2009; Woods et al., 2007).

In a systematic review of all randomized controlled clinical trials published between 1990 and 2012, researchers set out to assess the effectiveness of AAT upon various mental and behavioral problems involving not only studies with therapy dogs but also those applying other animals like dolphins, birds, farm animals (cows), rabbits, cats, ferrets, and guinea pigs (Kamioka et al., 2014). As shown, animals in general may provide a holistic therapy through patients' interaction with animals in nature. However, dog therapy remains the most validated form of AAT, mostly because of their advanced training skills, prosocial nature, and cognition, which makes dogs superior in dealing with depression and adverse life events that may evoke depressive reactions (Bernabei et al., 2013; Cirulli et al., 2011; Dietz et al., 2012; Dimitrijević, 2009; Fine, 2010; Friedmann & Son, 2009; Grimm, 2014; Headey, 2003; Johnson et al., 2002; McConnell, 2007; Penkowa, 2014; O'Haire, 2010,2013; Serpell, 1996; Siegel, 1990; Wells, 2007,2011; Wood et al., 2007).

Dogs also ameliorate depression in patients suffering from AIDS (acquired immunodeficiency syndrome) or infection with HIV (human immunodeficiency virus), and dogs are second to none in keeping loneliness at bay (Dimitrijević, 2009; Oyama & Serpell, 2013; Siegel et al., 1999; Walsh, 2009a,b).

In case of nursing home residents who can't keep their own pets, a regular visit by a friendly dog can certainly make a difference. A study showed that an AAA group intervention lasting thirty minutes per visit and held once a week for a period of six weeks in total can change things to the better, as this AAA resulted in a significant reduction in residents' depression scores as compared to a control group that did not receive visits from the dog (Le Roux & Kemp, 2009). During the visit the residents could pet, talk to, or groom the dog, who interacted with them as he was on a leash.

This is confirmed by other studies that show how a dog's visit improves recipients' mood and significantly reduce depression levels (Friedmann & Son, 2009; Marcus, 2011; Wiggett, 2006).

In addition, an Italian research team demonstrated that dog therapy may significantly improve the health condition in cancer patients who are submitting to chemotherapy (Orlandi et al., 2007). When oncological patients receive chemotherapy in a room where they can play with or pet a friendly dog, they gain psychological and physical health benefits along with improved quality of life and significantly reduced depression levels as compared to their matched controls consisting of cancer patients receiving chemotherapy without the company of furry friends (Orlandi et al., 2007).

Considering that most cancer patients have to go through long periods of receiving chemotherapy, it is no wonder that their quality of life is deeply influenced both with regards to physical and psychological aspects. That's why depression and anxiety often follow. This is exactly where dogs work miracles, as they offer unconditional support, love, security, joyous play, comfort, and social contact. That's why dogs are able to genuinely alter the outcome for the patients (Fine, 2010; Friedmann & Son, 2009; Orlandi et al., 2007; Siegel et al., 1999; Walsh, 2009a; Wood et al., 2007). As explained later in this chapter, scientists have begun to unravel the neurobiological mechanisms by which dogs improve the human mind and mood, and they involve specific biochemical and cellular changes conveyed when one is exposed to a furry friend.

PTSD

PTSD is closely connected with both anxiety and depression, as each of the conditions often occur simultaneously or lead to one another (Howard, 2014). In contrast to depression and anxiety, PTSD is one of very few psychiatric conditions in which the traumatic cause can be identified since the condition emerges in the aftermath of war, trauma, violent assault, rape, a serious accident, terrorist incident, natural disaster, bereavement, or any other kind of major life threat. Even if most patients will recover,

PTSD lasts for several months or years following the incidence, and most will experience anxiety or depression in any case.

When a traumatic or life-threatening event takes place, the normal human reaction pattern involves sudden flashbacks, nightmares, and intrusive memories of the terrible episode (Howard, 2006; Miller, 2010). As much as the symptoms are terrifying, they are also part of a normal reaction of our nervous system. That's why tolerance is the foremost and cardinal prerequisite.

To facilitate optimum coping skills, one may spend time with loved ones, focus in favorite activities, avoid alcohol, and get outside in nature. A coping repertoire that is much easier if you have a dog. However, your furry friend will not only encourage appropriate coping behavior. He or she will likely transform your life as the result of well-known psychosocial and emotional effects (Fine, 2010; Marcus, 2011; Penkowa, 2014).

Whether it's a pet dog, service dog, or therapy dog, the companionship, emotional support, and bond between the dog and the patient make up the greatest assistance anyone can provide simply by means of the dog's presence (Milller, 2010; Serpell, 1996).

Accordingly, studies show how dogs excel as stress buffers that counter PTSD, as shown in a wide range of mental health consumers, including victims to assaults or sexual abuse and especially military combat soldiers and army veterans (Barker & Dawson, 1998; Beck et al., 2012; Fike et al., 2012; Fine, 2010; Miller, 2010; Oyama & Serpell, 2013; Parish-Plass, 2008; Yount et al., 2012; Walsh, 2009a). Various types of AAI programs have facilitated successful rehabilitation of PTSD patients, partly because of the dog's antidepressant effects and their ability to relieve anxiety (Fike et al., 2012; Fine, 2010; Friedmann & Son, 2009; Miller, 2010; O'Haire, 2009; Yount et al., 2012; Walsh, 2009b; Wisdom et al., 2009).

An important aspect in any dog's PTSD treatment success is that the traumatic incident has most likely been caused by a human. That's why other people may act as a PTSD trigger rather than a support provider. A friendly dog is rarely seen as a threat or PTSD inducer. Instead the furry guy wagging his tail is perceived as a reliable, comforting, and safeguarding partner.

For the very same reason getting a PTSD-specialized service dog is often the optimum solution and the most straightforward way to help reclusive victims get out of their homes, visit public places, go to recreational areas, and use public transportation even when they have been isolated for very long periods (Miller, 2010). In patients with PTSD service dogs prevent panicking and provide emotional support and a much-needed feeling of safety, which in postcombat soldiers in particular is a necessary element for coping with a return to civil life. An important aspect here is that returning veterans may have severe problems sleeping or fear other people, and in such cases the dog may be the only way to cope since the dog can be trained to alert his or her owner to potential suspects, intruders, or threats in the environment (Fine, 2010; Goodavage, 2012; Miller, 2010). For any soldier who has faced battlefields, including the terrible risk of unstable explosives, booby traps, and akin devices, getting through the night or walking the public streets are not feats to be taken for granted. Consequently, being able to trust that the dog will alert you in case of any dangers or looming strangers provides a new leash to a bearable life (Beck et al., 2012; Fike et al., 2012; Goodavage, 2012; Miller, 2010).

> Further details on PTSD-specialized dogs can be obtained at the following websites:
> http://www.servicedogseurope.com/3956-2/ptsd-anxiety-depression,
> http://www.mentalhealthdogs.org/Psychiatric-Service-Dogs.html, and
> http://www.pawsitivityservicedogs.com/ptsd.html.

On the subject of recovery and rehoming after deployment, a clinical research-based organization called Warrior Canine Connection (http://warriorcanineconnection.org) has pioneered the field by recruiting convalescing veterans and teaching them how to train service dogs in order to provide their fellow veterans with a furry companions (Yount et al., 2012). The process of training the dogs is not only done to the benefit of the recipient of the dog. Hence, when warriors have to teach the dog how to feel safe and remain calm, even in the case of startling incidents, they have to believe it themselves, and so their teaching of the dogs becomes self-therapy. During upsetting or unexpected events like hearing sirens, fireworks, or cars backfiring, the soldiers need to calm and praise the dog. Doing so, they can't turn inward or have flashbacks to their trauma, as they will instead focus on someone outside themselves, get distracted by a wagging tail, and thereby remain focused on the overall purpose of helping a fellow veteran (Yount et al., 2012). All along when service dog training is put into practice, it will help the soldiers go outside their homes, walk in public places, experience touch, communicate, and exchange emotions with the dog, which will promote their ability to seek contact with other people and their dogs.

In addition, the veteran dog trainers report that their experience from showing positive emotions to the dogs while they praise and reward them has improved their family lives and parenthood. In the end what makes the Warrior Canine Connection a win-win game is the overall goal of offering disabled postcombat soldiers a specially trained service dog that can provide mobility assistance, safety, friendship, and increased quality of life (Beck et al., 2012; Fike et al., 2012; Yount et al., 2012).

Schizophrenia

More than fifty years ago, two Americans, a professor of psychology named Dr. Boris Levinson and a psychiatrist named Dr. Harold Searles, each described how dogs benefitted those suffering from mental diseases like schizophrenia, an effect mediated by dogs' inborn ability to show unconditional affection and empathy and spread unreserved joy (Levinson, 1962; Searles, 1960).

Since then, a number of researchers have supported the idea of dogs helping patients with schizophrenia as well as other mental disorders, as dogs can relax and soothe these patients in ways other humans simply cannot (Barak et al., 2001; Chu et al., 2009; Cirulli et al., 2011; Nathans-Barel et al., 2005). Many schizophrenics are overly suspicious and paranoid, and they generally lack confidence and trust toward the psychiatric system. A dog, on the other hand, doesn't have any hidden agenda. Nor does he or she ask to get anything in return. Even the most anguished and psychotic patients will not be able to convince themselves that the dog is conspiring against them. In view of that, a dog can make schizophrenic patients slow down and feel less stigmatized, while their interactions with the dog can help the patients seek social contact, recover their self-control, and return to a perception of reality (Beck & Katcher, 1983; Fine, 2010; Miller, 2010; Walsh, 2009a; Wells, 2011).

In a clinical study of hospitalized psychotic patients suffering from schizophrenia, schizoaffective disorder, or other schizophrenic psychoses, the therapeutic effect of a single thirty-minute AAT session was compared to that of a control intervention consisting of the hospital's standard therapy, which included recreational music, art, or educational activities (Barker & Dawson, 1998).

The results showed that psychotic and schizophrenic patients who spent thirty minutes together with the therapy dog experienced a significant reduction in their anxiety-related symptoms, as compared to the control intervention, which had no significant effect upon the patients. Hence, the therapy dog's effect upon patients' anxiety levels was twice as big as the effect of the control treatment.

The study also revealed another important aspect. The therapy dogs applied not only reduced symptoms in psychotic and schizophrenic patients. These furry therapists also benefitted those with other types of psychiatric diseases like mood disorders (bipolar and depression) and a range of cognitive, personality, or somatization disorders (Barker & Dawson, 1998). The effect of dog therapy has to be weighed against the control therapy with the purpose of comparing the outcomes. Interestingly the control treatment only influenced anxiety in patients with mood disorders, while it had no significant effects upon other diseases such as psychoses, schizophrenia, and cognitive, personality, or somatization disorders. As a result, therapy dogs' therapeutic range and their clinical application are obviously increased relative to the control (Barker & Dawson, 1998).

The proposed mechanisms behind the therapy dogs' success include a distraction of the patients' thoughts, making them focus on the outside world and perceive reality instead of getting trapped inside their heads where reality is shattered. The dogs also convey a feeling of safety, rapport, and support, to which is added the impact of touch, as patients were petting, stroking, and patting the dogs. These mechanisms are suported by the way dogs affect the brain's biochemistry, and ultimately this will induce a relaxed and reassured state of mind (Barker & Dawson, 1998; Cirulli et al., 2011; Fine, 2010; Nagasawa et al., 2009a,2015; Odendaal & Meintjes, 2003).

> "There is no psychiatrist in the world like a puppy licking your face."
> —Ben Williams.

Schizophrenic patients can also by means of a dog's company achieve significant improvements in several psychosocial parameters, such as social appropriateness, interactions with other people, reintegration into society, more personal engagement, and increased motivation, while they experience less apathy, less anhedonia, better adaptation to the environment, and better quality of life (Bernabei et al., 2013; Dimitrijević, 2009; Knisely et al., 2012; Miller, 2010; Muñoz Lasa et al. 2013; Walsh, 2009a; Wells, 2011). Overall, data show how dogs, both when they are part of formal AAT or AAA programs and when they are pets, can alleviate schizophrenic symptoms and reduce health expenditures. Consequently, pet owners are less likely to develop schizophrenia as compared to those who do not own pets (Becker, 2002; Muñoz Lasa et al. 2011; Penkowa, 2014; Wisdom et al., 2009).

Hence, in a study of middle-aged, institutionalized patients with chronic schizophrenia, a weekly session of AAI for a total period of nine months improved significantly the rehabilitation of the patients who regained their living skills with regards to domestic activities, housekeeping, and personal health (Kovács et al., 2004). Affective social behaviors, such as gestures, eye contact, and facial expressions, also improved as did the patients' cognitive and language skills, including the abilities to concentrate and communicate (Kovács et al., 2004). This is supported by another study of elderly schizophrenic patients residing in a closed psychogeriatric institution. In this study, they were followed for twelve months, during which they received AAT once every week (Barak et al., 2001). Each patient in the AAT group could choose either a therapy dog or a cat, while the control patients got to read and/or talk about the news bulletin. The control intervention happened simultaneously with the AAT group's weekly four-hour session with their therapy animals. The outcome was assessed in a blinded manner, and the data showed that AAT significantly improved schizophrenic patients' social and adaptive functioning when compared to those of the control group (Barak et al., 2001). According to the authors, the therapy animals acted as role models for the patients with regards to their personal hygiene and levels of self-care. The patients had to take care of their animals by means of grooming, bathing, and feeding them during the sessions.

AAT also improved significantly the elderly patients' social contact, including politeness, appropriateness, and friendliness toward others. Their communication and conversations with strangers also improved. This effect is in itself an interesting detail since geriatric patients with schizophrenia are characterized by an extraordinarily big deficiency in social functioning. Moreover, AAT was successful regarding increased mobility by walking outdoors, as patients walked the animals outside of the clinic. AAT also heightened well-being and strengthened patients' activities of daily living, as determined relative to the outcome of the control intervention (Barak et al., 2001). Having said this, it is obviously a major flaw of the study that the authors did not compare the outcome of dog-versus-cat sessions since it likely would have revealed some interesting differences (Fine, 2010; Friedmann & Son, 2009).

One of the most difficult symptoms to treat in these patients is anhedonia, a diminished capacity to experience pleasure from activities that are usually found enjoyable. Anhedony, which is a core clinical feature of schizophrenia, does not respond to the standard therapy, and to address this challenge, an Israeli research group conducted a study aiming at evaluating a therapy dog's effect on anhedony in middle-aged, chronic schizophrenics (Nathans-Barel et al., 2005). Patients met with the therapy dog, a golden retriever, for one hour every week during a period of ten weeks in total. Durinig the AAT, patients would pet, interact, groom, and talk to the dog. They also took the dog outside for a walk on the hospital grounds. The control group did not meet the dog, as they instead had to gather and talk about animals (mainly dogs). They also went outside for walks in order to match the activity level of the experimental AAT group (Nathans-Barel et al., 2005).

This experiment reveals how a therapy dog can significantly ameliorate anhedony in schizophrenia, as the AAT group showed a significant enhancement of their hedonic tone (level of pleasure) when they were compared with controls. Moreover, the therapy dog also benefitted patients' use of leisure time, motivation, and life quality. Additional positive results derived from the dog included improved mood, empathy, and feelings of attachment. Patients who missed the dog in between the weekly sessions enthusiastically looked forward to the next dog session, even though their attitudes toward treatment were usually very negative (Nathans-Barel et al., 2005).

Fortunately dogs don't have any age limits with regards to changing our lives, as they also benefit children and adolescents with psychiatric diseases, including schizophrenia (Beck & Katcher, 1983; Cirulli et al., 2011; Fine, 2010).

The first therapist to use dogs in the treatment of mentally ill children was Dr. Boris Levinson, who quite by accident noticed how his own dog Jingles reached a severely disturbed child when humans couldn't (Levinson, 1962,1965). It started as Dr. Levinson one day left the withdrawn, uncommunicative child in his therapy room, and while nobody noticed, Jingles decided to step in. When the doctor returned, much to his surprise he found the hitherto silent, reclused, and unreachable kid talking to Jingles. This illustrates the very core of pet therapy in that a dog may be the only one calling forth speech and spirit from mute or lost souls. Sometimes people can safely approach an animal even when they have given up on humans.

Following this incident, Dr. Levinson discovered that when his canine co-therapist joined the psychotherapy, the children's resistance vanished, while communication, trust, and rapport became possible and allowed therapy to take place. Accordingly, Dr. Levinson coined the term "pet therapy" and began writing scientific papers on the subject as exemplified by his experience with Jingles. At first colleagues literally laughed at him and made jokes about Jingles's role. They even asked if he would pay Jingles part of his fee. Today nobody is laughing.

Even back then, though he was ridiculed, Dr. Levinson sent out questionnaires to his colleagues and asked them about their possible use of animals in psychotherapy. Much to his surprise, it turned out that more than one third used animals in their clinics and that more than 58 percent recommended their patients get pets for building better mental health (Beck & Katcher, 1983; Cirulli et al., 2011).

Since then, the use of a dog's nuzzle when it's most needed has only increased (Fine, 2010; Grimm, 2014; Hare & Woods, 2013).

Since the era of Jingles, other extraordinary canines have provided their devotion, soft touch, and uncritical friendship to those in need. A most diligent example of the cocker spaniel Graham has been described by the researchers Norine Bardill at Florida State University and Sally Hutchinson, PhD, at University of Florida Health Science Center. When Graham was eight months old, he moved into a psychiatric, sixteen-bed, closed unit with children and adolescent patients aged eleven through eighteen years old. In the unit Graham resided twenty-four hours a day and had free-range access to the inpatients and staff members who took care of him together, though ultimately the staff was responsible for feeding, grooming, and walking him. His achievements were reported by the time he was two years old, and as described by the Florida researchers, Graham was the main act by his ability to transform the psychiatric unit's atmosphere and ameliorate patients' diseases, which included schizophrenia and various other diagnoses (Bardill & Hutchinson, 1997). First of all Graham made patients more trusting and positive about their hospitalization, which is important since most patients are forced into the unit. In this way, by wagging his tail and greeting people, Graham redefined not only patients' attitudes but also their families' impressions of the unit. Importantly the merry cocker spaniel also made youngsters feel safe, protected, and placed in good hands, which helped to alter their negative perception of the staff. This is vital since mentally ill kids and adolescents in general represent a challenge to the personnel (Kruger et al., 2004).

> Quotations from patients: "Sometimes you can talk to him when you can't talk to anybody else. He doesn't judge you." "When I have problems with people I just sit down with Graham. He's such a good listener." "When I was mad at staff and everyone, I had Graham … Sometimes he helps me more than all you staff people do" (Bardill & Hutchinson, 1997).

To some of the kids, Graham replaced absent relatives and negative emotions or fear, as he provided unconditional devotion, sincere friendship, and uncritical company to these patients who talked to Graham in ways they never talked to humans (Bardill & Hutchinson, 1997).

Moreover, Graham distracted patients in a positive way that made their suspicion, anxiety, or temper fade away just as he alerted the staff when a kid deteriorated or had nightly seizures.

This kind of acceptance and listening with empathy and intimacy is a virtue of dogs, especially while the speaking person gets full and silent attention, which only very few modern people can match (Fine, 2010; Kruger et al., 2004). Hence, having a resident therapy dog as bright as Graham not only paves the way to better psychiatric wards but also allows us to reach severely disturbed youngsters who may otherwise remain unreachable for therapy.

Hence, the dog's nonjudgmental, highly affectionate, patient, and nonthreatening nature makes children feel safe, loved, protected, and understood, whereby they perceive and embrace therapy more positively (Bardill & Hutchinson, 1997; Beck & Katcher, 1983; Fine, 2010; Kruger et al., 2004; Cirulli et al., 2011).

This also illustrates how a dog's mechanisms of therapeutic actions are different depending on the age of the recipient, as therapy dogs benefitted elderly and middle-aged schizophrenics in other ways involving mainly extroversion, improving social communication and outdoor activities. These are fundamentally different to the ways a dog can heal children and teenagers.

Besides their ability to improve psychiatric outcomes, therapy dogs will most likely also decrease the length of hospitalization, consumption of psychopharmaceuticals, and the health-care costs (Beck & Katcher, 1983; Fine, 2010; Kruger et al., 2004; Oyama & Serpell, 2013).

Autism Spectrum Disorder

When a baby is born, hopeful parents will anticipate its developmental pattern. Normally babies will smile and gaze at faces by six weeks of age. They get hold of sufficient motor control to sit up at six months, while they typically speak a few words and can walk on their own when they reach one year of age or soon thereafter. Their cognition, language, and emotions will continue to develop, and soon the toddlers have an understanding of their surroundings, other individuals, and social interactions as they engage in make-believe play and communication with family and friends.

However, not all kids follow this program, particularly not those suffering from pervasive neurodevelopmental disorders, such as autism spectrum disorders, which mainly include autism and Asperger's syndrome.

The word *autism* is derived from the Greek *autos*, which refers to *self*, and in this context the term is used to describe the isolated self (social withdrawal) representing one of the three primary disabilities— impaired social skills, impaired communication, and repetitive or unusual behaviors (Grandin & Johnson, 2005). Individuals with autism mainly suffer from social impairment, as they have difficulties understanding and communicating with other people in part because their language as used in a social interaction is abnormal. The sense of hearing is also disturbed in autism, whereby the brain's processing of spoken words as used in our colloquial language is anomalous (Fine, 2010; Gervais et al., 2004; Grandgeorge & Hausberger, 2011). Hence, normal verbal communication with others is severely impaired in autistic individuals. That's why they often end up being isolated from other kids, an outcome that only serves to further aggravate their problem. Moreover, theory of mind (sense of empathy and mind reading) capacity and their intuitions about other people are deficient (Grandgeorge & Hausberger, 2011; Muñoz Lasa et al. 2013; O'Haire, 2013; Olmert, 2009). To exemplify the social impairment, autistic children are insusceptible to contagious yawning, and they avoid eye contact and do not approach others spontaneously (Grandin & Johnson, 2005; Helt et al., 2010).

Since animals do not rely on verbal communication, they are in general quite successful with autistic people, as they share the tendency to apply sensory information like touch, smell, vision, body language, and sound instead of verbal speech. The lacking theory of mind relating to autism does not cause as big a problem when autistic people interact with animals as it does in case of interpersonal contact. Dogs in particular are highly suitable for interacting with autistic persons, as they communicate by means of their body language, whereby emotions and intentions are revealed without the use of words. Accordingly, both encounters with therapy dogs and deployment of service dogs provide significant benefits for autistic people (Fine, 2010; Grandin & Johnson, 2005; Martin & Farnum, 2002; O'Haire, 2013).

The American scientists Dr. Joan F. Goodman and Dr. Laurel A. Redefer at the University of Pennsylvania performed an early study of therapy dogs applied in the treatment and management of autism spectrum disorders (Redefer & Goodman, 1989). Dr. Goodman and Dr. Redefer described how a furry friend provides powerful stimuli compensating for autistic children's developmental deficits, leading to improved contact seeking with both dogs and people as well as a reduction in the kids' social withdrawal.

Accordingly, people with autism spectrum disorders may relate socially and emotionally to a dog, allowing them to experience a feeling of being appreciated and accepted in spite of their developmental, cognitive impairments and lack of social skills.

The scientific understanding of autism has grown, and though there are still some controversy, autism is causally associated with abnormal brain chemistry (Lam et al., 2006; Olmert, 2009; Corbett et al., 2008; Spratt et al., 2012). Hence, the regulation and signaling of certain neurohormones like cortisol (stress hormone) and oxytocin (prosocial hormone) are altered in autism. Cortisol is increased, while oxytocin is decreased. Such a biochemical imbalance may explain why individuals with autism spectrum disorders show abnormal stress responses as well as a lack of social and emotional bonding (Aoki et al., 2015; Domes et al., 2007,2010,2013; Grandgeorge & Hausberger, 2011; Lam et al., 2006; Meyer-Lindenberg et al., 2011; Olmert, 2009; Viau et al., 2010).

The role of imbalanced cortisol secretion in autistic children has been open to discussions, though more recently research data converge on the finding that cortisol is significantly increased during its circadian fluctuations, a factor that contributes to autistic children's abnormal stress reactions as well as their difficulties in adapting to change (Lam et al., 2006; Corbett et al., 2008; Spratt et al., 2012; Viau et al., 2010). Normally stress hormones are kept in check by the hormone oxytocin, but for autistic individuals this means double trouble because their oxytocin secretion and signaling are compromised (Olmert, 2009).

Individuals with autism spectrum disorders suffer from reduced oxytocin levels in their circulating blood, as their oxytocin molecules also display an abnormal structure that does not correspond to normal oxytocin (Green et al., 2001; Olmert, 2009). This is consistent with the finding that autistic individuals display alterations in their brain, in particular in the area named the hypothalamus, one of the most important regions in terms of oxytocin synthesis (Kurth et al., 2011; Olmert, 2009).

As explained later in this chapter, oxytocin is a powerful hormone and signaling molecule mediating social bonding, devotion, attachment, and stoical calmness (Bartz et al., 2011; Handlin, 2010). Two professors Dr. Johannes S. J. Odendaal and Dr. Roy A. Meintjes at the University of Pretoria in South Africa studied the dog's effect upon human biochemistry and vice versa, and they learned that oxytocin is increased significantly in both species when they interacted for fifteen to thirty minutes, and it applies whether it's an unfamiliar or familiar dog (Odendaal, 2000; Odendaal & Meintjes, 2003). Ever since then, the research of Dr. Odendaal and Dr. Meintjes has had huge influence upon any researcher studying canine-human interactions and bonding, and so their work belongs to the most important publications in this millennium. Consequently other researchers have confirmed how levels of oxytocin increase in humans and dogs as a result of social interactions and gazing at each other (Beetz et al., 2012b; Handlin, 2010; Handlin et al., 2011; Miller et al., 2009; Nagasawa et al., 2009a,b,2015). This rise in oxytocin levels caused by dog exposure may explain why people with autism spectrum disorder benefit from interacting with friendly dogs. Hence, a dog's company has been shown to notably ameliorate many of the autistic symptoms, as dog exposure improves prosocial behaviors, mood, stress reactivity, and contact seeking in autistic individuals (Aoki et al., 2015; Fine, 2010; Grandin & Johnson, 2005; Martin & Farnum, 2002; O'Haire, 2013; Olmert, 2009). Accordingly, kids with autism prefer to interact with dogs rather than with objects or other people (Beetz et al., 2012b; Prothmann et al., 2009).

Because dogs are a source of sensory-based, nonverbal stimulation and interaction, they may also elicit better development of cognitive abilities in autistic children (Grandgeorge & Hausberger, 2011). This was initially demonstrated by Dr. Levinson's pioneering work, which indicated how therapy dogs could promote language skills in children with autism (Levinson, 1962). Moreover, dogs easily hold the attention of kids with autism who as a general rule calm down when they are around the dogs.

Besides, when the kids play with the dog, they release excess energy, which also contributes to calming children.

These findings are confirmed by other studies, and the scientific data point to a range for benefits for autistic people, as dogs may convey improved skills in terms of social behavior, communication, mood, language, and cognition (Beetz et al., 2012b; Fine, 2010; Grandgeorge & Hausberger, 2011; Grandin & Johnson, 2005; Martin & Farnum, 2002; O'Haire, 2013; Olmert, 2009; Redefer & Goodman, 1989).

The notion that dogs' ability to increase human oxytocin might be a crucial mechanism behind their impact upon autism has gained substantial support from medical placebo-controlled trials, which tested pharmaceutical oxytocin treatment of autistic people and controls (Aoki et al., 2015; Domes et al., 2007,2010,2013,2014; Watanabe et al., 2014). Hence, scientists at the University of Freiburg in Germany have administered oxytocin to individuals with autism spectrum disorders, including Asperger's syndrome (Domes et al., 2013,2014), and the data have since then been replicated by other researchers (Aoki et al., 2015; Watanabe et al., 2014). These studies show that oxytocin administration rectifies the autistic symptoms.

However, as the name autism spectrum disorder implies, the patients represent without a doubt a more heterogenous population than imagined, and most likely there are different subtypes of the disorder, which expectedly request differential interventions and caretaking. However, in terms of oxytocin regulation, the company of a furry friend is certainly the safer choice and more fun as compared to pharmaceutical oxytocin administration, which otherwise may be an option in some subgroups of patients (Aoki et al., 2015; Domes et al., 2007,2010,2013,2014; Watanabe et al., 2014). Nevertheless, science supports that dogs might represent the most suitable and complete method for alleviating autism spectrum disorders, as dogs not only target oxytocin levels but also provide several other biochemical and behavioral benefits (Beetz et al., 2012b; Fine, 2010; Grandin & Johnson, 2005; O'Haire, 2013; Viau et al., 2010). So therapy or service dogs are highly suitable for being incorporated into the interventions applied for autism spectrum disorders.

Safety of Service and Therapy Dogs

While dogs are highly beneficial for autistic individuals, their welfare might be at risk if they are left all alone with autistic children. If you are considering getting an autism service dog for your child, you need to first recognize the parental responsibility that follows and beware of a number of physical stressors to the dog. Mainly parents must at least make sure that (1) the dog gets sufficient rest and recovery time after being with the kid, (2) there is a certain amount of predictability in your daily routines, and (3) the dog is provided with adequate, daily recreational activities. Parents also need to avoid putting the dog in danger, as autistic kids may unintentionally poke, harm, stress, or abuse the dog. Studies show that autism service dogs bond primarily with the parents and less so with the often unpredictable autistic child. That's why parental failure to respond to the dog's needs and welfare may adversely influence the outcome (Burrows et al., 2008).

Pain

Pain is a huge burden to mankind, particularly in cases of uncontrollable pain because of cancer or chronic conditions. Unfortunately chronic pain conditions are rarely cured, and pharmaceutically there are no truly successful treatment options. A major problem with prescription painkillers is unacceptable side effects and addiction problems. For this reason patients with chronic pain are often weighed down because of the various consequences of being in pain, such as decreased mobility, agitation, increased isolation, depression, sleepless nights, hampered rehabilitation, malnutrition, and increased visits to the physician or admission to hospitals (Fine, 2010; Marcus, 2011; Howard, 2014). Thus, chronic pain victims are afflicted in ways that not only relate to the physical, neurological problem but also to the experience of suffering. Being in pain all the time eventually changes the person's life on a psychological, social, emotional, personal, and/or spiritual level, and this is often followed by some financial and practical concerns. Consequently it is not enough to focus only on the physical component of pain if one is aiming to help these patients who in frequency outnumber all other types of neurological patient groups (Becker, 2002; Fine, 2010; Greenberg et al., 2012; Serpell, 1996).

Today more and more patients with pain request nonpharmaceutical approaches to health care and in particular in the managing of chronic pain, a condition that would otherwise lead to daily intake of medications and the burden of adverse side effects. Nonpharmaceutical approaches may either replace drugs, reduce the need for painkillers, or be used in conjunction with medications as a multimodal strategy to control pain. Before we look into the painkilling effects conveyed by dogs, a few other nonpharmaceutical methods (recreational therapies) such as music and massage deserve to be mentioned, as they are also backed up by research and becoming increasingly popular for pain management (Dobek et al., 2014; Furlan et al., 2010). However, the pain reduction as a result of these recreational therapies is primarily evident during or immediately after the therapy session, after which the benefits fade away (Furlan et al., 2010). Yet these methods are slightly more effective against pain than other popular trends or methods like acupuncture, which according to research also causes severe side effects involving increased aches or bleeding (Furlan et al., 2010). Accordingly, if burdened by chronic pain, other interventions are welcome, and this is where the method of four paws comes in. More and more scientific evidence has emerged in support of using dog therapy against pain conditions, as dogs have the power to change not only the pain itself but also the psychological elements of pain, such as the suffering component of being in chronic agony (Becker, 2002; Engelman, 2013; Fine, 2010; Marcus et al., 2012).

First of all a friendly dog can reduce pain transmission by changing our biochemistry and hormone levels as demonstrated more than a decade ago (Odendaal, 2000; Odendaal & Meintjes, 2003). Hence, research confirms that fifteen to thirty minutes of human-dog interactions make our bodies release significantly increased amounts of endorphins (also known as "the body's own morphine" or endogenous opioids) while our neurophysiological pain processes are counteracted (Motooka et al., 2006; Odendaal, 2000; Odendaal & Meintjes, 2003). In other words, we respond by means of biochemistry, physiology, and neurobiology in response to our furry friend, and as a bonus, pain is ameliorated. This effect was obtained when subjects interacted with their own dogs as well as therapy dogs, though the highest and fastest effects arose when they were interacting with their own pets (Odendaal, 2000; Odendaal & Meintjes, 2003). This reflects that it is not only a matter of plain contact, as the emotional bond seems to fuel the painkilling potential too.

Another benefit experienced by pet owners is the dog's inborn ability to recognize when it hurts or when life seems unbearable. In those moments owners report how their dogs draw closer to cuddle and comfort them, and such kind of spontaneous attentiveness and its timing will soothe most people more than any drug is able to (Becker, 2002; Engelman, 2013; Fine, 2010; Marcus, 2011). Dogs are not scared of being close even in our darkest moments, which reflects yet another canine virtue that is not always shared by our human fellows.

Mutts, Music, and Massage

A vast range of complementary and/or alternative interventions are claimed to reduce chronic pain, which remains a major societal challenge, as conventional drugs only provide limited benefits, in part because of their serious side effects. Turning to clinical research, three complementary therapies stand out as efficient painkilling interventions—mutts, music, and massage. While dog therapy is a most efficient painkiller that matches the effects of codein and paracetamol, you may also benefit from listening to music or getting a good massage (Braun et al., 2009; Dobek et al., 2014; Furlan et al., 2010; Marcus et al., 2012,2013).

A prospective study showed how adopting a dog could cut down pain and related health troubles in the order of 50 percent as seen for headaches, back pain, pain in the joints, and likewise troubles relating to the stomach, ears, and/or sinuses (Serpell, 1990,1991). For comparisons people either without pets or who adopted cats were compared to those who adopted dogs. In every case examined only those who chose the dogs obtained long-lasting benefits and a significant pain reduction (Serpell, 1996). Along with this, other researchers confirmed that dogs can reduce pain and distress in their owners as compared to those who did not own dogs.

Studies of patients admitted to hospital, palliative clinics, or long-term care facilities also support that therapy dogs can significantly reduce pain along with its suffering component as compared to the control measurements (Dietz et al., 2012; Engelman, 2013; Friedmann & Son, 2009; Headey & Grabka, 2007; Marcus, 2012a,b; Marcus et al., 2012; Miller, Oyama & Serpell, 2013). With the dogs' effects follow other benefits, such as a reduced need for psychoactive drugs, painkillers, and other medications, while health-care costs are cut down to 50 percent as compared to the control measurements (Geisler, 2004; Lust et al., 2007). Accordingly, some of the more complex, chronic pain syndromes like fibromyalgia or migraine are also ameliorated by AAT (Marcus, 2009; Marcus & Bhowmick, 2013; Marcus et al., 2013; Oyama & Serpell, 2013). Both fibromyalgia and migraine are prevalent, disabling, chronic pain conditions often found in female patients, and each disorder is characterized by an intricate collection of sensory, somatic, neurological, psychological, and/or emotional symptoms. Yet they are examples of disorders that are not easily managed by traditional, pharmaceutical medications. For that reason the demonstration of AAT as a successful therapy option for these patients has made a huge difference to these patients (Marcus & Bhowmick, 2013; Marcus et al., 2013). In fibromyalgia patients spending as little as twelve minutes with a therapy dog was enough to reduce significantly pain and distress in a clinically meaningful manner, while patients' moods were elevated by the dog when they were compared to matched control patients not receiving AAT (Marcus et al., 2013).

Children and adolescents may also benefit significantly from therapy dog visits during hospitalization, in particular since the admission may worsen fear, distress, and vulnerability in the kids (Beck & Katcher, 1983). In Minneapolis, a study showed convincing evidence that AAT was an effective painkiller for children as compared to the control intervention consisting of fifteen minutes of quiet relaxation (Braun et al., 2009). The study was privileged by its extraordinarily skilled therapy dog named Kat, an English springer spaniel that was thirteen years old at the time. With every single patient, Kat spontaneously chose to draw near the child, with whom this dog synchronized his breathing (Braun et al., 2009). Therapist Kat decreased pain significantly with the fifteen to twenty minutes for AAT sessions, and in fact, the pain reduction conveyed by Kat was four times greater than the effect of relaxation (Braun et al., 2009). In other words, within fifteen minutes Dr. Kat generated a painkilling effect that equaled the effect of pharmaceutical analgesics like acetaminophen (paracetamol) with and without additional codeine (Braun et al., 2009). Moreover, one of the kids obtained complete pain relief thanks to Kat, even though the child did not get any medication for three hours. Kat's painkilling action is quite remarkable, even though this particular English spaniel was undoubtedly a canine prodigy that will remain a role model to other therapy dogs.

At Children's Hospital San Diego, a study included children and adolescents aged five to eighteen years who were admitted for operations after which they experienced acute pain because of the surgery (Sobo et al., 2006).

The children got painkilling drugs as needed, and once during their postsurgery hospital stay, they received AAT by means of Lizzie, a nine-year-old West Highland white terrier who began her career as a therapist when she was three months of age. The researchers measured the children's pain levels before and after the single AAT session, which in most cases lasted eleven to twenty minutes. The results showed that a therapy dog significantly and rapidly relieved pain in children who had recent operations, both in terms of physical and emotional pain levels (Sobo et al., 2006). The authors concluded that AAT provided a complementary pain relief that added to the effects of the pharmaceutical treatments. Hence, therapy dogs may serve as an effective, rapid, and rather safe method for pain relief, and in case of postsurgical pain dogs may reduce the need for strong painkillers, such as morphine, which causes serious side effects and problems of addiction.

The study also explored the mechanisms of action, which involve the dog's positive distraction of the children who became sufficiently diverted yet comforted and relaxed by Lizzie. That's why their pain threshold changed significantly (Sobo et al., 2006).

At the University of Pittsburgh School of Medicine, Dr. Dawn A. Marcus has conducted several wisely designed studies of a therapy dog's impact upon patients' experience of chronic pain (Marcus, 2011,2013a).

One AAT study enrolled 382 participants consisting of (1) patients suffering chronic pain, (2) their family or friends (relatives) who accompanied the patients to the clinic, and (3) the clinical staff.

From each of the three groups of participants, a total of 286 individuals met the certified therapy dog, a five-year-old soft-coated wheaten terrier (male) named Wheatie, while ninety-six individuals from all groups served as controls and did not meet Wheatie (Marcus et al., 2012).

The experimental part took place in a waiting area as individuals within the AAT group (mainly patients and accompanying family or friends) encountered the therapy dog while they waited for the patients' scheduled appointments with a health-care professional. The clinical staff, however, could also interact with Wheatie during his working hours.

The control group (also including patients, their relatives, and staff members) had to remain in a waiting room devoid of a dog (Marcus et al., 2012). Two interesting details within this study design deserve attention. One is the inclusion of nonpatients, such as the patients' relatives (family and friends) and members of staff who are likely free of symptoms. The other interesting detail is the timing and the way AAT is implemented. The therapeutic intervention (i.e., the dog) is encountered independently from the patient's appointment, and as the study didn't require informed consent from participants, the AAT group did not exactly know in advance that they could choose to wait with or without Wheatie. Nor did they know exactly why he was present or what they could obtain from him. This aspect limited the risk of a placebo effect, as it ensured participants weren't prejudiced in favor of a potential painkilling effect of AAT.

In case of a consenting process, participants would have been told about aims, expected outcomes, and anticipated pain relief. By avoiding that, participants were expected to rate their pain levels as unbiased as possible.

The study concluded that the AAT group benefitted in several ways compared to the controls, as shown by measuring different health parametres in patients, relatives, and staff. Measurements were collected before and after participants entered the AAT waiting room or the control waiting area (Marcus et al., 2012). The conclusions made from these data were clear-cut as explained below for each group of participants.

Patients

After patients encountered Wheatie, they showed significantly reduced pain as well as significantly less fatigue, stress, aggravation, anxiety, sadness, and irritability, while they also reported a significant increase in calmness, cheerfulness, and pleasantness. The pain relief was substantial despite the fact that patients presented a variety of chronic pain conditions, such as back and/ or neck pain, neuropathic pain, arthritis, migraine, fibromyalgia, and other types of chronic pain that are normally rather difficult to treat (Marcus et al., 2012). In contrast, there were no measurable effects to gauge in the controls who spent their waiting time without a dog.

Relatives

What's no less interesting is that the relatives consisting of patients' family or friends who encountered Wheatie did also experience significant improval of the same health parameters—pain, fatigue, stress, aggravation, anxiety, sadness, irritability, calmness, cheerfulness, and pleasantness.

In this group the baseline pain scores were logically much less those of the patients, and yet relatives had a 25 percent reduction in their aches. Their benefits were substantially larger in terms of their levels of stress, anxiety, and sadness, which were cut down by approximately 50 percent. The relatives of the control group did not experience any changes because of the time spent in the waiting area without a dog (Marcus et al., 2012).

Staff

This group did not experience pain, but they did obtain effects of AAT in terms of all the other health parameters. Hence, the staff members who went to visit Wheatie showed significantly improved scores in fatigue, stress, aggravation, anxiety, sadness, irritability, calmness, cheerfulness, and pleasantness. Those staff members who chose to visit the waiting area without a dog only felt a change in calmness (Marcus et al., 2012).

Some of the participants had diagnosed depression or suffered from anxiety disorders as well. Despite these extra health challenges, these participants would still obtain significant improvements in all their scores because of the dog interaction (Marcus et al., 2012).

The latter observation illustrates how magnificent dogs are, as they obviously deal with all the patient's different concomitant problems at once, something a medical drug could never do.

In terms of their pain regulatory mechanisms, dogs may modulate pain levels based upon their roles in the three major communication systems within our body—the nervous system, the endocrine (hormone) system, and the immune system. Functionally the nervous system talks with the endocrine system (a field referred to as psychoneuroendocrinology) and with the immune system (psychoneuroimmunology) (Bonaz & Bernstein, 2013; Howard, 2014).

Hence, when a dog influences our nervous system, it leads to biochemical changes in the body's hormones, which exert feedback actions upon the nervous system, and this psychoneuroendocrine signaling will in turn alter the biochemistry of our pain response (Braun et al., 2009; Howard, 2006; Odendaal, 2000; Odendaal & Meintjes, 2003). Likewise, as we experience nervous system changes because of the dogs in our lives, the mentioned biochemical changes along with altered hormonal signaling will ultimately spill over to the immune system, which is intricately communicating with the brain. Molecules released by the immune system are key players in the pain reaction (Bonaz & Bernstein, 2013; Elenkov et al., 2000; Howard, 2014; Serpell, 1996; Ziemssen & Kern, 2007).

To be more specific, exposure to a friendly dog causes us to secrete increased levels of beta-endorphins (as mentioned previously), and while these hormones work as the body's own morphine, promoting the feeling of painless well-being, they are also signaling agents within the immune system. Endorphins increase our immune defense responses, and so in the end these mechanisms all converge on inducing pain relief (Braun et al., 2009; Elenkov et al., 2000; Howard, 2014; Motooka et al., 2006; Odendaal, 2000; Odendaal & Meintjes, 2003; Ziemssen & Kern, 2007).

Pharmaceuticals may only surpass AAT in one aspect, namely the notorious, unwanted side effects.

Even the milder, over-the-counter painkillers like aspirin, ibuprofen, paracetamol, and codeine, just to mention a few cause a range of adverse effects.

Hence, medications like aspirin and ibuprofen may lead to abdominal pain, risk of bleeding, heartburn, stomach or intestinal ulcers, tinnitus, vomiting, blurred vision, respiratory problems, dizziness, nausea, edema, allergies, and skin rashes, just to mention some of the possibilities on a very long list of side effects. This is also a matter of dosage and sensitivity, but many prefer to be safe rather than sorry and may opt for the furry solution to the problems of pain.

Disaster

Nobody is truly prepared for disasters, which most often strike without warning, and they leave devastating trails of destruction in their wakes. Though survivors can to some degree fend for themselves and may even be armed with the right equipment and information, most disaster-hit individuals do not get through on their own when they meet an unexpected, sudden, and overwhelming disaster.

While there may not be any outwardly visible signs of physical injuries, most disaster-hit citizens carry a serious emotional toll that may tarnslate into psychiatric problems. Shortly after disaster strikes, many will be in a state of shock and denial, which are typical, self-protective, and very strong emotional responses that make you feel numb or disconnected from life. In the last decades both the United States and Japan have been hit by natural disasters and/or major terrorist or shooting attacks, and both nations have shown the world how to take advantage of the healing power of rescue and therapy dogs. These occasions have also taught us that it takes a dog to make a human connection in the midst of a public catastrophe (Shubert, 2012b). Consider the efforts made in New York City in the aftermath of the terrorist attacks on September 11, 2001, where close to five hundred animals and their handlers were recruited for rescue, relief, and remedy purposes in New York, New Jersey, and Virginia. More recently the International Therapy Dog Association in Japan announced the opening of a new center for disaster-hit dogs that were abandoned after the Fukushima nuclear accident in March 2011. The center promised to train and turn these dogs into therapy dogs.

This is likely inspired by other initiatives like Therapy Dogs International, an organization founded in 1976 in New Jersey that has provided disaster stress relief programs for major catastrophic events like the Oklahoma City Bombing, September 11, 2001, and Hurricane Katrina.

On such occasions, dogs are better than anything else in providing stress relief and consolation for the victims, their families, and the rescue workers. In order words, you should look to the canine side if you want to witness a true master of disaster. Hence, despite the fact that people are in great pain or in shock and therefore not able to process necessary information, they are still drawn to and comforted by the dogs, who also are more likely to make them talk again. That's why these dogs might be imperative in order to reestablish communication and trust (Shubert, 2012b). In many ways dogs provide the comfort and calmness that the victims and their families need at a time when most other people would either feel uncomfortable in providing it or would be occupied with the disastrous event and the collateral damage. The dog fills a gap in the rescue work.

How Dogs Touch the Human Brain and Mind: Mechanisms of Action

Every second in life more than a million chemical reactions go on in your brain, and one of its prime functions is being its own chemist.

The brain cells release hundreds of transmitter molecules and identified bioactive agents. Some are involved in mood, memory, learning, bravery, sleep, arousal, motivation, reward, friendliness, and openness, while others turn things the other way, as they make you feel worried, sad, doomed to failure, sedated, angry, malicious, revengeful, or aggressive (Breggin, 2013; Howard, 2014). However, modern man is somehow not always capable of inducing the most appropriate brain processes. Because of health hazards, we sometimes need a helping hand or paw to balance our brain's biochemistry or cellular activity. This is where those furry friends enter the stage.

When we bond with dogs, we respond in a number of neurobiological ways that involve several processes ranging from the smallest nanoscaled particles to the increasing complexity of systems, organs, and whole-body physiology.

Hence, spending time with dogs leads to changes in elementary particles, molecules, and cells, and changes occur in specific brain regions, functional centers, and systems like the brain-hormone communication axis (psychoneuroendocrinology) and the autonomous nervous system. By means of the brain's role in regulating the body's homeostasis, dogs also affect our internal organs. For instance, exposure to a dog reduces the adrenal glands' secretion of stress hormones and calms the heart. That's why dogs seem to be able to do what medications can't, as dogs benefit our whole-body physiology (Barker & Wolen, 2008; Fine, 2010; Marcus, 2011; Odendaal & Meintjes, 2003; Penkowa, 2014 Stanley-Hermanns & Miller, 2002).

Accordingly, as scientists quantify measurable biological changes inside the human brain tissue, it is no wonder that owners experience how a dog may transform one's mind, cognition, and mood.

The Mechanisms behind the Dog's Effect on the Human Brain

- Elementary Chemistry (The concentration of oxygen)
- Biochemistry (Molecules: transmitters, hormones, and cytokines)
- Cells (Frontal lobe neurons, mirror neurons)
- Brain Centres (Amygdala)
- Psychoneuroimmunology/endocrinology (Hypothalamic-pituitary-adrenal axis)
- Nervous System (Autonomic shift to parasympathetic mode)
- Physiology (Blood pressure, pulmonal pressure)
- Psychology (Emotions and mood)
- Cognition (Task solving, stamina)

Oxygen has atomic number eight on the the periodic table of the elements, and considered by mass, it is the most abundant element in the human body. Oxygen is primarily required for respiration in order to survive, and at the very core of this fundamental necessity for life lies the dog. Hence, when we interact with dog, our oxygen levels are increased significantly as shown by measuring the blood's oxygen saturation in patients with and without the company of a dog (Cole et al., 2007; Orlandi et al., 2007).

The dog's molecular influence upon these was kick-started by the South African professors Johannes S. J. Odendaal and Roy Alec Meintjes at the University of Pretoria. Dr. Odendaal and Dr. Meintjes discovered how pet dogs and therapy dogs increased the release of dopamine, oxytocin, prolactin, beta-endorphins, and beta-phenylethylamine, which in general are feel-good molecules transmitting positive emotions such as reward, bonding, affectionate interaction, well-being, relief, motivation, energetic drive, and attachment behaviors (Odendaal, 2000; Odendaal & Meintjes, 2003).

On top of this Dr. Odendaal and Dr. Meintjes also showed that dogs block the release of stress hormones (cortisol) in the body, whereby arousal and the fight-or-flight response are cushioned while your thoughts are kept away from current tensions and anxiety.

These molecular dog actions are fundamental in our understanding of dog therapy and why dogs indeed are able to cause measurable changes in the human brain and mind. Since the biochemical research field was ignited in South Africa, other scientists have brought their focus to the field and begun exploring the molecular mechanisms of dog therapy (Beals, 2009; Cole et al., 2007; Fine, 2010; Friedmann & Son, 2009; Handlin, 2010; Handlin et al., 2011; Marcus, 2011; Nagasawa et al., 2009a; Odendaal, 2000; Odendaal & Meintjes, 2003; Penkowa, 2014).

In terms of antistress effects of a dog, the findings of Dr. Odendaal and Dr. Meintjes have been further investigated, and it turns out that a dog not only counters cortisol but also reduces other stress-activating hormones/neurotransmitters like epinephrine and norepinephrine (Cole et al., 2007).

The stress buffering effect of the dog may very well be a core feature of the way dogs reduce the risk of getting severely ill (Fine, 2010; Friedmann & Son, 2009; Howard, 2014; Krause-Parello et al., 2012; Serpell, 1996). An individual with chronically increased stress hormones is being held in a continuous fight-or-flight condition, which hampers the immune system and makes us prone to disease just as it takes its toll on the brain, cognition, and the mind (Servan-Schreiber, 2011). The constantly activated stress response causes a range of deleterious effects, including impairments of the most important cells to the immune defense, increased arousal, tensions, and anxiety, and at some point, depending on the individual's coping skills and resilience, the condition may lead to a depression and/or dementia (Howard, 2006; Penkowa, 2014; Servan-Schreiber, 2011). Hence, a decrease in the stress response, as seen when a dog's around, can spare you from a lot of wear and tear, which in the end may spare you from some serious diseases of the brain and mind. What's also interesting to note is that it barely takes fifteen minutes in the company of a dog before it is possible to measure the mentioned molecular changes (Odendaal, 2000; Odendaal & Meintjes, 2003). And there's more. These benefits are easy to reach, as they simply require any dog's presence whether it is our own pet dog or a dog belonging to someone else or a professional therapy dog (Aoki et al., 2012; Beals, 2009; Cole et al., 2007; Handlin, 2010; Handlin et al., 2011; Nagasawa et al., 2009a; Odendaal, 2000; Odendaal & Meintjes, 2003).

Nevertheless, the bond with a pet dog is naturally stronger than the affiliation to an unfamiliar dog, and so some of the molecular changes may occur faster when you interact with your own dog as compared to a stranger's dog, even if the benefits take place in either case (Cole et al., 2007; Handlin, 2010; Nagasawa et al., 2009a,b; Odendaal & Meintjes, 2003). Hence, the more we pet, play, and/or genuinely love our dogs, the greater changes occur more rapidly, whereby healthiness, happiness, relaxation, and resilience are coming our way. This should not hold you back from enjoying the company of an unfamiliar dog though because research supports that people's basic attitude toward dogs (as measured by means of the Pet Attitude Scale score) does not influence their the health benefits. This reflects the fact that dog therapy leads to both physical, biological, and psychological changes (Charnetski et al., 2004; Fine, 2010; Marcus, 2013a).

In addition to hormones and neurotransmitters, dogs also influence other brain biochemicals, such as the case with the protein chromogranin A, a biomarker synthesized and released from the adrenal glands in response to stressful conditions of the brain. Hence, the higher the levels of chromogranin A, the more distress in a patient.

In the saliva of demented patients receiving either six AAT sessions or serving as controls (without AAT), researchers determined the levels of chromogranin A before and after the intervention (Kanamori et al., 2001). The study showed that chromogranin A generally increased by 19 percent in the control patients, while patients receiving six sessions of AAT displayed a reduction in chromogranin A. In fact, AAT tended to reduce chromogranin A levels by 57 percent (Kanamori et al., 2001).

> Your brain is not as much a computer as it is a pharmacy.

In addition, exposure to dogs in early life results in increased levels of interleukin-10, which is a multifunctional cytokine, ie. a messenger between cells. In the injured brain and spinal cord, interleukin-10 plays important roles to protect the neurons against degeneration and cell death (Penkowa et al., 2005; Thompson et al., 2013). So interleukin-10 is released in the brain along with a set of vital growth factors and survival-promoting molecules that improve the brain's repair and functional recovery (Penkowa, 2006,2010; Penkowa et al., 2005). Research shows how exposure to a dog in early life makes our cells increase the synthesis and secretion of

179

interleukin-10 when compared to controls who either are cat owners or live without furry pets (Gern et al., 2004). Hence, the increased interleukin-10 levels induced by dog exposure may explain why dogs can facilitate a better course or outcome of disorders of the brain and/or mind.

The benefits obtained from a dog are also reflected in cellular changes of the brain, whereby the neural activity in specific areas like the frontal lobes or amygdala is modified (Cheshire, 2013; Marcus, 2011; Penkowa, 2014). Such cellular changes affect how we experience life, how we feel, and how we choose to behave just as they extend to our responses to injuries, threats, bereavement, pathogens, allergens, diseases, disasters, medications, surgery, and any other kind of event (Howard, 2014; Serpell, 1996). To distinguish cellular from molecular changes, science indicates that cellular reactions occur the moment our eyes fall upon a dog, while the changes in the brain's molecular meshwork set in after some minutes of interaction with the dog (Cole et al., 2007; Handlin, 2010; Nagasawa et al., 2009a,b; Mormann et al., 2011; Odendaal & Meintjes, 2003; Penkowa, 2012; Walsh, 2009a,b; Wells, 2009,2011).

> The brain is divided into anatomical areas, of which the most obvious are the four lobes—the frontal, parietal, occipital, and temporal lobes. The outer surface of the lobes comprises the cerebral cortex, which consists of numerous neuronal cell bodies (grey matter). The human cortex is folded and that's why you see all those wormy, wrinkled convolutions, when you look at a brain. The folding of the human cortex is important because it greatly increases the brain's surface area, and so humans have a relatively big cortex, though it is limited by the size of our skull. To each area in the brain a set of functions can be ascribed (Kandell, 2013).

The frontal lobes are the seat of consciousness and rationality, as they have roles within cognition, perception, language, self-control, intelligence, self-worth, learning, memory, personality, and all higher mental and mindful processes (Howard, 2014). Hence, it is highly relevant to know that a dog's presence increases neural activity in the cortex of the frontal lobes as shown in human brains by means of a method called near-infrared spectroscopy (Aoki et al., 2012). The same study also showed that therapy dogs ignite brain activity in most parts of the frontal cortex. The dog-mediated change is highly interesting because the frontal cortex is considered to be the most advanced regions in terms of human consciousness and cognition. This part of the brain deals with complex thoughts and emotions, including decision making, judgment, planning, conceptualizing, personality, morality, and self-control. The frontal lobes also handle complex emotional thoughts, such as remorse and ethics (Kandel et al., 2013).

This is interesting with regards to mental disorders like depression in which the patients display reduced activity in the frontal cortex (frontal lobes). That's why the increased frontal activity triggered by a dog might serve as a kick-starter explaining how dogs ameliorate depression (Kameyama et al., 2006; Le Roux & Kemp, 2009; Siegel et al., 1999).

Another cell type of the human brain that's activated by a dog's company is the mirror neuron, which is the neurobiological foundation of empathy, cohesion, social insight, awareness, and bonding (Bekoff, 2007; Hare et al., 2002; Reid, 2009; Silva & de Sousa, 2011; Udell & Wynne, 2011; Udell et al., 2010,2011). Just as dogs can read our minds by means of their mirror neurons, we are able to interact on an emotional and psychosocial level with dogs, thanks to our mirror neurons. Hence, when we are accompanied by a friendly, tail-wagging dog, we tend to pick up on the dog's innate joy, harmony, calmness, mindfulness, and happiness, and for that reason life simply feels better when a furry friend is around (Beck & Katcher, 1983; Fine, 2010; Marcus, 2013a; Walsh, 2009a,b).

The amygdala is the driver of the brain's alarm circuit. Hence, innate, primary emotions such as fear or the fight-or-flight state are ignited when the amygdala activates the autonomous nervous system (the sympathetic part), whereby reflex-like, rapid, and automatic alarm reactions take place in order to secure survival (Howard, 2006). The amygdala along with the other components of the brain's limbic system are parts of the evolutionary ancient brain, the emotional brain (Kandell et al., 2013). Because of its role in the autonomous alarm circuit, an unbalanced or dysfunctional amygdala has been linked to neuropsychiatric disorders, such as PTSD, anxiety, and panic disorders (Greenberg et al., 2012; Hariri & Whalen, 2011). However, for the amygdala to initiate the neural circuits leading to fight-or-flight, transmitter molecules like norepinephrine and epinephrine are needed for the activation of the sympathetic nervous system (acting like the gas pedal triggering the fight-or-flight response), whereby the person gains the energy needed to either fight or flee for his or her life. These changes happen so rapidly that the person won't be aware of them, and that's why people may react to danger even before they are fully aware of what they are doing. Along with the fight-or-flight reaction performed by the sympathetic nervous system, the amygdala activates the second component (the psychoneuroendocrine part) of the alarm system. There is a release of hormones by the hypothalamic-pituitary-adrenal (HPA) axis, whereby the hypothalamus and its pituitary gland release hormones that make the adrenal glands secrete cortisol (stress hormone) into the blood stream. The HPA axis signals to keep the sympathetic nervous system on high alert (Ulrich-Lai & Herman, 2009).

As mentioned earlier, a friendly dog's presence inhibits both norepinephrine and epinephrine levels as well as cortisol release through the HPA axis (Cole et al., 2007; Odendaal, 2000; Odendaal & Meintjes, 2003). Thus, the amygdala's alarm calls, including both the sympathetic nervous system's fight-or-flight response and the HPA axis's cortisol secretion, are effectively blocked when you're together with a furry friend. That's why dogs make us calm down and keep us cool instead of morphing into frenzied madmen (Barker & Wolen, 2008; Ernst, 2012; Fine, 2010; Friedmann & Son, 2009; Le Roux & Kemp, 2009).

The reason why dogs are superior to most other available stress- and anxiety-relievers is that they not only inhibit the previously mentioned alarm circuits but also promote neurobiological processes and parasympathetic activity that acts in concert to turn off the amygdala's ignition of the fight-or-flight state, which is of major importance since stress counteracts good health and inhibits recovery processes in the body (Bonaz & Bernstein, 2013; Ernst, 2013; Howard, 2014; Olmert, 2009; Penkowa, 2012; Servan-Schreiber, 2011).

This is achieved by dogs' induction of increased oxytocin and prolactin levels, as these hormones turn off the amygdala's alarm buttons to make us feel calm, safe, sociable, trustful, relaxed, amiable, and affiliated with others (Handlin, 2010; Handlin et al., 2011; Larsen & Grattan, 2012; Olmert, 2009). In fact, the augmented release of oxytocin and prolactin promotes a broad range of advantageous cellular and molecular pathways in the brain, including activation and mobilization of the neural stem cells, which represent the brain's resident source of new neurons, repair, and regeneration (Greenberg et al., 2012; Howard, 2006; Larsen & Grattan, 2012; Leuner et al., 2012; Penkowa, 2006,2010; Penkowa et al., 1999). By recruitment of the brain stem cells, dog therapy might provide an even more broad strategy than previously thought, as stem cell activation opens up a whole plethora of new applications for patients suffering from traumatic brain injury and neurodegenerative diseases (Howard, 2014; Kandel et al., 2013; Penkowa, 2006,2010).

Dogs May Promote Brain Stem Cells

Stem cells hold the capacity to produce an indefinitely amount of new cells, which can develop (differentiate) into practically any kind of cell type in the body. The neural stem cells constitute the brain's resident stem cells, and they are able to replace and renew dying or damaged cells in the brain.

Dog exposure also increases significantly other brain biochemicals like dopamine, beta-endorphins, and beta-phenylethylamine (Odendaal, 2000; Odendaal & Meintjes, 2003). Each of these potent neurotransmitters contributes in itself to the dog's amelioration of particular neuropsychiatric diseases, and the fact that even brief dog exposure increases all of them simultaneously may explain why dogs have such profound impact upon our health. As explained earlier in this chapter, Parkinson's disease is directly caused by a lack of dopamine. Yet data indicate that levels of phenylethylamine are also too low in people with Parkinson's disease and depression (Wolf & Mosnaim, 1983). Moreover, endorphins are also lowered in a range of conditions, including chronic pain and depression (Howard, 2006). Thus, the fact that dog exposure leads to concurrent increases in circulating dopamine, beta-endorphins, and beta-phenylethylamine might be one of several therapeutic mechanisms that explain why dogs are so excellent for our health (Odendaal, 2000; Odendaal & Meintjes, 2003).

Just as important, dogs elicit the most powerful relaxation response by evoking also the parasympathetic nervous system, which functions in opposition to the sympathetic nervous system's fight-or-flight response (Cheshire, 2013; Levine et al., 2013; McConnell, 2007; Olmert, 2009; Serpell, 1996). Accordingly, being in a parasympathetic state equals to a "repair, rest, and digest" condition, and so it is a requisite for brain recovery, functional restoration, and rehabilitation (Howard, 2006).

Interestingly dog exposure makes us shift into the parasympathetic state. That's why being with dogs allows us to repair, recharge, and rebuild mind and body, which is one of the key mechanisms explaining why dog owners in general are more resilient, less ill, and better to recover when they are compared to people without dogs (Aiba et al., 2012; Arhant-Sudhir et al., 2011; Cheshire, 2013; Cole et al., 2007; Ernst, 2013; Marcus, 2011; Penkowa, 2014; Serpell, 1996). In elderly people who walk or look after another person's dog, the parasympathetic nervous activity is elevated during times when they are together with the dog relative to those periods when they are without the dog (Motooka et al., 2006).

These data indicate that a dog increases the parasympathetic tone, while it diminishes sympathetic activity (i.e., stress, arousal, and the fight-or-flight state). This is of huge importance with regards to practically any human disease, risk factor, or adverse health circumstance, as in general these conditions are always followed by an increased sympathetic activity (i.e., an imbalance in the autonomic nervous system), which impairs recovery and healing (Aiba et al., 2012; Cheshire, 2013; Ernst, 2012,2013; Serpell, 1996; Servan-Schreiber, 2011; Ulrich-Lai & Herman, 2009).

To gain resilience and increased capacity to resist diseases, the parasympathetic activity must exceed the sympathetic stress (fight-or-flight) reaction in order for the individual to enter the parasympathetic state also known as "rest and digest" (Bonaz & Bernstein, 2013; Olmert, 2009; Howard, 2014).

So a shift from sympathetic to a more parasympathetic mode is also an important mechanism behind the dog's ability to balance other organs and bodily functions since the heart rate and the blood pressure decrease as soon as the parasympathetic tone dominates over the sympathetic one. This reflects how the autonomous nervous system determines not only our states of mind or brain functions but also whether our bodies are in a fight-or-flight mode or allowed to rest and digest (Aiba et al., 2012; Cheshire, 2013; Howard, 2014; Levine et al., 2013).

Though the amygdala acts as a key driver of the brain's alarm circuit, this almond-shaped mass is also involved in other brain functions, such as emotional memory, learning, behavior, and perception (Greenberg et al., 2012; Hariri & Whalen, 2011; Howard, 2014). As an example of this, the amygdala is continuously screening for any changes in other people's expressions, moods, or behaviors, which might be important to us, and so the amygdala is vital in our moment-to-moment judgment of our friends and relatives, as it enables us to learn from various social encounters and to read people's faces.

Hence, the amygdala is responsible for a variety of survival skills, vigilance, and emotional reactions to others, which explains why it is connected extensively with most other brain regions (Kandell et al., 2013). One of such skills allocated to the amygdala relates to individual attentiveness with regards to our surroundings including being aware of whom to find when, how, and where in the neighborhood or nearby milieu. It is naturally of great importance for a human to know where to locate the nearest guardian (or foe) in case of emergency situations or if a hostile intruder is underway. In line with this notion, researchers published that the human brain contains a subset of neurons situated only in the right-sided amygdala that selectively and specifically responds to the sight of a furry animal (Mormann et al., 2011). Consequently these animal-specific or -sensitive neurons are readily activated also when we see furry animals in photographs, which reflects just how much our brains were shaped by evolution in order for us to not miss out on visual information relating to dogs. Accordingly, it is not surprising that even today dogs can easily seize our attention. We see them when we are walking in the streets. They automatically catch our eyes and distract our thoughts from whatever we were doing. This mechanism also points to the huge value dogs have held throughout our coevolution.

Moreover, research into the amygdala's response to different emotional inputs and stimuli shows that an increase in the activity of the right amygdala leads to significantly reduced levels of depression (Desbordes et al., 2012). This finding is of paramount importance, as it explains why dogs seem to provide the best mood enhancer and antidepressant treatment.

To sum up the amygdala, science supports that subsets of the amygdala's neurons (those involved in the alarm circuit) are deactivated by a dog's company, while other neurons of the right-sided amygdala are activated by the sight of a dog. The first part helps to explain the dog's calming, stress-relieving, and comforting effects upon us, while the latter mechanism sheds light on the dog's ability to make us happy and put smiles on our faces, even in times of sorrow or bereavement when we would rather opt for depression. When dogs increase the activity of our right amygdala, they also distract our thoughts and make us forget about troubled life (Fine, 2010; Olmert, 2009; Mormann et al., 2011). Accordingly, dogs have differential influence upon different parts of the amygdala, which reflects the specific nature of the dog's health effects, thereby indicating that AAT might work in more multifaceted yet exact and complex manners than anyone would have guessed. In particular, this may explain why dog therapy is flourishing since the multimodal mechanisms of healthy actions are likely to surpass the effect of a medical drug that most often targets one single molecule in our bodies, and considering the complexity of any human individual, such a narrow target will not be enough to heal something as complex as a human being.

Besides, the mentioned neurobiological mechanisms influenced by the dogs in our lives do in fact also reflect how evolution has shaped the brain in a way that engaged the amygdala in more nuanced functions than simply providing a switch-on button for the fight-or-flight reaction.

From all the previously mentioned mechanisms of neurobiological action, we can ascertain the fact that dogs profoundly influence the human mind by affecting emotions, resilience, and cognition.

If we are supposed to be able to think and solve complex tasks, improve learning and memory, or simply work in a brain-powered manner, it's mandatory to be in a parasympathetic mode since only then can our sapient brain work properly. Hence, anyone who is stressed or anxious will not be able to really use that big brain.

To feel good, feel confident, and to be able to live up to our highest expectations, we have an obligation to maintain balance and harmony, and the very best way to do it is to be next to a furry friend. Hence, as explained earlier in this book, when we touch a dog's soft fur, pet or play with him or her, laugh at his or her silly moves or playing, take care of the dog and most importantly, feel that deep bond between us, then—and to some of us perhaps *only* then—may we have life's opportunity to feel truly fulfilled, whole, happy, loved, and resilient.

The Autonomous Nervous System

One of the major ways for a dog to alter our brains is by means of balancing the autonomous nervous system, which on the whole regulates and directs our mental, emotional, cognitive, and behavioral state. The autonomous nervous system is named so because it functions automatically and independent from our consciousness like a reflex that starts without any intention or planning behind it. The autonomous nervous system handles the functions of our internal organs—the heart, blood vessels, bladder, stomach, glands, airways, and intestines, just to mention a few. To illustrate the autonomy of this system, we are not aware or in control of sudden changes in our heart rate, blood pressure, oxygen use, or digestion, as these processes are regulated by the autonomous nervous system.

The body, however, cannot be separated from the brain and mind, as changes in our bodies are reflected by activity changes in our nervous system and vice versa (Libet, 2006). So the autonomous nervous system also has control over the brain and mind, in particular our emotional responses and cognition.

Before we go any further into the autonomous nervous system, we should split it into its two principal parts, the sympathetic nervous system (sympaticus) and the parasympathetic nervous system (parasympaticus), which operate independently and contradictory. First of all each system induces a specific and principal state of our brain, mind, and body. We are said to be in either a sympathetic or parasympathetic tone when one or the other is dominant. When the sympathetic nervous system is dominant, we display the fight-or-flight reponse (the acute stress reponse), which is our quick survival response system elicited by stressors and physiologically driven by the release of major stress hormones like adrenaline and cortisol (Howard, 2014; Kandel et al., 2013). Hence, sympaticus makes us able to either flee or battle in order to get out of a threatening situation alive, and so being in a sympathetic tone corresponds with arousal, energy generation/expenditure, increased blood pressure and heart rate, and inhibition of digestion, and most importantly, it shifts the brain and mind into a highly aroused state whereby we react emotionally instead of rationally. We perceive everything and everyone around us as a potential threat or enemy. In other words, the survival instinct has set in. Fear is exaggerated. Cognition and second thoughts have vanished as we see everything through the filter of possible danger.

In terms of evolutionary biology, the fight-or-flight response was only meant as a quick fix, meaning the sympathetic tone should not be dominant except in emergency situations. Thus, it is of vital importance to obtain a parasympathetic tone as soon as we have either escaped or defeated our enemy. However, today's people are getting more and more stressed without the option of either fleeing or going into a physical fight to end the problem since most stressors and *enemies* in modern life are not real, physical threats like a hungry saber-toothed tiger eager to have you for dinner. Nowadays the fight-or-flight response is activated by common stressors like bad bosses, bullying, or marital problems, problems that tend to last many months or more often years. Thereby people are stuck in a sympathetic overdrive. That is why they develop chronic stress syndrome, which carries a high risk of complications like major depression and/or dementia.

To end the fight-or-flight mode requires activation of the parasympathetic system, which acts like the brakes bringing body and mind back to the baseline. Unless your life is acutely threatened, parasympaticus is the ideal state to be in, as it normalizes body and mind in order to allowing you to function, think, and behave in a stress-free and rational manner. The parasympathetic tone is also required to repair, regenerate, recover, reload, and rewire physically and psychologically. That is why it is also termed the "rest and digest" response. Our brain, cognition, memory, learning abilities, judgement, reflection, intelligence, and other higher functioning only operate properly or to their full potential when we are not frightened. That is when we are dominated by the parasympathetic system. The same goes for our social and emotional state, as parasympaticus facilitates social behavior, empathy, emotional well-being, and attenuated stress (Greenberg et al., 2012; Howard, 2006; Kandel et al., 2013). Consequently when people seek medical help for their health problems, the first thing that needs to be achieved is the balance of their autonomous nervous systems in the direction of parasympaticus because as long as you are stuck in sympaticus, neither health nor happiness may improve, no matter what else is done. Therefore, an intervention that effectively shifts the balance toward a parasympathetic state is a most welcomed one if you ask health-care workers, and this is exactly where the dog enters the scene. Hence, merely living with a dog results in an autonomous nervous system that is dominated more by the parasympathetic system and is less involved in the fight-or-flight response (Aiba et al., 2012; Arhant-Sudhir et al., 2011; Cheshire, 2013; Cole et al., 2007; Ernst, 2013).

Yet there may well be additional mechanisms behind the canine effects, but because of today's relatively limited understanding of the complexity of the human brain, these additional mechanisms of actions are yet to be revealed.

Even though neuroscientific research has expanded radically during the last decades and even though neuroscientists have had many breakthroughs, there are still many more questions than answers with regards to the functioning of the brain cells, even more so when considering the human mind and its various mental and/or emotional states.

However, even though we still don't fully understand the human brain and mind, we are slowly getting closer and closer, and that's as good as it gets.

Even if we don't yet understand every tiny bit and detail behind it, nobody denies the dramatic influence a dog may have upon our lives.

As explained in this book, the different dog-mediated effects upon the human brain and mind are amazing, and yet they seem to be even more relevant and needed when we are succumbing to neurological or psychiatric diseases. Consequently our canine companions significantly impact our well-being and quality of life, and dogs ameliorate neurological, developmental, and psychiatric conditions, which all remain incurable. That's why they continue to be a major burden upon humankind (Barker & Wolen, 2008; Fine, 2010; Friedmann & Son, 2009; Knisely et al., 2012; Marcus, 2011; Muñoz Lasa et al., 2011; O'Haire, 2010).

CHAPTER 6

Dogs Promote Cardiovascular Health

After years of mounting media coverage of dogs' beneficial health effects, not least with regards to dog owners' improved survival after a heart attack, the health benefits of pet ownership caught attention from the National Institutes of Health and the American Heart Association (Kulbertus, 2013; Levine et al., 2013). The latter summoned experts to analyze pets' health effects upon the human heart and the risk of cardiovascular diseases, and in 2013 a scientific statement was released by the expert panel led by Dr. Glenn N. Levine, professor of medicine at Baylor College of Medicine and director of the Cardiac Care Unit at Michael E. DeBakey Medical Center in Houston (Levine et al., 2013).

> "Owning a dog could reduce your risk of heart disease."
> —The American Heart Association

The conclusions stated that dog ownership associates with reduced risk of cardiovascular disease and that owning a dog likely has a causal role in decreasing the risk of heart diseases. The statement on behalf of the American Heart Association was endorsed by the American Association of Cardiovascular and Pulmonary Rehabilitation, the American Society of Hypertension, the American Society for Preventive Cardiology, the National Heart Foundation of Australia, the Preventive Cardiovascular Nurses Association, and the World Heart Federation (Levine et al., 2013).

Who would have guessed that dogs made it all the way to become a highly commended intervention praised by the American Heart Association and the National Institutes of Health? Well, dog owners might not be surprised, whether they are also scientists or not.

Dogs Are the Heart of the Matter

Those who share their lives with dogs know by heart how wagging tails can provide positive benefits on health and well-being, and by now anyone interested in cardiology knows how dogs may transform their owners' survival rates after heart attacks. Hence, when compared to people without pets, dog owners enjoy lower blood pressure, lower levels of cholesterol and triglycerides in the blood, less coronary heart disease, and improved outcomes after heart conditions (Anderson et al., 1992; Arhant-Sudhir et al., 2011; Barker & Wolen, 2008; Cole et al., 2007; Enmarker et al., 2012; Fine, 2010; Friedmann & Son, 2009; Friedmann & Thomas, 1995; Friedmann et al., 1980, 2011).

Accordingly, dogs influence both the course and outcome of already established cardiovascular diseases, and dogs reduce many of the various risk factors promoting cardiovascular problems. These risk factors include hypertension (elevated blood pressure), too high blood levels of lipids like cholesterol (hypercholesterolemia) and triglycerides (hypertriglyceridemia), and other hazards, such as smoking, uncontrollable stress and negative feelings, and a lack of physical activity (exercise).

These are all controllable risk factors, and to this end, a dog might just be the easiest way to find what's needed for changing your lifestyle and reducing the risks of getting heart disease.

How to Win a Heart

The more owners love and care for their dogs, the better health gains they get with regards to the risk of cardiovascular diseases. Medical research shows how the mere showing of empathy, support, and unselfishness toward someone else incurs a significant reduction in the risk factors leading to cardiovascular diseases (Schreier et al., 2013). Owners who enjoy kissing their dogs also benefit from higher levels of cardioprotective hormones than owners who never kiss their dogs (Handlin, 2010). In fact the more you kiss or cherish your dog, the more health gains you get. Even if you don't wanna kiss your dog, you may boost a hormonal surge of oxytocin by gazing more at your furry friend or even better, by gazing and petting Fido more frequently (Nagasawa et al., 2009a,b; Payne et al., 2015).

With regards to smoking, a survey showed that pet owners who smoke become motivated to quit their bad habit when they learn how harmful secondhand smoke is for their pets, who suffer at least as much or likely more than humans from passive smoking (Bawazeer et al., 2012; Milberger et al., 2009; Roza & Viegas, 2007).

Accordingly, public health campaigns against smoking would likely benefit from stating just how much harm secondhand smoke causes to our pets, who will suffer from breathing problems, allergies, discomfort, stinging eyes and airways, nausea, skin diseases, respiratory and cardiovascular diseases, eye diseases, and cancers as a result of living in a smoker's home (Milberger et al., 2009).

From a personal point of view I find the Animal Welfare Act to be far from adequate in this regard, as today's level of knowledge regarding adverse effects of active and passive smoking is not compatible with the fact that people may keep animals in a smoker's home.

A Whine Just in Time

The reason we have witnessed a burst in the research field of AAT and AAA has to do with a most cited pioneering scientific study performed by

Dr. Erika Friedmann, who is a professor at the University of Maryland's School of Nursing (Friedmann & Thomas, 1995; Friedmann et al., 1980).

Dr. Erika Friedmann has opened the world's eyes to the fact that a dog can change human survival after a heart attack (acute myocardial infarction or AMI) or cardiovascular disease. So our furry friends are capable of much more than changing our lifestyles, emotions, or levels of risk factors, as owning a dog is directly linked to the balance between being dead or alive (Friedmann & Son, 2009). The survival-promoting effect of dog ownership is not dependent on the severity of the disease or other relevant physiological or demographic parameters that could otherwise contribute to the effect. Hence, it is an effect evoked by the mere owning of a wagging tail, and it is worth to count on, since the people who doesn't own dogs have a four times higher mortality rates in dog owners. For some yet unknown reasons cat ownership could not convey reduced mortality or reduce the risk of a rehospitalization when cat owners were compared to the outcome of dog owners (Friedmann & Thomas, 1995). Hence, the risk of dying was 6.7 percent for those without dogs as compared to a mortality risk of 1.15 percent in dog-owning patients.

Already back in 1980, Erika Friedmann and colleagues conducted a study of patients with either AMI or angina pectoris (a medical term that describes momentary chest pain occurring when the heart is not getting enough blood and oxygen). They compared the one-year survival chances of pet-owning versus non-pet owning patients (Friedmann et al., 1980). The conclusion was that 28 percent of people who did not own pets died within one year after the admission to hospital, while only 6 percent of pet owners died within one year. The study also ruled out that the effect was caused by dog owners' exercise when they walked their dogs, whereby the survival effects conveyed by pets is caused by the human-animal bonding, social affiliation, and companionship rather than walking exercise (Friedmann et al., 1980). Since then, the same researchers have followed up on their findings, and they've demonstrated that the increased survival of pet owners is not only valid for the first year but for four years after the heart disease (Friedmann et al., 2011).

Milena Penkowa, M.D., Ph.D., DMSc

Heart Healthy Dogs

The link between dogs and heart health has been confirmed by other clinical trials showing how pet dogs improve a range of cardiovascular risk factors, such as depression, diabetes, stress reactions, hypertension, hypercholesterolemia, hypertriglyceridemia, and other hazards (smoking, sedentary lifestyle, etc.) (Arhant-Sudhir et al., 2011; Barker & Wolen, 2008; Fine, 2010).

A milestone study was conducted at the University of California, where researchers investigated the effect of AAT upon hospitalized patients with advanced heart failure (Cole et al., 2007). The patients were divided in three groups that received either a twelve-minute visit from a volunteer with a therapy dog or a twelve-minute visit from the volunteer only. Before, during, and after the intervention, information was collected by measuring cardiovascular parameters, including blood pressure, stress hormone levels, and anxiety. The conclusions were that as little as a single twelve-minute visit with a therapy dog resulted in a significant improvement of the pulmonary blood pressure, decreased levels of stress hormones (epinephrine and norepinephrine), and reduced anxiety, which were direct consequences of the therapy dog's presence (Cole et al., 2007).

Likewise, studies have proven how dogs decrease not only the blood pressure but also heart rate, referring to the number of heartbeats per minute (Allen et al., 2001,2002; Friedmann & Son, 2009). In fact, it only takes fifteen minutes in a dog's company before your blood pressure will drop, and it's possible both with your own pet dog and an unfamiliar dog (Odendaal & Meintjes, 2003). And there's more. You don't have to exercise with the dog to obtain this effect. You can simply sit down and make yourself comfortable while you pet him or her for fifteen minutes. Along with the reduced blood pressure comes an antistress effect upon the mind and body. This is due to the dog's ability to reduce stress hormones and shift the autonomous nervous system from a sympathetic state to the parasympathetic counterpart (Barker & Wolen, 2008; Cole et al., 2007; Odendaal & Meintjes, 2003). Functional improvement in the endothelial cells (the cells lining the blood vessel wall) is also a likely contributor to the dog's cardiovascular benefits, whereby the risk of cardiac and/or circulatory dysfunction is reduced (Arhant-Sudhir et al., 2011).

White Coat and Some Fur

If you're a parent worried about your kid's health, you should know that the mentioned antistress and cardiovascular effects may also apply to children (Fine, 2010). You may even take it further if you have a fearful child or one who doesn't like to be examined by physicians since bringing a dog to the session will make your child relax. All the while their systolic blood pressure, arterial pressure, and heart rate will go down too (Nagengast et al., 1997). In contrast, when children are examined by a doctor without being joined by the dog, the kids display behavioral distress and physiological anguish, including high blood pressure and increased heart rate, a state reflecting a fight-or-flight state (Nagengast et al., 1997). This is also the case with adults because in approximately half of the population, the blood pressure surges when measured in a doctor's office, while it is normal at home, a phenomenon called white coat hypertension, which is certainly disturbing a lot of today's measurements of blood pressure (Labinson et al., 2008). Hence, by having a dog in the clinic, the patient benefits, and the result of the doctor's work also benefit. In fact, the health professional staff may also benefit in other regards from having a dog around since studies show how a brief (five minutes) interaction with the dog reduces cortisol levels and arousal in the health-care professionals and staff (Barker et al., 2005; Fine, 2010). Such an antistress effect upon the health-care workers might cause profound benefits for a range of other aspects during their workday and the quality of care they offer to their patients. This aspect finds support also in other sectors and organizations, as workplaces that allow their employees' pet dogs to be present during the workday benefit a great deal (Wells & Perrine, 2001). Hence, when owners bring their pets to work, the dogs are shown to prevent stress, increase productivity, decrease absenteeism, and increase job satisfaction not only for their owners but for the all the employees (Barker et al., 2012; Fitzgerald & Danner, 2012). Despite the scientific evidence backing up dogs in the office, many organizations still limit employees' dogs at work. However, according to CNBC (http://www.cnbc.com/id/101396437) several major companies like Google, Amazon, Procter & Gamble, Ben & Jerry's, and Zynga allow pets. Moreover, Amazon keeps their own dog park, where employees' dogs may roam and have fun, while Procter & Gamble provide free dog food. However, Zynga is likely the most procanine workplace, as Zynga employees may take their dogs to the "wooftop" dog park and enjoy lunch in the cafeteria's dog-friendly "barking lot," and the company even offers a dog health insurance. What's also hard to beat: Zynga was named after a dog.

Canine Cardioprotection

An Australian study set out to compare cardiovascular risk factors in pet owners versus people without pets, for which they recruited 5,741 participants (4,957 with and 784 without pets) who visited the Baker Medical Research Institute in Melbourne (Anderson et al., 1992). The study concluded that pet owners had significantly lower systolic blood pressure and less fat (triglycerides) in their blood as compared to participants without pets. Male pet owners also had significantly reduced cholesterol levels. This result was obtained despite the fact that all participants had similar body mass index (BMI), smoking habits and socioeconomic profiles. Adding to this, pet owners reported eating a less healthy diet with more meat and takeaway food than non-pet owners, and yet their risk of getting heart disease was lower (Anderson et al., 1992).

One of the most essential research studies of dogs' cardiovascular and behavioral benefits was performed by Dr. Karen Allen at the State University of New York at Buffalo and her collaborators. By means of a cunning test, they compared the health effects resulting from being accompanied by either a subject's pet dog, friend, or spouse, as compared to being alone when the subject was exposed to a very stressful test that elicit the sympathetic nervous system (i.e., the fight-or-flight response) (Allen et al., 1991, 2002). It turned out that the pet dogs were significantly better at reducing heart rate and blood pressure in their owners than were either the friend or the spouse who in contrast to the dog increased tension in the subjects.

Hence, stress responses were stronger and task performance poorer in participants who were either alone or accompanied by anyone other than the dog. Not only did the dogs counter severe stress reactions in their owners, but they also eliminated their emotional perception of stress

(Allen et al., 1991, 2002). When subjects reacted to the stressful test during the experiment, only their dogs made them recover more quickly as compared to the situation without their dogs. The latter is important with regards to the subject's risk profile, as faster recovery (i.e., the return to a parasympathetic and relaxed state) is associated with diminished risk of future heart diseases.

The studies by Karen Allen's research group reached a very interesting level as they investigated how much a pet's presence could add to the effects of medical drugs, such as the antihypertensive pharmaceutical called Lisinopril. Lisinopril is an inhibitor of the angiotensin-converting enzyme (ACE), whereby the drug blocks the renin-angiotensin system, which would otherwise constrict the blood vessels leading to increased blood pressure. Hence, Lisinopril reduces effectively the blood pressure, and so it was used in Karen Allen's study of hypertensive individuals. The participants were exposed to psychologically stressful tasks (mental arithmetic and speech tasks) that naturally evoke the sympathetic nervous system and increase cardiovascular reactivity (i.e., raise blood pressure and heart rate) (Allen et al., 2001). In this context half of the participants were assigned to acquire a pet, either a dog or a cat, as the researchers wanted to find out how much a pet's company could do in terms of preventing arousal and cardiovascular reactivity induced by the stressful tasks. The other half of the participants did not get a pet and served as controls to the pet-acquiring group.

The results showed that lisinopril treatment in general reduced participants' resting blood pressure, but during the stressful tasks the drug didn't help much, as blood pressure, heart rate, and the renin-angiotensin system's stress reactivity increased. Yet the pet-owning participants showed a different response, as they remained relaxed during the stressful tasks, in that their blood pressure, heart rate, and renin-angiotensin system's activity remained low both when they were stressed by the mental arithmetic or the speech task as well as during resting time. Hence, pet owners were impervious to the stress exposure as compared to the group of people who did not own pets and who went into the fight-or-flight state because of the stressful situation (Allen et al., 2001).

The lessons learned from this cunning experiment embrace that the dog's cardiovascular benefits are conveyed by the same molecular mechanisms as those of ACE-inhibiting pharmaceuticals (i.e., reducing the blood levels of renin, a hormone causing hypertension). The study also showed that the dog is even more efficient in terms of stress reduction and cardiovascular protection than ACE-inhibiting pharmaceuticals.

> A dog surpasses the cardiovascular effects of modern antihypertensive medications.

The mentioned research by Karen Allen points toward the dog's emotional and mind-altering effects, which are also supported by others who demonstrate that the dog conveys more cardiovascular protection when subjects are petting it inside their home than it does during a walk (Motooka et al., 2006).

Hence, even though walking the dog is highly beneficial for your heart and general health, you don't want to miss cuddling up to your dog.

How Dogs Touch the Human Heart: Mechanisms of Action

The biological mechanisms underlying the dog's impact upon the human cardiovascular system most likely involve an interplay of physiological, social, neuroendocrine, emotional, and biochemical factors (Cirulli et al., 2011; Fine, 2010; Knisely et al., 2012; Marcus, 2011; Penkowa, 2014).

To many people the quality of our social relationships might seem far off in terms of the risk of getting a cardiovascular disease, but the truth is it's not. In fact, it is critically involved in maintenance of health (Uchino et al., 1996). Hence, our social bonds and emotional levels of affiliation toward others are playing an important role in cardiovascular regulation and mortality (Serpell, 1996). Hence, being physically isolated from social contact is directly linked to increased mortality, as shown by a study set out to follow 6,500 British citizens in the period from 2004 to 2012 where they correlated mortality and social isolation (Steptoe et al., 2013). Hence, the death rates of highly isolated participants were 21.9 percent as compared to a 12.3 percent mortality rate seen in those characterized by little isolation. As already mentioned, a dog provides excellent social and emotional support and friendship, and this is a key aspect with regards to cardiovascular protection and resilience, and it contributes to the survival chances after cardiac attacks (Friedmann et al., 2011; McConnell et al., 2011; Uchino, 2006).

Moreover, increased cardiovascular reactivity to stress (i.e., showing elevated blood pressure and heart rate during stressful tasks) is a crucial risk factor in the development of cardiovascular disorders (Friedmann & Son, 2009; Uchino et al., 1996). As described earlier, nobody can counteract cardiovascular reactivity to stress as much as a furry friend. In fact, the dog's stress-buffering capacity is beyond that of medicine even when it's compared to the most frequently prescribed type of medication for hypertension. In line with this, the dog's effect also surpassed the stress-absorbing effect of being with a good friend (Allen et al., 1991,2001,2002; Arhant-Sudhir et al., 2011; Barker & Wolen, 2008; Cole et al., 2007). Moreover, dogs may benefit cardiac health also through their emotional influence on us, as dogs increase feelings of safety, belonging, purpose in life, morale, attachment, and being needed by others, which are all factors that increase resilience and benefit the cardiac physiology (Johnson et al., 2002; Katcher & Beck, 1983; Olmert, 2009).

Any change in emotions or mentality is bidirectionally linked to bodily changes in physiology and biochemistry, as neither the human mind nor body works as an isolated entity (Arhant-Sudhir et al., 2011; Barker & Wolen, 2008; Cirulli et al., 2011; Cole et al., 2007; Friedmann & Son, 2009; Johnson et al., 2002; Odendaal, 2000; Walker et al., 2000). This is supported in numerous cases, and in particular when considering patients with mood disorders, as having a depression is in itself a risk factor for cardiovascular diseases (Abreu-Silva & Todeschini, 2014). Hence, the dog's antidepressive action is not only making people smile again but also protecting them against heart attacks.

Hence, the psychological comfort we get from a dog is mirrored by physiological mechanisms regulating the cardiovascular system, as a friendly dog-human interaction alters our heart rhythm, respiration (oxygen saturation), blood pressure, mean arterial pressure, pulmonary vessel pressure, skin conductance, and temperature (Allen et al., 1991; Barker & Wolen, 2008; Cole et al., 2007; Fine, 2010; Friedmann & Son, 2009; Marcus, 2013a; Motooka et al., 2006; Odendaal, 2000; Orlandi et al., 2007; Walker et al., 2000). In fact, these physiological changes occur quite rapidly since we only have to spend five to twenty-four minutes (fifteen minutes on average) with a furry friend before our blood pressure plunges (Odendaal, 2000; Odendaal & Meintjes, 2003). Other studies support the rapid health effect, as a single session of twelve minutes with a friendly dog is enough to improve most parameters (Cole et al., 2007).

The physiological changes are part of a systemic biological response to dogs, which also comprise biochemical changes involving hormones, transmitters, and secretory molecules acting on the cardiovascular system (Fine, 2010; Friedmann & Son, 2009; Marcus, 2013a; Penkowa, 2014). Stress hormones like cortisol, epinephrine, and norepinephrine, which in general arouse and put a strain on the cardiovascular system, are reduced within twelve to fifteen minutes of human-dog interaction (Cole et al., 2007; Odendaal, 2000; Odendaal & Meintjes, 2003). Likewise, neuroendocrine molecules like oxytocin, beta-endorphin, prolactin, beta-phenylethylamine, and dopamine are rapidly increased by a dog's company, and these hormones are implicated in the cardiovascular system and regulation of the sympathetic nervous system's fight-or-flight reaction (Handlin, 2010; Handlin et al., 2011; Nagasawa et al., 2009a,b; Odendaal, 2000; Odendaal & Meintjes, 2003; Olmert, 2009; Petersson, 2002). For instance, oxytocin act directly upon the blood circulation and the cardiac muscle cells, as shown both in healthy individuals and patients with heart diseases (Grewen & Light, 2011; Gutkowska & Jankowski, 2008; Petersson, 2002). Hence, oxytocin administration may be used in the treatment or prevention of heart diseases with loss of cardiac muscle cells, such as an AMI. Oxytocin regulates several heart functions, including cardiac stem cells that can be used to repair, regenerate, or reinforce damaged cardiac tissue (Gutkowska & Jankowski, 2008; Jankowski et al., 2012). Moreover, chromogranin A and three peptide hormone derivatives (vasostatin-1, catestatin, and serpinin) of chromogranin A serve as molecular regulators of cardiovascular functions during health and disease, and by its influence upon the chromogranin A system, the dog have yet another way of improving our cardiovascular health (Kanamori et al., 2001; Tota et al., 2014).

From all the mentioned physiological, biochemical, social, neuroendocrine, psychological, and emotional mechanisms by which a dog alters our cardiovascular system, it becomes clear that the dog holds a major key to the heart of the matter, namely the autonomous nervous system (Marcus, 2013a; Motooka et al., 2006; Penkowa, 2014). Hence, all the scientifically validated changes caused by the dog act in accordance with a shift toward the parasympathetic nervous system (the "rest and digest") state instead of being trapped in the sympathetic nervous system's fight-or-flight reaction. At the end of the day the dog's influence leads to a calm, balanced, happy, and harmonious state that overall reduces the risk of dying from cardiovascular problems (Friedmann & Thomas, 2003; Friedmann & Son, 2009; Motooka et al., 2006).

CHAPTER 7

Dogs and the Immune System

The immune system consists of the highly specialized white blood cells (leukocytes) that are produced by stem cells of the bone marrow. The newly formed leukocytes enter the circulation in order to survey, scavenge, and protect us against diseases, tissue damage, and infections from bacteria, virus, parasites, or other types of microorganisms (Abbas et al., 2014). Ultimately the immune system's most specialized cells, the lymphocytes, also serve to eliminate any cells that display permanent damage or detrimental mutations or malformations, especially cells that have transformed into malignant tumor cells. To fulfill these roles, the leukocytes apply an armory of signaling molecules. For instance, antibodies (immunoglobulins) produced by the B lymphocytes, which are crucial when other immune cells (such as T lymphocytes and natural killer (NK) cells) are activated. Together these specialized cells perform an orchestrated attack that ultimately kills invading microorganisms, mutated cells, or any other unwanted component (Abbas et al., 2014).

Accordingly, if the immune system doesn't function normally, the host's health is at risk. If the leukocytes are less active than needed, such as in case of immunodeficiencies, repeated and life-threatening infections may occur. Immune system deficiency may be the result of either inherent genetic diseases or acquired conditions, such as AIDS (aquired immunodeficiency syndrome), or it may be due to side effects caused by medicine (Abbas et al., 2014). Moreover, chronic stress conditions and/or depression are also associated with an insufficient immune defense (Elenkov & Chrousos, 2006; Penkowa, 2012; Sternberg, 2006).

On the other hand, immune disorders can also be rooted in the opposite problem, namely autoimmune or inflammatory diseases, in which the leukocytes are continuously hyperactive, whereby they unfortunately attack your own body. This is the case in dreaded diseases such as diabetes mellitus, multiple sclerosis, rheumatoid arthritis, asthma, and systemic lupus erythematosus.

Likewise, allergies are due to a fateful mistake. The leukocytes misjudge a harmless molecule and interpret it as a dangerous and offending substance (allergen). From then on the immune system is overactive and raises its defenses every time it encounters the allergen, which most often consists of pollen, dust mites, molds, animal dander, insect stings, food allergens, and various industrial additives that are components that normally don't cause immune activation (Abbas et al., 2014). Some fifty million Americans have allergies, and because of their overactive leukocytes, they suffer a bevy of unpleasant symptoms, such as wheezing, sneezing, swelling, itching, nasal congestion, and running eyes.

Unfortunately having a hyperactive immune system does not mean your immunity is better or stronger. Both allergy and autoimmune diseases are due to a mistaken immune system. That's why the normal, warranted immune defenses to infections, injuries, diseases, or harmful changes in cells are likely to be chronically disrupted (Abbas et al., 2014; Federico et al., 2007). Accordingly, having either a hyperactive or a deficient immune system carries a risk of gearing the journey to malignant cancer development (Federico et al., 2007).

According to this, the major point is that a healthy and properly activated immune system is crucial for any individual's health profile both in the short and in particular in the long run. In this regard our furry friends once again are a blessing since they provide us with healthy hearts, minds, and brains. However, the dog is also our immune system's best friend. As described, living with dogs improves our immune defense reactions. That's why dogs protect us from infections, diseases, and allergies (Fine, 2010; Fujimura et al., 2014; Gern et al., 2004; Marcus, 2011,2013a; Penkowa, 2012; Serpell, 1996).

Milena Penkowa, M.D., Ph.D., DMSc

Dogs Boost Your Immune System

Living with dogs or simply being around a friendly dog for a short while can significantly improve our immune defense. Even a short exposure to a dog influences the activity of leukocytes and improves their release of protective antibodies (Charnetski et al., 2004). As a result, dog owners' immune systems are stronger. That's why they are less burdened by infectious diseases and allergies as compared to people without pets or with pets other than dogs (Gern et al., 2004; Penkowa, 2014; Rock et al., 2003; Serpell, 1990,1991,1996).

The most groundbreaking study was performed by Dr. Carl J. Charnetski, who is a professor in the Department of Psychology at Wilkes University. Dr. Charnetski and his colleagues were the first to investigate a dog's molecular impact on the human immune system, as they studied college students before and after the students petted a dog for eighteen minutes (Charnetski et al., 2004). As controls, other students were assigned to either pet a stuffed toy dog or to sit comfortably on a couch for eighteen minutes. Before and after the experiment the levels of protective antibodies, such as immunoglobulin A (IgA) produced by the B lymphocytes, were measured in the saliva of the college students. The conclusion from their analyses was that only those participants who petted the real dog (a sheltie) yielded a significant increase in their IgA antibodies (Charnetski et al., 2004). Hence, petting a stuffed toy dog (which had the same shape, size, and texture as the sheltie) or relaxing on the couch did not lead to significantly improved levels of antibodies. The college students were also examined by means of the Pet Attitude Scale in order to see whether their immune functions were related to their feelings toward pets. Interestingly their basic attitudes regarding pets were not affecting the immune system benefits derived from the dog (Charnetski et al., 2004). The latter aspect indicates that it is not as much a psychological impact but rather a matter of physiological and biochemical mechanisms that are responsible for the dog's immunobiological benefits. This notion is further supported by a study where medical researchers from University of Wisconsin-Madison and University of Chicago analyzed participants genetically, and they demonstrated that the dog influences the human immune system by genotype-specific mechanisms (Gern et al., 2004).

Hence, the dog's immune effects interact with your genetics and the ways your DNA is arranged in specific genes relevant to the leukocytes, which underscores that dogs not only make us feel better but make us react better as well.

> Did you know that owning a dog might be the easiest way to boost your immune system? Science supports that living with a furry friend reduces the risk of infectious, allergic, inflammatory, and autoimmune disorders.

Canine Allergy Fighters

Contrary to popular belief (myth), mounting medical research reveal how living with a dog confers significant protection against various allergic disorders, including asthma, eczema, rhinitis, atopic dermatitis/atopy, wheezing, and seasonal allergies from pollen and likewise airborne allergens, as demonstrated in both children and adults (Almqvist et al., 2003; Bufford & Gern, 2007; Bufford et al., 2008; Chen et al., 2008; Lødrup Carlsen et al., 2012; Mandhane et al., 2009; Ownby et al., 2002; Salo & Zeldin, 2009; Serpell, 1990,1991,1996; Simpson, 2010).

The notion of dogs preventing allergies was already proposed by Dr. James A. Serpell decades ago. He showed how dog adoption could significantly reduce the rates of allergy in the newly fledged owners, an effect that could not be matched by the control situation (cat acquisition or no pet adoption) (Serpell, 1990,1991). Similar antiallergic benefits are obtained in puberty, as teenagers may reduce their risk of allergy later in life by getting pets (Mandhane et al., 2009). This study also supports how dog-specific allergic sensitization is rather uncommon since dog exposure stimulates proper maturation of the immune system, whereby the leukocytes' mistaken reaction toward allergens is counteracted (Simpson & Custovic, 2005). Accordingly, living in a household with dogs is not causing allergy to furred pets. In fact, science shows that keeping dogs results in quite the opposite (Almqvist et al, 2003;. Bufford & Gern, 2007; Linneberg et al., 2003; Mandhane et al., 2009; Ownby et al., 2002).

Living with two or more dogs is even more protective against allergy than living with only one single dog, which reflects that dogs' effect upon our immune system is dose-dependent just as is the case with most medical drugs (Ownby et al., 2002; Simpson, 2010). The dose-dependency finds support in a prospective study of 474 children who were followed from birth to the age of six to seven years, during which time they were tested for allergies and levels of allergic IgE antibodies (Ownby et al., 2002).

The fact that dog ownership is not equal to immune hyperresponsiveness and allergic sensitization might come as a surprise since many people mistakenly think that dogs increase the risk of allergy, which shows just how difficult it is to kill a myth. And a myth it is. Dogs in your home do not lead to increased allergic disorders. On the contrary, they do just the opposite as shown by a continuously growing amount of evidence published in research papers (Anyo et al., 2002; Bertelsen et al., 2010; Chen et al., 2008; Epstein et al., 2011; Hesselmar et al., 1999; Lowe et al., 2004; Lødrup Carlsen et al., 2012; Mungan et al., 2003).

However, the reason the myth persists might to some degree be due to the allergic risk associated to other furry pet types, for instance cats. When compared to dogs' effects, cats exert a range of opposite effects on our immune system (Bertelsen et al., 2010; Epstein et al., 2011; Linneberg et al., 2003; Rock et al., 2003).

Hence, the cat (but not the dog) is among the four most common sources of allergens, the three others being house dust mites, grass pollen, and the fungus Alternaria alternata (Arshad et al., 2001). Being sensitized to these four allergens is strongly linked with the incidence of allergic diseases. When selecting those in a population who react to cat allergens, two out of three (66.7 percent) also suffer from asthma, eczema, and/or allergic rhinitis (Arshad et al., 2001). In fact, exposure to cats in early life may increase children's risk of developing allergic conditions, in particular asthma, eczema, and bronchial hyperresponsiveness later in their childhood, while the opposite is the case with dog exposure (Bertelsen et al., 2010; Epstein et al., 2011; Rock et al., 2003). However, considerable controversy exists with regards to cat allergens, while in the case of dogs growing data support how dog exposure is a significantly protective factor against allergy and asthma (Marcus, 2011; Penkowa, 2014; Serpell, 1990,1991; Simpson, 2010). In fact, numerous scientific studies have now pinpointed how keeping dogs significantly reduces immune-related malady and in particular asthma and allergic disorders, including atopy, eczema, rhinitis, seasonal allergies to pollen, and atopic dermatitis (Almqvist et al., 2003; Bufford & Gern, 2007; Bufford et al., 2008; Chen et al., 2008; Fujimura et al., 2014; Gern et al., 2004; Lødrup Carlsen et al., 2012; Mandhane et al., 2009; Ownby et al., 2002; Salo & Zeldin, 2009; Serpell, 1990,1991; Simpson, 2010).

> If you are a dog owner, your risk of allergy or an infection is drastically reduced as compared to people with cats or without pets (Serpell, 1990,1991). Hence, dogs prevent us from getting colds, flus, and problems with ears, eyes, stomaches, bladders, and sinuses. And there's more. When you are acquiring a dog, it only takes one month before you can enjoy long-lasting health benefits (Serpell, 1996).

Pregnancy Guide: Get a Dog

Further support for this comes from studies of expectant mothers living with pets and in particular dogs during pregnancy since they deliver babies who show significantly reduced levels of allergic IgE antibodies (Aichbhaumik et al., 2008). Moreover, prenatal dog exposure (by means of pregnancy combined with dog ownership) leads to healthier offspring since the children of dog-holding mothers enjoy significantly better health and far less immune disorders, such as allergies and asthma (Ezell et al., 2014).

Dogs provide other immune benefits as well since the rates of urinary tract infections in expectant mothers are reduced by dog exposure compared to the rates of pregnant cat owners (Stokholm et al., 2012). Moreover, living with a dog did not lead to significant increases in the frequency of urinary tract infections as compared to expectant mothers without pets. In contrast, mothers who kept cats during pregnancy showed a statistically significant increase in infection rates relative to those without pets (Stokholm et al., 2012).

The healthy impact of keeping dogs during pregnancy has also been demonstrated by other clinical researchers, as childhood health parameters and rates of allergies and asthma are improved significantly in cases of prenatal exposure to dogs, i.e., in case the expectant mother kept one or more dogs (Ezell et al., 2014).

Fur and Forest Therapy

On top of this there's another benefit for dog owners and/or dog walkers since studies show how an outdoor trip to a forest may increase both the numbers of lymphocytes in the blood circulation, the immune defense performed by the NK (natural killer) cells, and the cellular production of anticancer proteins that protect us from developing malignant tumors (Li & Kawada, 2011; Li et al., 2010). And if you don't feel like it next time your furry friend wants to go outdoors, you ought to know that the mentioned immune benefits obtained by the forest outing did in fact last for more than seven days after the trip. In addition, science has shown that children with asthma and allergic diseases, such as atopic dermatitis, benefit significantly from a forest recreational trip (Seo et al., 2014). Hence, clinical researchers in Korea recruited a group of forty-eight kids with either asthma or atopic dermatitis who were transferred from their urban homes to a national recreational forest for an outdoor leisure trip. After the forest trip the group displayed significant improvements in a range of clinical, biochemical, and respiratory parameters, indicating better immune system functions and less allergic reactions (Seo et al., 2014). So we all ought to go more often to nature's fields. In fact, they are the best places to enjoy life with our furry friends. And there's more. You might even get exercise while you are having some forest fun with Fido.

Organ Transplantation

Organ transplantation is used to replace the recipient patient's damaged or absent organ by means of an organ donor. While it may sound simple, It Is a complex area of modern medicine because the recipient's immune system may reject the donor's organ and cause transplant failure. This is why the immune system of the recipient patient has to be medically suppressed before the new organ is implanted. However, the type of immune suppression induced in these patients carries a high risk of life-threatening complications, such as invasive infections (Abbas, 2014).

According to the described immune benefits of dog exposure, it is not far-fetched to anticipate that dog ownership may alter the course and outcome of organ transplantation when compared to those of recipients without dogs.

Yet no major clinically controlled study publication exists regarding transplantation in dog-owning recipients versus patients without dogs. Nevertheless, a clinical study led by professor Annette Boehler at the Division of Pulmonary Medicine at the University Hospital Zurich in Switzerland examined the course and outcome of lung transplantation in pet owners compared to those who did not own pets (Irani et al., 2006). While the study certainly is interesting, it also holds a major weakness since it doesn't differentiate between ownership of dogs and other pet animals, as the data from all owners regardless of their type of pet were pooled into one group. Thus, the different and sometimes opposing health effects of each pet type are masked.

Despite this bias, the study showed that pet ownership in general improves significantly the patients' physical and psychological health as compared to lung transplanted patients without animals (Irani et al., 2006). The pet benefits were found after they controlled for all other possible factors, such as demographics, baseline health, and type of diagnosis before the transplantation.

Interestingly 76 percent of owners had contact with their pets for several hours every day, and 91 percent fed their pets themselves. That's why their exposure to animals can be deemed noticeable. Pet owners showed significantly higher scores concerning optimism as compared to those without pets. This is interesting since all patients usually express higher optimism after the transplantation procedure. So did the patients without pets, but pet owners surpassed their level by far (Irani et al., 2006).

Likewise, all patients reported increased life satisfaction after transplantation, but once again the pet owners significantly exceeded the satisfaction of patients without pets. In several parameters measured—energy/zest for life, freedom from anxiety, independence, living conditions, family life, relationships, social support, and sexuality—there were no areas in which patients without pets did better than pet owners (Irani et al., 2006).

These differences occurred despite that levels of fitness and mobility were similar in pet and non-pet owners, and so the pet benefits could not be ascribed to simple confounders like differences in daily exercise. Moreover, clinical anxiety and depression were much lower (about halved) in pet owners after transplantation. Even when lung-transplanted pet owners' moods, minds, and mental health are compared to those of the average background population (normal people without diseases), transplanted pet owners display better mood and decreased incidents of depression (Irani et al., 2006).

The study conducted at the University Hospital Zurich may cast huge impact upon health-care approaches and clinicians in particular, as the Swiss research contradicts those who warn immunocompromised patients against keeping pets. Other scientists and clinicians have also reported that the health benefits derived from pets and dogs in particular support that transplanted patients should not be warned against keeping pets, even if animal exposure logically carries a risk of zoonotic transmission (Avery et al., 2013; Kotton, 2007). Hence, if patients are taught how to best handle and interact with their different types of pets, among whom dogs are considered to be significantly safer than cats, reptiles, and birds, they should know that there is no scientific evidence arguing against pet ownership (Avery et al., 2013; Irani et al., 2006; Kotton, 2007).

In agreement with this, the reported incidence of zoonoses is not higher in transplanted patients as compared to other groups (Kotton, 2007). In fact, the percentage of transplant recipients who were hospitalized at least three times and the percentage who needed two or more antibiotic treatments per year were both increased in non-pet owners as compared to transplanted pet owners (Irani et al., 2006). The latter reflects that pet ownership led to less severe and fewer infections in transplanted patients. This is not to say that zoonotic transmission from pets won't happen. Instead the point is that there are huge differences between the risk carried by different types of animals (Avery et al., 2013; Kotton, 2007). Besides, what's likely the most essential risk factor with regards to zoonoses is human conduct since owners' behavior and daily feeding or cleaning habits around their pets are the cornerstone that can dramatically reduce if not decide the risk of pathogenic transmission (Avery et al., 2013; Kotton, 2007).

According to the research described hitherto, it makes sense that pets and in particular dogs are no longer considered as risk factors to be avoided by immunocompromised patients, a notion supported by the Centers for Disease Control and Prevention. Accordingly, a report on pets and organ transplant patients was published by the Centers for Disease Control and Prevention, and in it species-specific guidelines are issued (http://www.cdc.gov/healthypets/specific-groups/organ-transplant-patients.html).

This is supported by a Swedish study of lung transplant recipients, as it demonstrated hospital departments and their water supplies to be the primary source of pathogenic bacteria in particular the much-dreaded, multiresistant bacterium Pseudomonas aeruginosa that causes high morbidity and mortality rates (Johansson et al., 2014). Even though it is considered to be relatively safe to keep dogs, there are other species who might pose a risk according to scientific studies. Hence, following organ transplantation, close contact with cats (especially young cats), reptiles, exotic pets, monkeys, aquarium water, rodents, birds, and ill animals is discouraged, and so is the cleaning of cat litter boxes, fish tanks, and bird cages if patients are to adhere to a safe way of living (Avery et al., 2013; Irani et al., 2006).

Finally antiseptic standards and daily hygienic habits of the health-care professionals, in particular regular hand washing and the use of gloves among the staff, are likely to represent areas that need to be improved, and perhaps this should be prioritized before anything else.

While the study described here is of huge interest and relevance, it has to be underscored that perhaps it did not reveal the full potential of the health benefits derived from a dog since the dog's health impact would likely become diluted or masked because of the pooling of all pet owners into one group (Irani et al., 2006).

Hence, knowing that different types of pets cause very different health effects (Bertelsen et al., 2010; Epstein et al., 2011; Gern et al., 2004; Linneberg et al., 2003; Penkowa, 2014; Rock et al., 2003; Serpell, 1990,1991), the pooling of all pet owners throws in a huge bias in the Swiss study. For this reason we may have yet to see the magnitude of dogs' health and immune benefits during and after a solid organ transplantation.

Milena Penkowa, M.D., Ph.D., DMSc

Regulation of Immune Molecules

The dog's ability to improve the human immune system in diverse ways and settings as described previously relates to several mechanisms of actions, which are only beginning to be explored in detail.

First of all the fact that fifteen minutes together with a therapy dog can make our production of IgA antibodies increase significantly is of great importance to human health (Charnetski et al., 2004). This pioneering work has been a research landmark impacting the scientific community and facilitating the hype regarding the view of AAT and dog ownership as a therapeutic intervention. Since then, other data have revealed how as little as five minutes of AAT is able to increase IgA levels in health-care professionals as compared to other soothing interventions, such as twenty minutes of quiet resting (Barker et al., 2005). Hence, after five minutes with the therapy dog, IgA levels in the saliva of health-care professionals had increased to 105.7 percent relative to their baseline levels (levels before AAT), while in the control intervention (twenty minutes of relaxation) salivary IgA dropped to 83.1 percent of baseline levels. While it may be surprising how dogs impact our body and mind's biochemistry, scientists have known for decades how dogs efficiently improve specific biomedical parameters, such as blood pressure and mental arousal, and that dogs surpass the effects of other health (Beck & Katcher, 1983; Jenkins, 1986). Nonetheless, the increase in human IgA production because of dog exposure is an important health promoter because IgA represents the most abundant type of antibody defense system in our body. That's why it is particularly abundant in all the body's mucosal linings (for instance in the respiratory and digestive tracts), where IgA forms a line of defense protecting us from invading microorganisms and toxins (Cerutti et al., 2011). According to this, if you suffer from IgA deficiency, which is the most common antibody-related immunodeficiency, you are burdened by higher than average rates of infectious diseases as seen mainly in the respiratory, gastrointestinal, kidney, or urinary tracts (Abbas et al., 2014).

In contrast, exposure to dogs reduces yet another type of antibody called the IgE, which rises as part of certain disorders of the immune system. IgE has a detrimental role because of its involvement in allergy (Ownby et al., 2002; Fujimura et al., 2014).

In addition, dogs boost the immune system by means of molecular changes involving some of the previously mentioned hormones, such as beta-endorphin, dopamine, oxytocin, and prolactin, which all are potent signaling factors in the immune system (Penkowa, 2014; Rojas Vega et al., 2012; Sarkar et al., 2010,2012). The dog's ability to reduce significantly the stress hormone cortisol also has a major impact on the immune benefits since cortisol suppresses the immune defense reactions (Abbas et al., 2014; Odendaal, 2000; Odendaal & Meintjes, 2003).

Hence, dopamine balances the overall activity of lymphocytes, as it activates the inactive cells while already activated lymphocytes are downregulated (Sarkar et al., 2010). Thereby, dopamine makes sure that the lymphocytes remain properly engaged in the body's defense reactions.

Endorphins, on the other hand, increase the number of leukocytes, including both NK cells and macrophages, the cells that engulf, digest, and remove unwanted and/or decaying material (debris) (Sarkar et al., 2012). Thereby, a stronger immunity is yielded against all kinds of debris, including degenerated or dying cells, cancer cells or infectious microorganisms. In addition, enhancing macrophages may also promote our tissue regeneration and repair processes after damage or injuries (Abbas et al., 2014; Penkowa, 2014).

Likewise, prolactin has several roles in the human immune system, as it stimulates development and maturation of the immune cells, promotes cell renewal, and activates specific lymphocytes during both health and diseases (Freeman et al., 2000; Rojas Vega et al., 2012). The importance of prolactin is also reflected by its role in organ transplantation, as the hormone plays a role during recipient patients' potential graft reaction or acceptance of the implanted donor organs (Freeman et al., 2000).

In addition, dogs may also boost the immune system by affecting other hormones, particularly through the reduction of stress hormones like cortisol, which has several harmful effects on the immune defense responses (Elenkov & Chrousos, 2006; Sternberg, 2006). Mainly cortisol impairs the immune defense by inhibiting proper migration of the leukocytes, which thereby are prevented from reaching intruding microorganisms or keeping debris from building up in the body. Cortisol also disrupts repair processes, wound healing, and recovery. That's why living in distress takes its toll on our health (Irwin, 2008; Ziemssen & Kern, 2007). As a result, people with severe or unending stress conditions, including PTSD, are burdened by the associated high increase in stress hormones. That's why their immune defenses and repair capacity ultimately are exhausted. The phenomenon of immune exhaustion has for many years been known to exist also with regards to depression and loneliness (lack of social networks), which in due course will also impede significantly an individual's immune system and resilience (Serpell, 1996).

For such reasons their stress-relieving and antidepressive effects along with the dog's role as an attachment figure offering social and emotional support are vital elements with regards to dogs improving of our immune system and overall health (friedmann and Son, 2009; Marcus, 2011; Penkowa, 2014; Serpell, 1996; Virués-Ortega & Buela-Casal, 2006).

Inasmuch as dogs are naturals, when it comes to balancing our immune system, another explanatory aspect is that the immune system of dogs and humans are very much alike with regards to genetic organization, defense mechanisms, antimicrobial activities, and tissue distribution of immune molecules and cells (Abbas et al., 2014; Leonard et al., 2012).

Canines and Cytokines

Cytokines are the prime messenger molecules of the immune system. Leukocytes communicate with one another by means of releasing specific cytokines. There are hundreds of different cytokines that all have distinct actions and targets, and so by a precisely controlled release of certain types of cytokines in a certain concentration during a certain time period, each leukocyte may communicate a distinct message to one or more of the other leukocytic cell types, allowing for the immune system to generate a coordinated, robust, and appropriate defense reactions to any given targets, such as foreign bodies or pathogenic microorganisms. Likewise, cytokines are also responsible for appropriate limitation of the immune cells, whereby inflammatory reactions can be brought to an end at the right time and place. The latter is just as important as the activation of an immune reaction, as the host would otherwise display hyperresponsiveness and thereby suffer from chronic inflammation, autoimmunity, or allergies.

Therefore, it is of huge importance that scientific studies have demonstrated how dog exposure leads to significant changes in the synthesis and timely release of distinct series of cytokines (Bufford et al., 2008; Fujimura et al., 2014; Gern et al., 2004). Accordingly, a dog's company not only alters the previously mentioned hormones and transmitters, as dogs also regulate some of the cytokines that control the immune system's activation and inactivation.

Cytokines consist of a broad class of secreted proteins acting as cell-to-cell messengers or signaling factors. Cytokines are divided into subclasses consisting of interleukins, chemokines, interferons, growth factors, and others (Abbas et al., 2014). Among these, the interleukins (or the interleukin family of proteins) are of specific interest, as they are the messengers by which leukocytes communicate with one another. Different types of leukocytes also need to organize and coordinate each of their immune actions, and this is done by secretion of distinct interleukins, which regulate the behavior of other cells as well as the secreting leukocyte itself (Abbas, 2014). This is also reflected by the name *interleukin*, which come from *inter* meaning "communication in between" and *leukin*, which refers to the cellular source of these molecules, namely the leukocytes.

As shown by medical and clinical scientists, growing up with a dog results in an increased release from the cells of different interleukins, such as interleukin-5, -10, and -13, each of which has specific functions within the immune system (Bufford et al., 2008; Gern et al., 2004). The regulation of interleukins by dogs is supported by other researchers showing how keeping dogs leads to reduced synthesis of allergy-related interleukins, for instance interleukin-4 (Fujimura et al., 2014).

The most dramatic effect of dog exposure is seen on the antiallergic cytokine interleukin-10, since the levels of interleukin-10 are significantly increased in response to a dog's company when compared to those living either with cats or without pets (Gern et al., 2004; Rock et al., 2003).

This is of crucial importance in order to understand better how dogs improve our immune system because interleukin-10 is a major and multifunctional regulator of leukocyte activity and specific immune functions (Bufford et al., 2008; Abbas et al., 2014; Moore et al., 2001). Thus, interleukin-10 serves to limit and terminate the activity of different subsets of leukocytes, whereby it can cease hyperactive immune responses, such as those causing allergic, inflammatory, and autoimmune diseases (Hilgenberg et al., 2014; Moore et al., 2001). Moreover, interleukin-10 is vital for the proper development and maturation of T lymphocytes, and so it has crucial immune functions in both health and disease, as interleukin-10 holds the key to allergen tolerance (Gern et al., 2004; Hilgenberg et al., 2014; Moore et al., 2001; Thompson et al., 2013).

Furthermore, dog exposure in the first year of life also leads to modest increases in kids' secretion of interleukin-5 and -13, which have both overlapping and distinct functions within the immune system (Gern et al. 2004; Rock et al., 2003). However, in other experimental studies the synthesis of allergy-related interleukin-4 and -13 was reduced after exposure to dog-related house dust (Fujimura et al., 2014). A reduction of interleukin-13 synthesis along with an increase in interleukin-10 secretion will most likely offer the most potent protection against a vast array of inflammatory and allergic disorders. However, the data on interleukin-13 may seem contradictory at a first glance, but in fact, the results aren't necessarily opposing since one study reports the levels of secreted proteins as measured in children's blood (Gern et al. 2004) while the other study measured murine lung tissue's activation of the gene coding for interleukin-13, in the sense that the gene is needed for cells to synthesize novel interleukin-13 (Fujimura et al., 2014). Certainly, this issue will be further clarified in near future as ongoing research into dogs' influence upon human cytokine regulation is becoming a scientific hot spot.

Nevertheless, nobody at this point can tell for sure what the exact roles of interleukin-13 are with regards to immune functioning, and the same goes for some of the other interleukins.

However, both interleukin-5 and -13 are therapeutic targets in asthma, although their precise functions within the immune system and during allergies remain to be fully elucidated (Bufford et al., 2008; Wechsler, 2014). Yet it is extremely exciting to follow the rapid progress of research discoveries made with regards to the dog's molecular impact on human health and immunity.

Hence, it is currently not totally clear to researchers how dogs' impact upon the different interleukins and other signaling factors in our body may fully explain how dog exposure reduce asthma, allergy, and chronic inflammation. Moreover, the full consequences of the differential interleukin regulation caused by dog exposure remain to be further scrutinized. Nevertheless, from the previously mentioned research, it's clear that dogs significantly alter the differential concentrations in the body of interleukins and hormones all the while they reduce the rates of allergic diseases, asthma, and other immune-related problems.

Another subclass of cytokines consists of the interferons, of which interferon-gamma is also modulated by dog exposure in early life (Bufford et al., 2008; Roponen et al., 2005; Simpson, 2010). This is supported by other studies showing momentous dog-derived regulation of interferons (Fujimura et al., 2014). This might explain why dog owners in general are less burdened by a vast array of different disorders (Serpell, 1990,1991,1996). Interferon-gamma is critical for our immune defense against both chronic and invasive infections and noninfectious diseases, which include some of dreaded conditions like tuberculosis, hepatitis, aplastic anaemia, cervical cancer, and psoriasis (Smith & Denning, 2014).

But how do dogs convey these molecular changes inside our body? Perhaps the answer to this is much more down to earth than we might have guessed.

Down to Earth, Divine Dirt, and Muddy Paws

Over the past century human behavior has changed as we have become more obsessed with hygiene. Today regular hand washing isn't enough, as we are now using sanitizer gels, antiseptic cleaners and disinfectant sprays as well as numerous antibiotic drugs (Penkowa, 2012). Logically having an infectious disorder and/or an immunodeficiency are legitimate reasons for such approaches, but except for that, could it be that modern society has gone overboard with regards to hygiene?

The Good, the Bad, and the Beneficial

Only a minority of all the known bacteria are harmful and disease-causing to humans. That's why they are termed pathogenic. Most bacteria are not pathogenic and nonhazardous to us, as they don't attack or invade our bodies, and they are rendered harmless by our immune system. Yet other types of bacteria like the gut's resident bacteria are valuable and essential for our health, and so they are actually beneficial.

Until fifty to a hundred years ago, we were primarily country people who grew up exposed to various germs, animals, and good old dirt from the farm or fields, which typically are nonpathogenic and therefore considered as "friendly filth." Back then we encountered vast microbial biodiversity, used less antibiotics, and practiced less hygiene. That's why the human body was richly colonized inside and on the skin surface with diverse populations of microbes serving beneficial roles and preventing invasion of pathogenic bacteria, fungi, vira, or parasites (Rook et al., 2014; Trasande et al., 2013). Back then and long before that, we didn't suffer much from allergies, asthma, or inflammatory bowel diseases since autoimmune and allergic disorders were uncommon, which is contrary to the state of things nowadays. Mounting research studies have suggested that our current obsession with hygiene and urban living without a daily dose of nature's friendly filth contribute to the current rates of immune-related disorders in the developed or Western societies. Hence, modern man's obsession with cleanliness has led to a reduction, displacement, or possibly even an extinction of the indigenous and beneficial microbes that used to be our healthy allies protecting us from immune malfunctioning, allergies, and asthma (Blaser, 2014; Rook et al., 2013,2014; Voreades et al., 2014).

This is not to suggest that good standards of hygiene are unimportant or that we should ignore pathogenic microorganisms causing epidemics, which still remain a major threat to global public health, not least of all in developing countries with limited access to clean water, medical aids, proper nutrition, vaccines, and health care.

In the most developed part of the world, we have stamped out the essential beneficial germs, as we have been obsessed with antiseptic products and increased our use of antibiotics. Today we are facing a situation where the friendly filth we require to educate and mature our immune system has been eradicated (Penkowa, 2012). And there's more. Our increased use of antibiotics has led to microbial adaptation (i.e., multiresistant superbugs that are deadly or impossible to treat), as seen in the case of MRSA (methicillin-resistant /multiresistant staphylococcus aureus), multidrug-resistant tuberculosis, and several other pathogenic bacteria (Rennie, 2012). Likewise, we are facing other global threats because of malaria and/or viral infections with Ebola, influenza, hepatitis B, and HIV.

In conclusion, good hygiene is about avoiding pathogenic microbes and infections while preventing transmission and epidemics. However, good hygiene is not a matter of being dirt-free and sweet-scented or making your home a shrine of hygiene (Penkowa, 2012). Good hygiene is about knowing when and where to act cleverly and only acting in situations or places that count (e.g., when greeting infected patients, when cooking or handling food, after using the toilet, after sneezing or coughing, and after having handled animals or touched any source to potentially harmful and pathogenic microorganisms).

Those of us who share our homes with one or more dogs know perfectly well how incompatible that is with a hygiene obsession or a passion for germ-free households. While most of your furry friend's daily provision of germs is not pathogenic, yet dog owners need to keep a rational hygiene standard, including hand washing after you have interacted with your pet, handled his or her equipment and toys, or prepared the food. When dogs or other animals are around immunocompromised or chronically ill patients, raised hygiene standards are obviously even more needed (Penkowa, 2012).

The reason for this focus on dirt, filth, and germs in our surroundings is to say that science has suggested that a significant causative link exists between dog exposure and an improved immune system, which seems to profit very much from those muddy paws (Almqvist et al., 2003; Bufford & Gern, 2007; Mandhane et al., 2009; Ownby et al., 2002; Salo & Zeldin, 2009; Serpell, 1990,1991,1996; Simpson, 2010).

This aspect relates to the so-called "hygiene hypothesis," which originally was put forth by Dr. David Strachan more than twenty-five years ago (Strachan, 1989). By his hypothesis Dr. David Strachan's suggested that early exposure to microorganisms (probiotics), a certain amount of infections, and friendly filth or dirt in general (be that mud, dust, soil, worms, germs, parasites, fungus, bacteria, virus, animal-derived components, fur, waste or dander and likewise material) can favorably challenge our immune system, leading to reduced risks of allergic diseases. Hence, living in an overly hygienic home will increase susceptibility to allergy because the lack of dirt and microorganisms will inhibit any normal development of the immune system (Strachan, 1989,2000). According to this, researchers propose that thanks to dogs, owners get exposed to muddy paws, dirt, microorganisms, and in particular endotoxins. That's why doggy household members enjoy better, more adaptive, and stronger immune systems relative to those living without animals (Fujimura et al., 2010; Gern et al., 2004; Penkowa, 2012; Simpson, 2010).

In other words, you may thank your furry friend for all his or her muddy paw prints in your living room, not to forget the dog hair, drool, bits, and pieces of chew sticks, bones, treats, chewing toys, dog beds, equipment, and any other dog stuff found in the furniture, on carpets, the kitchen floor, or in your bed since all these little souvenirs and the dust and dirt that follow will stimulate, advance, and boost your immune system— just as it may do with your patience (Penkowa, 2014; Simpson, 2010).

Trillions of Creatures and a Dog

You are probably sitting somewhere quiet as you read these lines, and most likely you think you know who else is present. But you are in fact totally outnumbered by some hitherto blind passengers since your body is home to trillions of tiny creatures, microorganisms that form a flourishing microbial ecosystem inside and on your body. They are particularly abundant in the gut and on the skin (Arrieta et al., 2014; Blaser, 2014). We are all housing ten times more microbial than human cells, as our body contains approximately ten trillion mammal cells, while we harbor around a hundred trillion bacteria (Tsai & Coyle, 2009). Thus, there are a hundred bacterial genes for every single human gene in us, and these microbial genes make up our so-called microbiome, to which thousands of different species of microscopic guests contribute. Our individual microbiome aids in nearly all aspects of human biology and health by interacting with the host, as demonstrated expansively with regards to the gut's bacterial ecosystem (Arrieta et al., 2014; Blaser, 2014; Voreades et al., 2014). In particular, researchers have demonstrated how our intestinal microbes influence human digestion, metabolism, and the risk of obesity (Arrieta et al., 2014; Tsai & Coyle, 2009). Hence, antibiotic treatment early in life is significantly linked with obesity later in life (Trasande et al., 2013). This is due to an all-inclusive killing of bacteria by the antibiotic drugs, which do not only fight pathogenic bacteria but also take out the beneficial microorganisms, and so the gut's colonization is hampered.

But even more significant is the gut microbiome's importance for the immune system and the risk of immune dysfunctions, such as those seen in allergic, inflammatory, and autoimmune diseases (Blaser, 2014; Trasande et al., 2013). To this end, the hygiene hypothesis offers an explanation as to the link between our intestine's microbial community and how well our immune system functions (Strachan, 1989; Voreades et al., 2014). Hence, correct development of immune tolerance is dependent on a healthy microbiome consisting of a proper mix of sufficient bacteria, viruses, and fungi (Arrieta et al., 2014; Blaser, 2014).

The emerging research field of the human microbiome's impact on health and disease points to a paradigm shift since microbes were previously cast as the villains in our battle for better health and longevity, while nowadays these microbial guests emerge as our ancient allies. Perhaps the single-celled microorganisms residing in our bodies might even be considered as microscopic members of the human-animal partnership that went through coevolution since the beginning of our common history as explained in chapter 1.

Nevertheless, as shown recently, the composition or the relative amounts of certain types of microbes are crucial for our susceptibility to immune dysfunction and a range of immune disorders, and so researchers are now targeting the factors that determine and shape an individual's microbial ecology. In brief, our environment and dietary habits are of huge importance, and in both cases a major factor here is our exposure to dogs, who naturally impact how many and which types of different microbes we encounter every day (Arrieta et al., 2014; Azad et al., 2013; Blaser, 2014; Trasande et al., 2013; Tsai & Coyle, 2009). Naturally this raises new concerns regarding the use of antibiotics or exaggerated use of chemicals in cleaning; however, it also reveals why living closely with dogs results in better health and resilience. Hence, dogs provide a rich source of various commensal microbes, immune-activating molecules, allergens, and other foreign particles, whereby owners' immune system is on a daily basis invigorated and kept in good health (Azad et al., 2013; Fujimura et al., 2010; Gern et al., 2004; Simpson, 2010). In fact, research shows that a dog's presence in your home influences significantly the microbial composition of the household dust and dirt (Fujimura et al., 2010). Hence, living with a dog ensures a significant increase in the bacterial richness and diversity of the household when compared to cat ownership or living without furry pets.

The research indicates that dogs increase the home's dust and in particular the dust's microbial diversity, and so our furry friends introduce us to some extra types of bacteria (Fujimura et al., 2010). Interestingly the study also showed that having dogs in the home leads to fewer fungi in the house dust and in particular less pro-allergenic fungal species associated with strong immune hyperresponsiveness, respiratory inflammation, and allergic disease (Fujimura et al., 2010; Penkowa, 2012). These results are supported by a study of pregnant pet owners who show a different bacterial flora relative to expectant mothers without pets (Stokholm et al., 2012).

To sum up this part, dog exposure primarily permits the maturation of a balanced, healthy immune system thanks to the dog's provision of more diverse and rich bacteria species, which has a beneficial impact on us much the same way as a vaccination helps us fight certain ailments (Fujimura et al., 2010; Gern et al., 2004; Simpson, 2010). Moreover, our exposure to dogs in the home might also provide our intestinal system with an advantageous gut microbiome, whereby we may uphold significant protection against a vast array of allergic, inflammatory, and autoimmune diseases (Arrieta et al., 2014; Azad et al., 2013; Blaser, 2014; Tsai & Coyle, 2009; Trasande et al., 2013). These consequences of living with a dog may also explain how your furry friend can convey specific and significant molecular changes to cytokines and immune defense molecules like interleukin-5, -10, and -13 as well as interferon-gamma and shift the balance of IgE versus IgG antibodies as explained previously.

The conclusive point here is that you should enjoy the essential assistance your dog provides, especially when the household is nothing but a collection of doggy dirt, dust, microbes, and dander covered in hair and muddy paw prints. While it may go against our idea of a nice home, it might actually be helpful in terms of your long-term health and resilience.

Laws of Muddy Paws

Next time you wipe down muddy paw prints and perhaps think that your dog isn't necessarily the cleanest family member, you should remember this: All the extra dirt and germs coming from your dog are helping you develop and boost a healthy immune system.

When the Dust Settles

Speaking of dog-related house dust, a brilliantly designed experimental study was conducted recently, and because of its groundbreaking results, it deserves our attention (Fujimura et al., 2014). The study was performed by a group of American medical researchers who took advantage of the fact that keeping dog equaled to a highly distinct milieu of household dust microbial exposure. Hence, from homes with and without dogs, researchers collected the indoor dust in tubes and transferred it to mice. For seven days these mice received a daily dose of either dog-related house dust or control (not dog-related) house dust (Fujimura et al., 2014). Afterward, the mice were sensitized to allergens, while they continued to receive either dog-related dust or the control dust twice per week for another two weeks. Following that, the mice were now challenged with the allergens, by which they were sensitized. At this time point in the study various interesting immune parameters were analyzed in the mice (Fujimura et al., 2014).

The experimental study showed three groundbreaking results. First dog-related house dust germs not only protected against allergen-mediated respiratory diseases (airway allergy) but also reduced airway inflammation in general and could prevent the abnormal transformation (metaplasia) of the airway goblet cells. Moreover, dog-related house dust exposure protected against pathogenic virus, whereby the dreaded airway infection with respiratory syncytial virus was prevented. Secondly exposure to dog-related house dust germs also led to a distinct change in the composition of the gut's microbiome, as resident bacteria restructure and increase specific beneficial germs (e.g., Lactobacillus) known to protect against a vast array of ailments. The fact that dog exposure increases the gut's content of helpful bacteria (like bifidobacteria) has also been publicized by other researchers (Azad et al., 2013). Moreover, the enrichment of the gut's microbiome is associated with genetic changes that related to improvements in carbohydrate metabolism, protein digestion, vitamin processing, hormone biosynthesis, drug metabolism, and disease resistance (Fujimura et al., 2014).

Thirdly, because of dog-related dust exposure, the amounts of distinct leukocytes (T lymphocytes and dendritic cells) are altered, and cell numbers of lymph nodes are reduced. So too, cytokines such as interleukin-4, -5, -13, and -17 plus interferon-gamma were decreased.

What makes this study groundbreaking is not only the impressive collection of results as presented in the research paper and its supporting information paper. The study is also groundbreaking because of its setup since the researchers could pin down how keeping dogs led to strictly biophysical benefits evoked without any contribution from psychological aspects.

Hence, the study only applied the house dust from the dog-owning households, while no live dogs were used as the intervention (Fujimura et al., 2014). Hence, any effects because of personal attitudes or feelings toward dogs (i.e., any psychological influence) can be ruled out, leaving us with the strictly biophysical benefits obtained by living in a household blessed with dogs.

Another strength of the study is the examination of laboratory animals, whereby researchers can get access to almost unlimited numbers of test individuals, and besides, there are no risks of getting biased results because of differences in diet, exercise, culture, races, etc., since laboratory animals are as homogenous as anything can be. That's why the groups exposed to different dust samples are perfectly suitable for comparisons, as we can be sure that any observed difference between the groups can only be explained by means of their different dust exposure. Since laboratory animals are fed, handled, and cared for in the exact same manner, a lot of the biases that otherwise and usually are associated with human test subjects are ruled out. While any experimental, laboratory finding in basic research will always have to ultimately be tested and verified in humans in order to one day get to market, one can never rely only on clinical testing in humans since people always live and behave quite differently and such lifestyle variations may logically affect or skew the obtained results. As such, it is valuable that the previously mentioned findings are drawn on both basic laboratory science with research animals as well as clinical trials with human participants or patients. However, there are most likely still some other and yet unidentified aspects that remain to be explored with regards to the dog's molecular and microbial immune mechanisms and the way they benefit human health.

The Mind-Body Connection

The field of psychoneuroimmunology explores the crosstalking that links our brain with the immune system, whereby they are forming a single functioning system (Bonaz & Bernstein, 2013; Howard, 2014). Thus, psychoneuroimmunology encompass the mind-body connection in health and disease. The brain can release hormones, transmitters, cytokines, and chemicals leading to reduced or enhanced immune defense reactions, while the opposite also happens, as immune cells may secrete and react to the same molecules as those of the brain, whereby the leukocyte-derived cytokines mediate specific changes of the brain and mind (Bonaz & Bernstein, 2013; Howard, 2006,2014). As any change in the brain's biochemistry tends to spill over to our mood, behavior, and immunity, the field of psychoneuroimmunology holds the key to explain a great deal of people's individual hardiness (Bonaz & Bernstein, 2013; Steinman, 2004; Sternberg, 2006). Moreover, it lights the torch in terms of explaining how psychological states affect immunity, healing, and the ability to recover after diseases. Accordingly, dogs may not only improve our immune system because of the mechanisms mentioned previously, as the dog's loyalty, love, and dedication to humans may indeed contribute on its own to the sturdy healthiness of dog owners. Hence, scientists have known for decades that individual levels of mental strength or fighting spirit along with assertiveness and will power profoundly affect the immune cells, such as the amounts of NK cells, and ultimately they affect the outcome of diseases (Howard, 2006). The mind's control over the body is evident from experiments where a placebo treatment leads to pain reduction that is similar to that of 8mg of morphine (Howard, 2014). Another example is seen in patients with AIDS in whom strong will power is associated with better immune system functioning (Howard, 2006,2014).

In that regard, the dog's ability to enhance well-being, self-confidence, and the feeling of being needed will beyond doubt contribute to the countless examples of improved health, resilience, and healing observed in dog owners as compared to those without pets (Fine, 2010; Grimm, 2014; Marcus, 2011; Penkowa, 2014).

Hazards of Pet Keeping and Feeding

Apart from the data on lung-transplanted patients as mentioned previously, scientific studies have also explored extensively the potential risks of zoonoses (i.e., infections passed from dogs to humans in case of different types of immunodeficiency, such as those in case of HIV/AIDS, severe burn injuries, and/or cancer patients treated with chemotherapy or radiation) (Fine, 2010; Hastings et al., 2008; Marcus, 2012b; Orlandi et al., 2007; Snipelisky & Burton, 2014; Steele, 2008).

In general, results indicate that the human health benefits from a dog outweigh the possible hazards, including the risk of zoonotic infections, even in case of elderly, debilitated, pediatric, and/or significantly immunocompromised patients, such as those with cancer (Fine, 2010; Friedmann & Son, 2009; Hastings et al., 2008; Hemsworth & Pizer, 2006; Johnson et al., 2002; Nahm et al., 2012; Orlandi et al., 2007; Penkowa, 2014; Steele, 2008). Thus, the clinical and psychosocial benefits overshadow the inconvenience of following certain important hygiene procedures that are recommended in case of immunodeficient owners or when therapy dogs visit immunocompromised inpatients (Fine, 2010; Irani et al., 2006; Nahm et al., 2012; Orlandi et al., 2007; Snipelisky & Burton,

2014). In return for sticking to a few daily routine practices, possible zoonotic diseases and transmission of potentially pathogenic organisms from the dog are prevented (Ernst, 2012,2013; Fine, 2010; Hemsworth & Pizer, 2006; Marcus, 2011; Penkowa, 2012).

As shown in a report from the Burn Intensive Care Unit and Burn Acute Care Unit at the Children's Medical Center Dallas, a therapy dog may visit more than three hundred patients yearly, and yet it does not cause infections (Hastings et al., 2008). Likewise, a very high safety level is found when therapy dogs are applied in emergency departments, in which 93 percent of patients and 95 percent of the medical staff reported that the dogs should be integrated in emergency units (Nahm et al., 2012).

This is in agreement with data collected from cancer patients visited by therapy dogs during their hospitalization and anticancer treatment (Bouchard et al., 2004; Caprilli & Messeri, 2006; Fine, 2010; Gagnon et al., 2004; Marcus, 2012b; Orlandi et al., 2007). Hence, when dogs and their handlers adhere to the standard guidelines for AAA/AAT in health-care facilities, the intervention carries no risk of infectious transmission from dog to patient (Lefebvre et al., 2008a; Marcus, 2012b). Even after thousands of encounters between therapy dogs and immunocompromised patients or in the case of dog-owning outpatients, there are no reports of zoonotic transfer or infectious diseases pertaining to the dog exposure (Banks & Banks, 2002; Ernst, 2012,2013; Fine, 2010; Hemsworth & Pizer, 2006; Marcus, 2012b; Orlandi et al., 2007; Penkowa, 2014).

Hence, when people adhere to standard procedures, it is most unlikely that AAT causes zoonoses or direct pathogenic transmission even in the most susceptible and immunocompromised patients (i.e., kids with severe burn injuries and patients with AIDS, malignancies, or any other critical disease placing them within emergency departments or intensive care units) (Ernst, 2012; Fine, 2010; Hastings et al., 2008; Johnson et al., 2002; Khan & Farrag, 2000; Lefebvre et al., 2008a; Nahm et al., 2012; Penkowa, 2012; Snipelisky & Burton, 2014; Stanley-Hermanns & Miller, 2002; Steele, 2008).

According to the mounting research, having therapy dogs visit inpatients is a very safe procedure leading to significant health benefits in practically any type of patient regardless of age, sex, disease, attitude toward pets, and various health parameters. Accordingly, when AAT standard procedures are followed, therapy dogs do not pose a risk with regards to the transmission of zoonoses, bites, or scratches (Cole et al., 2007; Ernst, 2013; Fine, 2010; Hemsworth & Pizer, 2006; Johnson et al., 2002; Kamioka et al., 2014; Marcus, 2011; Penkowa, 2014; Schantz, 1990; Snipelisky & Burton, 2014; Steele, 2008).

The immense numbers of research reports mentioned here do all lend credibility to the therapeutic use of dogs in clinical health care, as they converge with regards to the safety of AAT. Hence, the research studies did not detect significant hazards or adverse incidents despite the fact that thousands of different therapy dogs are working every day in many different countries worldwide. As described in several of the references mentioned here, hazards are minimized by means of the education, training, and certification of the dog and the handler.

Moreover, specific guidelines regarding the dog's sanitary and health-care standards along with regular vet examinations have to be followed. In brief, this is a matter of the dog's examination, nutrition, vaccination, cleaning, and screening (Fine, 2010; Khan & Farrag, 2000; Lefebvre et al., 2008a; Penkowa, 2012; Snipelisky & Burton, 2014).

Last but not least, any dog handler considering AAT programs and/or immunocompromised owners need to avoid feeding their dogs raw food and in particular raw meat.

Interestingly those lucky dogs who get to pick their own food, such as choosing between raw or cooked meats, generally and consistently prefer to have their meal cooked (Fogle, 1990; Houpt & Smith, 1981). When you think about it, it should come as no surprise considering man and his best friend's long and common journey of coevolution as depicted in chapter 1.

This is due to the fact that raw chow like BARF (bones and raw food) contains a variety of pathogenic bacteria that pose risks not only to the dog's health but in particular also to the people in the dog's immediate surroundings (Finley et al., 2008; Lefebvre et al., 2008b; Lenz et al., 2009; Lister, 1997; Strohmeyer et al., 2006; Weese et al., 2005).

> **BARF**
>
> "Tips for Keeping People and Pets Healthy and Safe from Germs in Pet Food," a publication by the Centers for Disease Control and Prevention, lays out why BARF should not be fed to your pet or handled by human hands without precautions (http://www.cdc.gov/ healthypets/resources/pet-food-tips_8x11_508.pdf).

The Myth of Hypoallergenic Breeds or Hospitals

If you suffer from an already established, symptomatic, and/or unmanageable allergy against furry animals and if you can't go through the vaccination immunotherapy to obtain desensitization, the acquisition of a dog is not a first-choice option. However, there are many people who have an allergy but still want dogs, and so while they may accept their diagnosis, they certainly defy the verdict and get dogs. For some it may work out if they adjust their antiallergic medication and comply with some precautions (Fine, 2010). But in case they get the dogs on the assumption that hypoallergenic breeds exist, they are in for a surprise since there are no such dogs.

> No scientific evidence exists for classifying certain dog breeds as hypoallergenic.

Nonetheless, pet stores and salesmen will likely still convince buyers that "nonallergic" or "allergy-safe" dog breeds are offered and that these critters allegedly don't shed dander, hair, or potential allergens. However, all dog breeds, also the hairless ones, do cast off dander, hair, and allergens (Ramadour et al., 2005; Vredegoor et al., 2012). In fact, we all encounter them every day whether we like it or not as explained below.

Because of their aerodynamic properties, allergens from animals are ubiquitously present in the human environment. They are airborne and will easily attach to clothing and other materials. That's why they are continuously spread around (Zahradnik & Raulf, 2014). Hence, animal-derived allergens are found everywhere on earth where humans are, including inside homes without any furry animals and in most schools, institutions, work stations, and public places (Kitch et al., 2000). And there's one more sector in which animal-derived allergens and in particular cat-specific allergens are present ubiquitously—hospitals and laboratories.

Surprisingly even within the health-care sector, we are all exposed to allergens from furry animals. That's why the mere thought of a purportedly allergen-free environment is flawed (Zahradnik & Raulf, 2014).

A study set out to evaluate the levels of released allergens from 288 dogs belonging to the following breeds: cocker spaniel, miscellaneous (non-cocker) spaniels, German shepherd, Pyrenean shepherd, poodle, griffon, labrador retriever, and Yorkshire terrier (Ramadour et al., 2005). Interestingly the study showed that the amount of allergens varied much between dog breeds and even within a single breed, as some variation comes from skin conditions of the day and gender. However, poodles and Yorkshire terriers were by far the worst in terms of very high levels of allergen production, while the hunting dogs (cocker spaniel and labrador retriever) produced the least allergens (Ramadour et al., 2005). The typical or average dog behaviors of these breeds may easily affect the results. Hence, hunting dogs are known for being very fond of water. That's why most of them happily jump into any small pond, river, lake, or the sea, whereby they will likely wash out more allergens as compared to the other dog breeds. This aspect is particularly obvious when one is comparing the average allergen levels of the cocker spaniel (very low) with those of the other (non-cocker) spaniels (medium levels). Hence, the English FT cocker spaniel represents the most distinctive gundog possessing unlimited hunting drive and excellence, and that fact may make this particular breed different as compared to other breeds. In the study the allergen levels of the non-cocker spaniels were three times higher than those of the cockers who by nature are keen on jumping into water (Ramadour et al., 2005).

However, frequent shampooing of dogs may have a detrimental effect with regards to allergen levels since such procedures are associated with skin conditions, most notably with seborrheic dermatitis, which significantly increases the dog's allergen levels.

Hence, the best doggy douche is the one that he or she takes care of himself in the outdoors.

CHAPTER 8

Dogs in the Fight against Cancer

Cancer comprises a big group of more than a hundred very different types of diseases. Yet they share some features that classify them as cancer, a term referring to their malignant (aggressive and malicious) nature.

Cancer starts with a series of mutations that ultimately transform a previously normal cell into an abnormal cancer cell. The cancer cells continue to produce new abnormal cell copies that grow out of control instead of eventually dying as they would if they were still normal cells. As the cancer cells grow, they invade other organs, and at some point they will also spread to distant body compartments, where they form metastases (disseminated satellites of cancer). If left untreated, cancers will usually cause serious complications and premature death. Malignant cancer cells have out-of-control growth patterns and spread metastases (Neal & Hoskin, 2009).

Not only in popular media and pet magazines but also in medical scientific journals, attention has been drawn more and more often to the fact that dogs can detect cancer in humans patients (Bjartell, 2011; Boedeker et al., 2012; Campbell et al., 2013; Church & Williams, 2001; Ehmann et al., 2012; Fine, 2010; Le Fanu, 2001; McCulloch et al., 2006; Penkowa, 2012; Sonoda et al., 2011; Williams & Pembroke, 1989; Willis et al. 2004).

Dogs do it primarily be means of a cancer-derived scent, which in itself is a sensation since nobody knew that cancer cells emitted tumor-specific odors or that they were detectable in remote parts of the patient's body than where the malignancy was originally located.

In that regard dogs have within the last decades contributed more than most of my colleagues to our current insight into human cancer and how malignant cells behave. And there's more. Dogs noses are beyond the capacity of any electronic, technological, or otherwise artificial kind of scent-detecting apparatus (Boedeker et al., 2012; Fine, 2010; Horvath et al., 2010,2013). Besides, the canine nose is much cheaper than any other method, even if they were equally suitable, and on top of it the dog works a lot faster (less than five seconds per patient) than any other methods would.

However, a dog's company may also significantly influence clinical outcome (prognosis) and ameliorate the burden of disease, such as the amount of pain suffered, fatigue, anxiety, and/or various complications caused by the cancer (Caprilli & Messeri, 2006; Friedmann & Son, 2009; Knisely et al., 2012; Marcus, 2012a,b,2013b; Penkowa, 2014). Just as important, a dog's company can improve the patient's hardiness by affecting energy levels, mood, optimism, confidence, and the motivation to cooperate with the staff, which all are factors that enhance your survival chances (Bouchard et al., 2004; Coakley & Mahoney, 2009; Fine, 2010; Marcus, 2011; Orlandi et al., 2007; Penkowa, 2012).

Accordingly, several clinical research studies of enrolled cancer patients have demonstrated that therapy dogs or sessions of happy dog interactions lead to improved quality of life, general health, life satisfaction, feelings of well-being, and cheerfulness as shown in both adult patients and children with cancer (Bouchard et al., 2004; Caprilli & Messeri, 2006; Gagnon et al., 2004; Larson et al., 2010; Serpell, 1996). In particular in children with cancer, these aspects are highly relevant since it has a huge impact on kids to be placed in a hospital bed as they are told about their potentially deadly diseases. Hence, 94 percent of parents and 96 percent of the health-care staff report that therapy dogs are beneficial for kids with cancer (Caprilli & Messeri, 2006) Besides, 84 percent of the health-care professionals stated that the dog was also good for the parents who suffer when their children were diagnosed with cancer (Caprilli & Messeri, 2006; Marcus, 2011). In that regard, the dog serves as a unique therapeutic intervention that may significantly facilitate the admission to the hospital, including its multiple stressors like uncertainty and anxiety as well as the burden of receiving chemotherapy.

This effect makes therapy dogs extremely valuable as part of an efficient anticancer strategy since the dog-induced improvements in well-being modulates the nervous, hormonal, and immune systems (Marcus, 2011,2012a,b,2013a; Oyama & Serpell, 2013; Penkowa, 2014). Ultimately resilience and endurance will increase, whereby the patient's overall chances of recovery and survival are increased (Coakley & Mahoney, 2009; Knisely et al., 2012; Marcus, 2011; Penkowa, 2012; Reiche et al., 2004).

Man's best friend doesn't stop here, as dogs may also excel with regards to cancer prevention (Tranah et al., 2008). Exposure to dogs reduces the risk of developing a cancer. (This will be explained in the next section.)

Cancer or Tumor?

Tumor and cancer are often used indiscriminately, which is rather misleading.

A tumor is defined as an abnormal lump of tissue, but a tumor may not always be cancer. When the tumor is not malignant, it is called benign, and in this case the tunmor is not cancer since cancer refers to malignant tumors only. While benign tumors may cause problems, they are seldom life-threatening, as they don't spread in the body (metastasize). Nor do they invade other organs (Neal & Hoskin, 2009). Tumor and neoplasm are synonymous, and when they are malignant, both are classified as cancer.

Dogs Protect against Cancer

It may come as a surprise, but cancer is primarily linked to our lifestyle and less to our genetic composition (Servan-Schreiber, 2011). This is why cancer can be prevented by means of a healthy way of life with eating a healthy diet, getting sufficient exercise and social support, and avoiding stress, smoking, and exposure to toxins (Servan-Schreiber, 2011). To the list of healthy habits should be added your furry friend, as dogs are able to reduce the risk of cancer, and they provide various benefits for those burdened by cancer (Anderson & Taylor, 2012; Becker, 2002; Brauer et al., 2010; Coakley & Mahoney, 2009; Fine, 2010; Friedmann & Son, 2009; Knisely et al., 2012; Marcus, 2011,2012a,b,2013a,b; Muñoz Lasa et al., 2011; Orlandi et al., 2007; Penkowa, 2012; Tranah et al., 2008).

While the immune system has the capacity to counter cancerous changes in our body, the most specialized cells of the immune system (the lymphocytes) may themselves undergo malignant transformation and convert into a lymphoma, a cancer rooted in the lymphocytes. Though there are different types and numerous subtypes of lymphomas, they share the tendency to hamper severely the immune system, as the malignant cells dislodge normal immune system cells, thereby depleting them (Hansen et al., 2000; Neal & Hoskin, 2009; Penkowa & Hansen, 1998). Malignant lymphoma cells are readily disseminated by means of both the lymph and the blood flow. When lymphoma cells enter the blood circulation, the condition is defined as leukemia, while the term lymphoma refers to cancer cells confined in the lymphatic system. Both in case of lymphoma and leukemia, the transformed, abnormal cells represent a lymphoid malignant disease (Hansen et al., 2000; Neal & Hoskin, 2009; Penkowa & Hansen, 1998; Penkowa et al., 2009).

Science shows that human-animal contact influences the possible development of malignancies, such as lymphomas, and results also indicate that your choice of animal does matter a great deal with regards to the risk of getting cancer (Fine, 2010; Penkowa, 2014). For instance, exposure to birds has no effect, but contact with cattle or pigs increases the risk. Furthermore, exposure to dogs reduces the incidence of lymphoma (Tranah et al., 2008). Pets other than dogs may mimic the dog's effect. Science also supports that anyone who owned a dog at some point in life has a significantly decreased risk of developing a malignant lymphoma at any point. Long-term ownership of dogs is inversely associated with cancer risk, or in other words, with longer periods of dog ownership, the risk of lymphoma gets smaller and smaller (Tranah et al., 2008).

The root cause of lymphomas is basically unknown, though an association exists between an abnormal immune system (being either immune deficient or allergic) and the development of cancer. Consequently patients with AIDS display increased rates of lymphomas (Hansen et al.,

2000; Penkowa & Hansen, 1998). The dog's ability to significantly benefit the immune system and prevent allergic disorders may indeed contribute to explaining why dog exposure protects us from cancers like the much-dreaded lymphoid malignancies (Tranah et al., 2008).

In fact, owning a dog not only protects against lymphomas, as dogs also benefit when cancer has occurred in other organs such as breast, lung, gastrointestinal system, head, and neck as well as in other regions (Orlandi et al., 2007).

A series of other research studies has demonstrated how dogs can help in different ways during the course of cancer (Anderson & Taylor, 2012; Becker, 2002; Brauer et al., 2010; Coakley & Mahoney, 2009; Fine, 2010; Friedmann & Son, 2009; Knisely et al., 2012; Marcus, 2011,2012a,b,2013a,b; Muñoz Lasa et al., 2011; Orlandi et al., 2007; Penkowa, 2012; Tranah et al., 2008). For instance, a dog provides comfort and support during the terminal phase of a cancer, during which dog owners rely very much on their pets (Larson et al., 2010). Yet dogs have several other ways of ameliorating different types of cancer, and these are described in the next section.

Anticancer Dog Therapy

Before we look into the way dogs act as a supplementary therapy against cancer, I first have to state very clearly that lifestyle approaches in general cannot cure an already established cancer, as malignant cells can only be killed efficiently by means of conventional, Western-style, science-based medicine, including chemotherapy, radiation, immunotherapy, bone marrow transplantation, and molecular genetics. However, when we receive such science-based anticancer therapy, it would be irrational not to supplement the treatment with complementary approaches that improve the condition and increase our chances of surviving (Becker, 2002; Marcus, 2011; Penkowa, 2012; Serpell, 1996; Servan-Schreiber, 2011).

What is likely the most pleasant and comforting kind of supplementary anticancer therapy is petting a friendly dog. Indeed, science has supported that cancer patients benefit from being visited by a therapy dog as compared to patients not exposed to a dog (Coakley & Mahoney, 2009; Fine, 2010;

Friedmann & Son, 2009; Marcus, 2011; Orlandi et al., 2007). Hence, cancer patients show reduced symptoms of anxiety, pain, depression, tension, stress, and fatigue, while their energy levels and mood are improved by the dog both when they are hospitalized and live as outpatients (Coakley & Mahoney, 2009; Fine, 2010; Friedmann & Son, 2009; Marcus, 2012a,b; Marcus et al., 2014; Orlandi et al., 2007). These benefits are highly relevant for cancer patients, who are often burdened by these additional problems due to getting diagnosed with cancer, uncertainty about the future and life in general.

Medical researchers have examined how dogs can serve as an adjunct to anticancer treatment in order to alter the course of cancer in both children and adult patients (Bouchard et al., 2004; Caprilli & Messeri, 2006; Fine, 2010; Knisely et al., 2012; Marcus, 2011; Marcus et al., 2014; Penkowa, 2014). As shown, dogs offer valuable contributions to the conventional anticancer treatment. Being visited by a therapy dog conveys physical (somatic), emotional, and psychosocial health benefits for patients with malignant diseases (Marcus, 2012a,b,2013b; Marcus et al., 2014; Orlandi et al., 2007; Penkowa, 2014). Hence, while cancer patients often show a worsening of symptoms and/or complications during their admission, those who were visited by therapy dogs avoided such aggravation (Marcus, 2011,2012a,b,2013b; Orlandi et al., 2007). For instance, the dog led to reductions in pain, nausea, vomiting, dyspnoea (impaired breathing and/or airway problem), and asthenia (weakness and lack of energy) in cancer patients treated with chemotherapy (Orlandi et al., 2007). Moreover, dogs also improve some general aspects, encouraging feelings of well-being, sociability, mood, quality of life, and better adaptation to the hospitalization and the fact that one has been diagnosed with cancer (Bouchard et al., 2004; Caprilli & Messeri, 2006; Knisely et al., 2012; Marcus, 2011; Marcus et al., 2014). This is supported by other scientific reports showing how dogs decrease patients' distress, lonesomeness, and melancholy, while a dog may also improve typical cancer-linked problems like insomnia or poor sleep, chronic pain, and loss of appetite (Marcus, 2012a,b,2013a,b).

Some of the most interesting information was obtained by an Italian research team that examined a total of 178 cancer patients receiving conventional anticancer therapy with or without the presence of a therapy dog (Orlandi et al., 2007). Half of the participants (eighty-nine patients) received chemotherapy without the company of a dog, while the other half (eighty-nine patients) enjoyed the company of a therapy dog, specifically a border collie or a Shetland sheepdog. The dog was present while patients were treated for their cancers, which included breast cancer, lung cancer, colorectal cancer, gastric cancer, head and neck cancer, and other types of malignancies.

Data were collected, and they consisted of both patients' history (subjective data) as well as clinical and paraclinical (objective) data. Patients who received chemotherapy with AAT experienced significant health benefits relative to those who did not get AAT (Orlandi et al., 2007). Hence, AAT led to significantly improved oxygen levels in cancer patients. In fact, they showed a 6 percent increase, while oxygen levels in the blood dropped by 4 percent in cancer patients who did not get AAT. AAT also led to significantly reduced depression and less side effects because of chemotherapy.

What's highly interesting about the results obtained by the Italian researchers is the fact that the dog's presence conveyed some health benefits that were different than those seen in other types of patients suffering from cardiovascular diseases. As a consequence the dog conveyed specific benefits to cancer patients but did not mimic those seen in patients with other diseases. In agreement with this, some of the common effects of AAT, such as reduced blood pressure, heart rate, and anxiety as mentioned in previous chapters, were not part of the dog's therapeutic repertoire in the Italian cancer study (Orlandi et al., 2007). This aspect along with the physical change in cancer patients' oxygenation indicates that AAT offers much more than merely emotional support or a one-size-fits-all approach. As suggested by the Italian researchers, the dog is likely to also help cancer patients by diverting their attention away from the disease (Orlandi et al., 2007).

Other researchers have also supported how therapy dogs and/or dog ownership add important health benefits to cancer patients (Becker, 2002; Fine, 2010; Friedmann & Son, 2009; Johnson et al., 2003; Knisely et al., 2012; Marcus, 2012b,2013b; Marcus et al., 2014; Muñoz Lasa et al., 2011). A small-scaled cancer study of thirty inpatients receiving radiation assigned the patients to three different treatment groups. One received twelve sessions of dog therapy, and one saw twelve control sessions as a supplementary treatment along with the radiotherapy (Johnson et al., 2008). The control sessions consisted of twelve visits by a volunteer or twelve sessions of quiet reading. The results showed a tendency for less anxiety and improved emotional health of cancer patients visited by the dog as compared to the control interventions (Johnson et al., 2008). However, there were only ten patients in each of the three groups, as to why the findings awaits further work. Yet patients rated their experience significantly better when they received AAT as compared to those offered sessions without AAT. Hence, 70 percent of patients perceived their anticancer program as being easier after the dog's visit, while this was only the case for 20 to 50 percent of those not receiving AAT (Johnson et al., 2008). In addition, cancer patients looked forward to the dog's visit as compared to the control sessions. So too, 90 percent of cancer patients receiving AAT got attached to the dog, while only 20 percent of patients felt attached to the volunteer (Johnson et al., 2008).

To sum up, dogs providing AAT or pet companionship are highly beneficial for cancer patients, as dogs lessen a broad range of physical and psychological symptoms linked to cancer. Thus, patients with cancer may benefit from adding dogs to their therapeutic regimens, as dogs can significantly boost the outcome of conventional medical anticancer strategies.

The Canine Mechanisms of Anticancer Action

Step by step, medical science has revealed that chronic stress facilitates cancer development because being in a fight-or-flight mode eventually weakens our antitumor immune defense. Hence, we need to avoid stressful lives in order to ward off cancer occurrence and malignant growth (Inbar et al., 2011; Reiche, 2004; Sarkar et al., 2012).

Consequently the ability to block the stress response is a key feature of the dog's anticancer mechanisms. Because of the dog's impact upon the major systems of our bodies as explained in previous chapters, exposure to dogs may enhance resilience and the DNA repair capacity, whereby potential cancer-promoting elements are eliminated. Hence, as dogs boost the human immune defense, they improve our tumor surveillance system that wards off malignancies (Bonaz & Bernstein, 2013; Elenkov et al., 2000; Howard, 2014; Marcus, 2011,2013a; Reiche, 2004; Serpell, 1996; Ziemssen & Kern, 2007).

Other common conditions found in modern man include depression, pain, anxiety, allergies, and the use of various drugs, and each of these may by themselves lead to immune deficiency and thereby an impaired natural defense against tumorigen changes (Cheshire, 2013; Inbar et al., 2011; Li & Kawada, 2011; McGregor & Antoni, 2009; Reiche et al., 2004). Therefore, when dogs ameliorate those disorders or reduce the need for medications, it also builds up our anticancer capacity.

In addition, dogs also work on the level of biochemistry, as they mediate molecular changes in transmitters, signaling agents, hormones, and cytokines as already explained earlier in this book, and these molecules significantly influence the immune defense reactions that may ward off cancer. In particular, the dog's ability to increase certain neurohormones, such as prolactin, endorphin, and dopamine, contributes to the immune system's tumor surveillance, and this also contributes to the fact that dog exposure is linked to reduced cancer occurrence (Freeman et al., 2000; Kovalitskaya & Navolotskaya, 2011; Meredith et al., 2006; Nouhi et al., 2006; Odendaal & Meintjes, 2003; Rojas Vega et al., 2012; Sarkar et al., 2012; Tran et al., 2010). For instance, prolactin inhibits a specific cancer-promoting molecule named proto-oncogene B-cell CLL/lymphoma 6 (abbreviated BCL-6) that acts as a driver of malignant cancer development and growth in humans (Freeman et al., 2000; Nouhi et al., 2006; Rojas Vega et al., 2012; Tran et al., 2010). Likewise, endorphins reduce the incidence of cancer by means of increasing certain anti-inflammatory cytokines while decreasing other inflammatory cytokines, whereby the tumor microenvironment and growth potential are efficiently thwarted (Kovalitskaya & Navolotskaya, 2011; Sarkar et al., 2012). Dopamine also deserves to be mentioned here since it blocks the survival and growth of cancer cells and in particular of transformed lymphocytes (lymphoma cells) (Meredith et al., 2006; Sarkar et al., 2010; Rubí & Maechler, 2010). In fact, even a small increase in dopamine levels specifically kills malignant lymphoma cells, while normal lymphocytes are spared (Meredith et al., 2006). This is an important characteristic of dopamine. On one hand, it explains why dogs are able to prevent lymphoma in their owners, and on the other hand, it indicates that dopamine offers an interesting target in the possible development of new strategic anticancer therapies.

However, dogs not only influence us on the biophysical and molecular levels. They also affect us psychologically by providing attachment figures, emotional support, comfort, empathy, and feelings of being connected and loved, aspects that promote recovery from cancer (Cheshire, 2013; Fine, 2010; Friedmann & Son, 2009; Johnson et al., 2003; Olmert, 2009; Reiche, 2004; Serpell, 1996; Walsh, 2009a,b). In particular, cancer patients may find it difficult to adapt to their often long course of hospitalization and anticancer therapy. Being distracted by friendly dogs should not be underestimated, even if the distraction only lasts for a moment because it allows the patients to momentarily forget about their disease and its consequences. Another benefit is the dog's strong ability to improve his or her owner's self-esteem, self-confidence, mood, audacity, and social behavior, which all work in the right direction with regards to survival chances (Beck & Katcher, 1983; Headey & Grabka, 2007; McConnell et al., 2011; Oyama & Serpell, 2013; Serpell, 1996; Servan-Schreiber, 2011; Wood et al., 2007).

Canine Cancer Diagnostics

The fact that dogs can sniff out cancer in humans became evident because of heroic pet dogs that paved the way for today's state of knowledge with regards to cancer sniffer dogs. In fact, these heroic canines are the reason for today's training of professional sniffer dogs that serve as diagnostic aids sniffing out diseases and in particular cancer (Bjartell, 2011; Boedeker et al., 2012; Campbell et al., 2013; Church & Williams, 2001; Ehmann et al., 2012; Fine, 2010; Le Fanu, 2001; Marcus, 2011,2012a,b; Penkowa, 2014; Sonoda et al., 2011; Welsh, 2004; Williams & Pembroke, 1989; Willis et al. 2004).

The first serious report of a dog alerting people to cancer was the one published in 1989 in the top-notch scientific journal *The Lancet,* as already mentioned in this book. In short, a mix of border collie and Doberman pinscher pet dog saved her owner's life by making her seek medical help at an early point when her malignant cancer could be cured (Williams & Pembroke, 1989).

The Pet Scan

Why would dogs be even the slightest bit interested in sniffing out a cancer in their owners? As in any other case, there has to be something, a reward of some kind in it for them.

Remember, your dog will always be thinking the very same as you and me whenever we interact. *What's in it for me?* So what's in it for dogs? To answer this, we have to go back to the first chapter, which explained how dogs and humans have coexisted and coevolved for more than a hundred thousand years. Humans provided warmth and protection during the nights by means of the campfire, which also was the key to the cooking of foods. Fire allowed canines and us to digest and nourish ourselves from much more calories than we would get on a raw diet. Hence, humans offered what it took to secure survival and become the fittest species in the Ice Age. In turn, canines could smell out and warn us against impeding danger, help us hunt and track down the prey to be cooked, and guard our families and belongings.In other words, man and dog took good care of each other. The point is that canines used their noses and their keen sense of smell for our benefit. Some would say our ancestors never would have made it without the help from dogs and their sense of smell.

So why would today's dogs want to sniff out cancer? Well, the answer might be as simple as this: If we are put in some kind of danger, the dog's own safety is at odds. If we are wounded or ill, it will directly compromise our ability to take care of the dog, as we wouldn't be able to guarantee his energy-rich food or provide a warm shelter.

The dog has adapted to the role of noticing even minor changes that may indicate trouble ahead or danger. So when you have a cut on the skin, practically any dog will smell his way to it and try to lick it clean. This is because he is noticing a change or something that deviates from the usual circumstances, which in itself is sufficient to motivate dogs to investigate the smell further.

Even such a minor cut could potentially mean that we are unable—one way or the other—to take proper care of the dog. And your furry friend would not like that to happen.

In nature, canines are hunters that are used to catching and killing prey, which most often would be the injured or weakest of the flock. Hence, the disabled, sick, or slowest prey gets caught first. Think of all the thousands of years when canines learned to sniff out the sick prey's scent and what happened when they got to eat it. They got hugely rewarded. In other words, sniffing out diseases in humans helps dogs catch their own prey in a manner of speaking, and all the while we get to catch an even bigger reward, reflecting how a sick scent is important to both man and his best friend.

No doubt there are other aspects to this issue, such as dogs being alert to anything they haven't encountered or smelled before, and so something new in their usual environment will usually draw their attention and investigational interest.

Since the first reports of early cancer detection by pet dogs, a number of similar cases have emerged. That shows that such lifesaving behavior from pet dogs is not at all rare. Hence, there are numerous anecdotes of dogs that all of the sudden became obsessed with particular patches on their owners. The owners would seek prompt medical advice only to find out that the patch contained cancer that had to be removed or otherwise treated (Church & Williams, 2001; Le Fanu, 2001; Marcus, 2011). In view of that, researchers have not surprisingly demonstrated that practically any ordinary household dog can be trained in a matter of weeks to successfully detect cancer (McCulloch et al., 2006).

Moreover, dogs are not only able to sniff out skin cancer. They are also equally adept at detecting cancer in internal organs, such as the bladder, stomach, intestine (colorectal), breasts, lungs, ovaries, kidneys, and prostate, which they do simply by smelling samples of either urine or exhaled breath collected from patients (Amundsen et al., 2014; Bjartell, 2011; Boedeker et al., 2012; Campbell et al., 2013; Church & Williams, 2001; Cornu et al., 2011; Ehmann et al., 2012; Marcus, 2011,2012a,b; McCulloch et al., 2006; Morgan, 2012; Penkowa, 2014; Sonoda et al.,

2011; Taverna et al., 2014; Welsh, 2004; Williams & Pembroke, 1989; Willis et al. 2004). Hence, cancer-sniffing dogs identify individuals with cancer without ever meeting the patients. Moreover, the sniffer dogs in training also encounter a range of control samples derived from patients with noncancerous diseases, which the dogs have no troubles weeding out from the cancer-positive samples. This reflects two important aspects. First a given cancer type releases its own characteristic scent signature, and secondly trained dogs can distinguish malignant scents from scents released by infection, inflammation, cell death, ischemia, bleeding, and/or scents caused by tobacco use, drugs, or toxins (Marcus, 2012b; McCulloch et al., 2006; Sonoda et al., 2011; Taverna et al., 2014; Welsh, 2004; Willis et al. 2004).

The Nose Knows

In a study of training cancer-sniffing dogs, the dogs kept alerting researchers to one of the control subjects. This seemed like a faulty behavior since this person did not have cancer, according to various conventional diagnostic tests. However, during the training sessions the dogs consistently identified this sample as a cancer. Despite the fact that this sample was not a cancer sample, the scientists got suspicious because of the dogs' impressive results in all other regards. Hence, they decided to repeat the diagnostic tests all over, and then they found a kidney carcinoma.

As shown in the mentioned clinical research studies, both pet dogs and professionally trained sniffer dogs provide several advantages as compared to the conventional procedures in particular because dogs detect even subtle amounts of cancer scents emitted in our breath or urine at very early times well before the clinical diagnosis would become clear. Therefore, dogs pave the way for early eradication and curative treatment leading to improved prognoses (Church & Williams, 2001; Cornu et al., 2011; Grimm, 2014; Le Fanu, 2001; Marcus, 2011,2012b; Morgan, 2012; Taverna et al., 2014; Welsh, 2004; Williams & Pembroke, 1989; Willis et al. 2004).

> Early cancer diagnosis is very important, and currently dogs do it best. Within the next decade we will likely see breath screenings available for cancer detection or follow-up on treated patients. Ultimately it will be a machine that is used for screening, but first scientists have to study closely the dog's snout, as it is the prototype model they have to imitate in order to build such a putative machine. Well done, Fido!

What's also very fascinating is the fact that the dog's diagnostic sensitivity and specificity, both of which are indicators of precision and validity, are notably higher than any other known test method (Cornu et al., 2011; Grimm, 2014; McCulloch et al., 2006; Sonoda et al., 2011; Taverna et al., 2014; Willis et al. 2004). Accordingly it is an impressive scientific reality that the dog's sense of smell is much more sensitive, fine-tuned, and exact to the target than any known technology, such as electronic noses or likewise scent-detecting machinery (Boedeker et al., 2012; Horvath et al., 2013; McCulloch et al., 2006; Sonoda et al., 2011; Taverna et al., 2014; Willis et al. 2004). Moreover, dogs are able to discriminate between only slightly different cancer types, such as ovarian cancer and other gynecological cancers, which is not only astounding but also very educational since it tells us that even the slightest difference in cancer cell types is reflected by a distinct scent signature, even when these cells belong to one functional unit in the body (Horvath et al., 2010,2013). Being able to tell the differential smells derived from an ovarian cancer and a cancer of the uterus is a feat only dogs have mastered.

The Road Ahead

Today researchers educate professionally trained cancer-sniffing dogs, and as science shows, most dog breeds are able to do well. However, it is not surprising that the hunting breeds have excelled because of their superior scent-detecting abilities along with their high stamina, energy levels, and working abilities. Thus, specific subtypes of certain gundog lines (e g , in particular the English FT cocker spaniel) has been shown by different scientists to be highly successful with regards to sniffing out cancer when compared to various other breeds (Marcus, 2012b; Penkowa, 2012,2014; Sakson, 2009; Willis et al.,

2004). However, other working spaniels, golden, and labrador retrievers are also very suitable, not to mention easy to train for this purpose.

As far as the cocker spaniel is concerned, various sources of information, including dog books, often describe the breed in a one-size-fits-all manner, which leaves the reader with the impression that the label "cocker spaniel" refers to a single breed of dog. This is, however, far from being correct.

The Cocker Spaniel

The name cocker spaniel is used for two different breeds—the English cocker spaniel known as a first-class, inexorable hunter and the American cocker spaniel known as an all-round, multipurpose dog.

Besides this, the two breeds have other protruding differences that make them physically and mentally dissimilar despite their common name.

Both breeds but in particular the English lines diverge into two genetic subtypes—the "field trial" (FT) cocker spaniel that is an extreme and supreme gundog and the "show" cocker spaniel that is bred for conformation and good looks in the show ring (Fogle, 1996).

If you opt for a family dog, you'd prefer the American cocker spaniel, while those looking for a gundog or a sporting dog will choose the English cocker spaniel. Unless you are absolutely certain that you on a daily basis can fulfill some extremely high-energy and intellectual needs, don't get a pure-bred English FT cocker spaniel. On the other hand, if you are up for it, this genetic strain is a never-ending journey of amazing achievements and in particular some serious hunting experiences. You won't face any dull days for a period of twelve to fourteen years.

Understandably the English FT cocker spaniel represents the original breed that earned the name "cocker," which derives from these dogs' matchless ability to sniff out and flush woodcocks (*Scolopax rusticola*), which as any hunter knows is the most challenging shot. No other trophy is held in so high esteem among European hunters as the woodcock. That's why the very best champions among the English FT cocker spaniels are ranked second to none. The very same character that makes them outperform other breeds during a hunt is also what makes them so brilliant at sniffing out cancer just as is the case in many other areas of civil service.

In line with this brief note on the different cocker spaniel breeds, it should be clear that any description of a cocker spaniel without further specification of his genetic strain or subtype may not represent a serious or in-depth source of information.

245

The risk of infection or zoonoses is also relevant when one is discussing the road ahead, particularly with regards to oncology (Lefebvre et al., 2008a; Marcus, 2012b). Thus, patients with cancer are often immunocompromised and carry a higher than usual risk of being infected with potentially deadly microorganisms. In particular this is the case when they receive chemotherapy or radiation, an issue that traditionally has hindered the introduction of AAT in oncology. However, as described in chapter 7, scientific data converge on how to avoid infectious transmission from dog to patient, and so standard guidelines for AAA/AAT in health-care facilities have been issued (Fine, 2010; Lefebvre et al., 2008a; Marcus, 2011,2012b). Accordingly, clinical research shows that dog interventions do not pose a threat to cancer patients, and there are no reports of zoonoses in cancer patients because of AAA/AAT. Dogs and their handlers merely need to adhere to the standard guidelines (Bouchard et al., 2004; Caprilli & Messeri, 2006; Fine, 2010; Gagnon et al., 2004; Marcus, 2012b; Orlandi et al., 2007). By now thousands of dog-patient encounters take place every year in many different countries, and despite this, therapy dogs have not increased the incidents of infections (Banks & Banks, 2002; Caprilli & Messeri, 2006; Friedmann & Son, 2009; Hemsworth & Pizer, 2006; Marcus, 2011,2012b; Orlandi et al., 2007, Penkowa, 2014).

REFERENCE LIST

4 Paws For Ability. [http://4pawsforability.org/mobility-assistance-dog/] (accessed on August 5, 2014).

Abbas AK, Lichtman AHH, Pillai S. Cellular and Molecular Immunology. Philadelphia PA: Elsevier Saunders. 2014.

Abbud G, Janelle C, Vocos M. The use of a trained dog as a gait aid for clients with ataxia: a case report. Physiother Can. 2014;66:33-5.

Abreu-Silva EO, Todeschini AB. Depression and its relation with uncontrolled hypertension and increased cardiovascular risk. Curr Hypertens Rev. 2014;10:8-13.

Adachi I, Kuwahata H, Fujita K. Dogs recall their owner's face upon hearing the owner's voice. Anim Cogn. 2007;10:17-21.

Adams DL. Animal-assisted enhancement of speech therapy: A case study. Anthrozoos. 1997;10:53-6.

Aiba N, Hotta K, Yokoyama M, Wang G, Tabata M, Kamiya K, Shimizu R, Kamekawa D, Hoshi K, Yamaoka-Tojo M, Masuda T. Usefulness of pet ownership as a modulator of cardiac autonomic imbalance in patients with diabetes mellitus, hypertension, and/or hyperlipidemia. Am J Cardiol. 2012;109:1164-70.

Aichbhaumik N, Zoratti EM, Strickler R, Wegienka G, Ownby DR, Havstad S, Johnson CC. Prenatal exposure to household pets influences fetal immunoglobulin E production. Clin Exp Allergy. 2008;38:1787-94.

Alexander CD. Bobbie, a Great Collie. New York: Dodd, Mead and Company. 1926.

Alladin A. The power of belief and expectancy in understanding and management of depression. Am J Clin Hypn. 2013;55:249-71.

Allen K, Blascovich J. The value of service dogs for people with severe ambulatory disabilities. A randomized controlled trial. JAMA. 1996;275:1001-6.

Allen K, Blascovich J, Mendes WB. Cardiovascular reactivity and the presence of pets, friends, and spouses: the truth about cats and dogs. Psychosom Med. 2002;64:727-39.

Allen KM, Blascovich J, Tomaka J, Kelsey RM. Presence of human friends and pet dogs as moderators of autonomic responses to stress in women. J Pers Soc Psychol. 1991;61:582-9.

Allen K, Shykoff BE, Izzo JL Jr. Pet ownership, but not ace inhibitor therapy, blunts home blood pressure responses to mental stress. Hypertension. 2001;38:815-20.

Almqvist C, Egmar AC, Hedlin G, Lundqvist M, Nordvall SL, Pershagen G, Svartengren M, van Hage-Hamsten M, Wickman M. Direct and indirect exposure to pets - risk of sensitization and asthma at 4 years in a birth cohort. Clin Exp Allergy. 2003;33:1190-7.

American Pet Products Association [http://www.americanpetproducts.org/press_industrytrends.asp] (accessed December 8, 2012)

Amundsen T, Sundstrøm S, Buvik T, Gederaas OA, Haaverstad R. Can dogs smell lung cancer? First study using exhaled breath and urine screening in unselected patients with suspected lung cancer. Acta Oncol. 2014;53:307-15.

Anderson W, Reid C, Jennings G. Pet ownership and risk factors for cardiovascular disease. Med J Aust 1992;157:298–301.

Anderson JG, Taylor AG. Use of complementary therapies for cancer symptom management: results of the 2007 National Health Interview Survey. J Altern Complement Med. 2012;18:235-41.

Andics A, Gácsi M, Faragó T, Kis A, Miklósi A. Voice-sensitive regions in the dog and human brain are revealed by comparative fMRI. Curr Biol. 2014;24:574-8.

Andreassen G, Stenvold LC, Rudmin FW. My dog is my best friend: Health benefits of emotional attachment to a pet. Psychology & Society. 2013;5:6-23.

Anyo G, Brunekreef B, de Meer G, Aarts F, Janssen NA, van Vliet P. Early, current and past pet ownership: associations with sensitization, bronchial responsiveness and allergic symptoms in school children. Clin Exp Allergy. 2002;32:361-6.

Aoki J, Iwahashi K, Ishigooka J, Fukamauchi F, Numajiri M, Ohtani N, Ohta M. Evaluation of cerebral activity in the prefrontal cortex in mood [affective] disorders during animal-assisted therapy (AAT) by near-infrared spectroscopy (NIRS): A pilot study. Int J Psychiatry Clin Pract. 2012;16:205-13.

Aoki Y, Watanabe T, Abe O, Kuwabara H, Yahata N, Takano Y, Iwashiro N, Natsubori T, Takao H, Kawakubo Y, Kasai K, Yamasue H. Oxytocin's neurochemical effects in the medial prefrontal cortex underlie recovery of task-specific brain activity in autism: a randomized controlled trial. Mol Psychiatry. 2015;20:447-53.

Arhant-Sudhir K, Arhant-Sudhir R, Sudhir K. Pet ownership and cardiovascular risk reduction: supporting evidence, conflicting data and underlying mechanisms. Clin Exp Pharmacol Physiol. 2011;38:734-8.

Arshad SH, Tariq SM, Matthews S, Hakim E. Sensitization to common allergens and its association with allergic disorders at age 4 years: a whole population birth cohort study. Pediatrics. 2001;108:E33.

Assistance Dogs International, Inc. About service dogs. 2012. [http://www.assistancedogsinternational.

org/service.php] (Accessed 15.04.2012).

Avery RK, Michaels MG; AST Infectious Diseases Community of Practice. Strategies for safe living after solid organ transplantation. Am J Transplant. 2013;13:304-10.

Awano T, Johnson GS, Wade CM, Katz ML, Johnson GC, Taylor JF, Perloski M, Biagi T, Baranowska I, Long S, March PA, Olby NJ, Shelton GD, Khan S, O'Brien DP, Lindblad-Toh K, Coates JR. Genome-wide association analysis reveals a SOD1 mutation in canine degenerative myelopathy that resembles amyotrophic lateral sclerosis. Proc Natl Acad Sci USA. 2009;106:2794-9.

Axelsson E, Ratnakumar A, Arendt ML, Maqbool K, Webster MT, Perloski M, Liberg O, Arnemo JM, Hedhammar A, Lindblad-Toh K. The genomic signature of dog domestication reveals adaptation to a starch-rich diet. Nature. 2013;495:360-4.

Aydin N, Krueger JI, Fischer J, Hahn D, Kastenmüller A, Frey D, Fischer P. Man's best friend: How the presence of a dog reduces mental distress after social exclusion. J Exp Soc Psychol. 2012;48:446-9.

Azad MB, Konya T, Maughan H, Guttman DS, Field CJ, Sears MR, Becker AB, Scott JA, Kozyrskyj AL. Infant gut microbiota and the hygiene hypothesis of allergic disease: impact of household pets and siblings on microbiota composition and diversity. Allergy Asthma Clin Immunol. 2013;9:15-24.

Bamidis PD, Vivas AB, Styliadis C, Frantzidis C, Klados M, Schlee W, Siountas A, Papageorgiou SG. A review of physical and cognitive interventions in aging. Neurosci Biobehav Rev. 2014;44:206-20.

Banks MR, Banks WA. The effects of animal-assisted therapy on loneliness in an elderly population in long-term care facilities. J Gerontol A Biol Sci Med Sci. 2002;57:M428-32.

Banks MR, Banks WA. The effects of group and individual animalassisted therapy on loneliness in residents of long-term care facilities. Anthrozoos 2005;18:396-08.

Bardill N, Hutchinson S. Animal-assisted therapy with hospitalized adolescents. J Child Adolesc Psychiatr Nurs. 1997;10:17-24.

Barak Y, Savorai O, Mavashev S, Beni A. Animal-assisted therapy for elderly schizophrenic patients: a one-year controlled trial. Am J Geriatr Psychiatry. 2001 Fall;9(4):439-42.

Barker SB, Dawson KS. The effects of animal-assisted therapy on anxiety ratings of hospitalized psychiatric patients. Psychiatr Serv. 1998;49:797-801.

Barker SB, Knisely JS, McCain NL, Best AM. Measuring stress and immune response in healthcare professionals following interaction with a therapy dog: a pilot study. Psychol Rep. 2005;96:713-29.

Barker SB, Pandurangi AK, Best AM. Effects of animal-assisted therapy on patients' anxiety, fear, and depression before ECT. J ECT. 2003;19:38-44.

Barker SB, Wolen AR. The benefits of human-companion animal interaction: a review. J Vet Med Educ. 2008;35:487-95.

Barker RT, Knisely JS, Barker SB, Cobb RK, Schubert CM. Preliminary investigation of employee's dog presence on stress and organizational perceptions. Int J Workplace Health Manag. 2012;5:15-30.

Bartz JA, Zaki J, Bolger N, Ochsner KN. Social effects of oxytocin in humans: context and person matter. Trends Cogn Sci. 2011;15:301-9.

Bauman AE, Russell SJ, Furber SE, Dobson AJ. The epidemiology of dog walking: an unmet need for human and canine health. Med J Aust. 2001;175:632-4.

Bawazeer S, Watson DG, Knottenbelt C. Determination of nicotine exposure in dogs subjected to passive smoking using methanol extraction of hair followed by hydrophilic interaction chromatography in combination with Fourier transform mass spectrometry. Talanta. 2012;88:408-11.

Beals EE. Emotional benefits of dog ownership: Impact of the presence of a pet dog on owners' responses to negative mood induction. New School University. 2009.

Beck AM, Katcher AH. Between pets and people: The importance of animal companionship. New York: G. P. Putnam's Sons. 1983.

Beck CE, Gonzales F Jr, Sells CH, Jones C, Reer T, Zhu YY. The effects of animal-assisted therapy on wounded warriors in an Occupational Therapy Life Skills program. US Army Med Dep J. 2012;Apr-Jun:38-45.

Becker M. The Healing Power of Pets. New York: Hyperion. 2002.

Beetz A, Julius H, Turner D, Kotrschal K. Effects of social support by a dog on stress modulation in male children with insecure attachment. Front Psychol. 2012a;3:352.

Beetz A, Uvnäs-Moberg K, Julius H, Kotrschal K. Psychosocial and psychophysiological effects of human-animal interactions: the possible role of oxytocin. Front Psychol. 2012b;3:234.

Bekoff M. The Emotional Lives of Animals: A leading scientist explores animal joy, sorrow, and empathy - and why they matter. California: New World Library. 2007.

Benbernou N, Robin S, Tacher S, Rimbault M, Rakotomanga M, Galibert F. cAMP and IP3 signaling pathways in HEK293 cells transfected with canine olfactory receptor genes. J Hered. 2011;102:S47-61.

Benbernou N, Tacher S, Robin S, Rakotomanga M, Senger F, Galibert F. Functional analysis of a subset of canine olfactory receptor genes. J Hered. 2007;98:500-5.

Bernabei V, De Ronchi D, La Ferla T, Moretti F, Tonelli L, Ferrari B, Forlani M, Atti AR. Animal assisted interventions for elderly patients affected by dementia or psychiatric disorders: a review. J Psychiatr Res. 2013;47:762-73.

Berns GS, Brooks AM, Spivak M. Functional MRI in Awake Unrestrained Dogs. PLoS One. 2012;7:e38027.

Berns GS, Brooks AM, Spivak M. Scent of the Familiar: An fMRI Study of Canine Brain Responses to Familiar and Unfamiliar Human and Dog Odors. Behav Processes. 2014;S0376-6357(14)00047-3.

Bertelsen RJ, Carlsen KC, Carlsen KH, Granum B, Doekes G, Håland G, Mowinckel P, Løvik M. Childhood asthma and early life exposure to indoor allergens, endotoxin and beta(1,3)-glucans. Clin Exp Allergy. 2010;40:307-16.

Bjartell AS. Dogs sniffing urine: a future diagnostic tool or a way to identify new prostate cancer markers? Eur Urol. 2011;59:202-3.

Black K. The relationship between companion animals and loneliness among rural adolescents. J Pediatr Nurs. 2012;27:103-12.

Blanchet M, Gagnon DH, Vincent C, Boucher P, Routhier F, Martin-Lemoyne V. Effects of a mobility assistance dog on the performance of functional mobility tests among ambulatory individuals with physical impairments and functional disabilities. Assist Technol. 2013;25:247-52.

Blaser MJ. The microbiome revolution. J Clin Invest. 2014;124:4162-5.

Bloom T, Friedman H. Classifying dogs' (Canis familiaris) facial expressions from photographs. Behav Processes. 2013;96:1-10.

Boedeker E, Friedel G, Walles T. Sniffer dogs as part of a bimodal bionic research approach to develop a lung cancer screening. Interact Cardiovasc Thorac Surg. 2012;14:511-5.

Bomers MK, van Agtmael MA, Luik H, van Veen MC, Vandenbroucke-Grauls CM, Smulders YM. Using a dog's superior olfactory sensitivity to identify Clostridium difficile in stools and patients: proof of principle study. BMJ. 2012;345:e7396.

Bonaz BL, Bernstein CN. Brain-gut interactions in inflammatory bowel disease. Gastroenterology. 2013;144:36-49.

Bouchard F, Landry M, Belles-Isles M, Gagnon J. A magical dream: a pilot project in animal-assisted therapy in pediatric oncology. Can Oncol Nurs J. 2004;14:14-7.

Brauer JA, El Sehamy A, Metz JM, Mao JJ. Complementary and alternative medicine and supportive care at leading cancer centers: a systematic analysis of websites. J Altern Complement Med. 2010;16:183-6.

Braun C, Stangler T, Narveson J, Pettingell S. Animal-assisted therapy as a pain relief intervention for children. Complement Ther Clin Pract. 2009;15:105-9.

Breggin PR. Psychiatric drug-induced Chronic Brain Impairment (CBI): implications for long-term treatment with psychiatric medication. Int J Risk Saf Med. 2011;23:193-200.

Breggin PR. Psychiatric Drug Withdrawal: A Guide for Prescribers, Therapists, Patients and Their Families. New York: Springer Publishing Company. 2013.

Breggin PR. Psychiatry's reliance on coercion. Ethical Hum Sci Serv. 1999;1:115-8.

Breggin PR. Toxic Psychiatry. Drugs and Electroconvulsive Therapy: The Truth and the Better Alternatives: Why Therapy, Empathy and Love Must Replace the Drugs, ... Biochemical Theories of the New Psychiatry. London, UK: HarperCollins Publisher. 1993.

Brown SW, Goldstein LH. Can Seizure-Alert Dogs predict seizures? Epilepsy Res. 2011;97:236-42.

Brown SW, Strong V. The use of seizure-alert dogs. Seizure. 2001;10:39-41.

Bufford JD, Gern JE. Early exposure to pets: good or bad? Curr Allergy Asthma Rep. 2007;7:375-82.

Bufford JD, Reardon CL, Li Z, Roberg KA, DaSilva D, Eggleston PA, Liu AH, Milton D, Alwis U, Gangnon R, Lemanske RF Jr, Gern JE. Effects of dog ownership in early childhood on immune development and atopic diseases. Clin Exp Allergy. 2008;38:1635-43.

Burrows KE, Adams CL, Millman ST. Factors affecting behavior and welfare of service dogs for children with autism spectrum disorder. J Appl Anim Welf Sci. 2008;11:42-62.

Burton A. Dolphins, dogs, and robot seals for the treatment of neurological disease. Lancet Neurol. 2013;12:851-2.

Burton FD. Fire: the spark that ignited human evolution. Albuquerque NM: University of New Mexico Press. 2009.

Buttner AP, Thompson B, Strasser R, Santo J. Evidence for a synchronization of hormonal states between humans and dogs during competition. Physiol Behav. 2015;147:54-62.

Call J, Bräuer J, Kaminski J, Tomasello M. Domestic dogs (Canis familiaris) are sensitive to the attentional state of humans. J Comp Psychol. 2003;117:257-63.

Camp MM. The use of service dogs as an adaptive strategy: a qualitative study. Am J Occup Ther. 2001;55:509-17.

Campbell LF, Farmery L, George SM, Farrant PB. Canine olfactory detection of malignant melanoma. BMJ Case Rep. 2013;2013. pii: bcr2013008566.

Canine Corner (blog by Dr. Stanley Coren). [http://www.psychologytoday.com/blog/canine-corner] (accessed March 5, 2014).

Canine Partners. [http://www.caninepartners.co.uk/] (accessed on August 5, 2014).

Caprilli S, Messeri A. Animal-assisted activity at A. Meyer Children's Hospital: a pilot study. Evid Based Complement Alternat Med. 2006;3:379-83.

Case L. Perspectives on domestication: the history of our relationship with man's best friend. J Anim Sci. 2008;86:3245-51.

Cattaneo L, Rizzolatti G. The mirror neuron system. Arch Neurol. 2009;66:557-60.

Centers for Disease Control and Prevention [http://www.cdc.gov/] (accessed August 5, 2014).

Centers for Disease Control and Prevention (CDC). Pets and organ transplant patients. [http://www.cdc.gov/healthypets/specific-groups/organ-transplant-patients.html] (accessed October 18, 2014).

Centers for Disease Control and Prevention (CDC). Tips for Keeping People and Pets Healthy and Safe from Germs in Pet Food. [http://www.cdc.gov/healthypets/resources/pet-food-tips_8x11_508.pdf] (accessed October 18, 2014).

Cerutti A, Cols M, Gentile M, Cassis L, Barra CM, He B, Puga I, Chen K. Regulation of mucosal IgA responses: lessons from primary immunodeficiencies. Ann N Y Acad Sci. 2011;1238:132-44.

Charnetski CJ, Riggers S, Brennan FX. Effect of petting a dog on immune system function. Psychol Rep. 2004;95:1087-91.

Chen CM, Morgenstern V, Bischof W, Herbarth O, Borte M, Behrendt H, Krämer U, von Berg A, Berdel D, Bauer CP, Koletzko S, Wichmann HE, Heinrich J. Influences of Lifestyle Related Factors on the Human Immune System and Development of Allergies in Children (LISA) Study Group; German Infant Nutrition Intervention Programme (GINI) Study Group. Dog ownership and contact during childhood and later allergy development. Eur Respir J. 2008;31:963-73.

Chen M, Daly M, Williams N, Williams S, Williams C, Williams G. Non-invasive detection of hypoglycaemia using a novel, fully biocompatible and patient friendly alarm system. BMJ. 2000;321:1565-6.

Cheshire WP. Highlights in clinical autonomic neuroscience: Autonomic correlates of social cognition. Auton Neurosci. 2013;174:5-7.

Chillot R. Louder than words. Psychology Today. 2013;46:52-61.

Church J, Williams H. Another sniffer dog for the clinic? Lancet. 2001;358:930

Christian H, Trapp G, Lauritsen C, Wright K, Giles-Corti B. Understanding the relationship between dog ownership and children's physical activity and sedentary behaviour. Pediatr Obes. 2013;8:392-403.

Chu CI, Liu CY, Sun CT, Lin J. The effect of animal-assisted activity on inpatients with schizophrenia. J Psychosoc Nurs Ment Health Serv. 2009;47:42-8.

Churchill M, Safaoui J, McCabe BW, Baun MM. Using a therapy dog to alleviate the agitation and desocialization of people with Alzheimer's disease. J Psychosoc Nurs Ment Health Serv. 1999;37:16-22.

Cirulli F, Borgi M, Berry A, Francia N, Alleva E. Animal-assisted interventions as innovative tools for mental health. Ann Ist Super Sanita. 2011;47:341-8.

CNBC [http://www.cnbc.com/id/101396437] (accessed on November 14, 2014).

Cohen-Mansfield J, Marx MS, Thein K, Dakheel-Ali M. The impact of stimuli on affect in persons with dementia. J Clin Psychiatry. 2011;72:480-6.

Cole KM, Gawlinski A, Steers N, Kotlerman J. Animal-assisted therapy in patients hospitalized with heart failure. Am J Crit Care. 2007;16:575-85.

Coleman KJ, Rosenberg DE, Conway TL, Sallis JF, Saelens BE, Frank LD, Cain K. Physical activity, weight status, and neighborhood characteristics of dog walkers. Prev Med. 2008;47:309-12.

Cook A, Arter J, Jacobs LF. My owner, right or wrong: the effect of familiarity on the domestic dog's behavior in a food-choice task. Anim Cogn. 2014;17:461-70.

Coppola CL, Grandin T, Enns RM. Human interaction and cortisol: can human contact reduce stress for shelter dogs? Physiol Behav. 2006;87:537-41.

Corbett BA, Mendoza S, Wegelin JA, Carmean V, Levine S. Variable cortisol circadian rhythms in children with autism and anticipatory stress. J Psychiatry Neurosci. 2008;33:227-34.

Coren S. How dogs think: Understanding the canine mind. New York, NY: Free Press. 2004.

Coren S. How To Speak Dog: Mastering the Art of Dog-Human Communication. New York, NY: Free Press. 2000.

Cornu JN, Cancel-Tassin G, Ondet V, Girardet C, Cussenot O. Olfactory detection of prostate cancer by dogs sniffing urine: a step forward in early diagnosis. Eur Urol. 2011;59:197-201.

Counsell CM, Abram J, Gilbert M. Animal assisted therapy and the individual with spinal cord injury.

SCI Nurs. 1997;14:52-5.

Courtney N, Wells DL. The discrimination of cat odours by humans. Perception. 2002;31:511-2.

Craven BA, Paterson EG, Settles GS. The fluid dynamics of canine olfaction: unique nasal airflow patterns as an explanation of macrosmia. J R Soc Interface. 2010;7:933-43.

Crompton AW, Musinsky C. How dogs lap: ingestion and intraoral transport in Canis familiaris. Biol Lett. 2011;7:882-4.

Custance D, Mayer J. Empathic-like responding by domestic dogs (Canis familiaris) to distress in humans: an exploratory study. Anim Cogn. 2012;15:851-9.

Dalziel DJ, Uthman BM, Mcgorray SP, Reep RL. Seizure-alert dogs: a review and preliminary study. Seizure. 2003;12:115-20.

Davis SJM, Valla FR. Evidence for domestication of the dog 12,000 years ago in the Natufian of Israel. Nature. 1978;276:608-10.

DeCourcey M, Russell AC, Keister KJ. Animal-assisted therapy: evaluation and implementation of a complementary therapy to improve the psychological and physiological health of critically ill patients. Dimens Crit Care Nurs. 2010;29:211-4.

de Godoy MR, Kerr KR, Fahey GC Jr. Alternative dietary fiber sources in companion animal nutrition. Nutrients. 2013;5:3099-117.

DeGreeff LE, Weakley-Jones B, Furton KG. Creation of training aids for human remains detection canines utilizing a non-contact, dynamic airflow volatile concentration technique. Forensic Sci Int. 2012;217:32-8.

Derr M. How the Dog Became the Dog: From Wolves to Our Best Friends. London, UK: Duckworth Overlook. 2012.

Desbordes G, Negi LT, Pace TW, Wallace BA, Raison CL, Schwartz EL. Effects of mindful-attention and compassion meditation training on amygdala response to emotional stimuli in an ordinary, non-meditative state. Front Hum Neurosci. 2012;6:292.

Desikan P. Rapid diagnosis of infectious diseases: the role of giant African pouched rats, dogs and honeybees. Indian J Med Microbiol. 2013;31:114-6.

Dietz TJ, Davis D, Pennings J. Evaluating animal-assisted therapy in group treatment for child sexual abuse. J Child Sex Abus. 2012;21:665-83.

Dimitrijević I. Animal-assisted therapy--a new trend in the treatment of children and adults. Psychiatr Danub. 2009;21:236-41.

Di Vito L, Naldi I, Mostacci B, Licchetta L, Bisulli F, Tinuper P. A seizure response dog: video recording of reacting behaviour during repetitive prolonged seizures. Epileptic Disord. 2010;12:142-5.

Dobek CE, Beynon ME, Bosma RL, Stroman PW. Music modulation of pain perception and pain-related activity in the brain, brainstem, and spinal cord: an fMRI study. J Pain. 2014;15:1057-68.

Domes G, Heinrichs M, Gläscher J, Büchel C, Braus DF, Herpertz SC. Oxytocin attenuates amygdala responses to emotional faces regardless of valence. Biol Psychiatry. 2007;62:1187-90.

Domes G, Heinrichs M, Kumbier E, Grossmann A, Hauenstein K, Herpertz SC. Effects of intranasal oxytocin on the neural basis of face processing in autism spectrum disorder. Biol Psychiatry. 2013;74:164-71.

Domes G, Kumbier E, Heinrichs M, Herpertz SC. Oxytocin promotes facial emotion recognition and amygdala reactivity in adults with asperger syndrome. Neuropsychopharmacology. 2014;39:698-706.

Domes G, Lischke A, Berger C, Grossmann A, Hauenstein K, Heinrichs M, Herpertz SC. Effects of intranasal oxytocin on emotional face processing in women. Psychoneuroendocrinology. 2010;35:83-93.

Douglas RH, Jeffery G. The spectral transmission of ocular media suggests ultraviolet sensitivity is widespread among mammals. Proc Biol Sci. 2014;281:20132995.

Dresler M, Sandberg A, Ohla K, Bublitz C, Trenado C, Mroczko-Wąsowicz A, Kühn S, Repantis D. Non-pharmacological cognitive enhancement. Neuropharmacology. 2013;64:529-43.

Driscoll CA, Macdonald DW. Top dogs: wolf domestication and wealth. J Biol. 2010;9:10.

Driscoll CA, Macdonald DW, O'Brien SJ. From wild animals to domestic pets, an evolutionary view of domestication. Proc Natl Acad Sci USA. 2009;106:9971-8.

D'Souza P, Jago C. Spotlight on depression: a Pharma Matters report. Drugs Today (Barc). 2014;50:251-67.

Dunbar RI. The social role of touch in humans and primates: Behavioural function and neurobiological mechanisms. Neurosci Biobehav Rev. 2010;34:260-68.

Duncan SL. APIC State-of-the-art report: the implications of service animals in health care settings. Am J Infect Control. 2000;28:170-80.

D'Urso A, Brickner JH. Mechanisms of epigenetic memory. Trends Genet. 2014;pii:S0168-9525(14)00058-4.

Edney AT. Companion animals and human health: an overview. J R Soc Med. 1995;88:704p-8p.

Edney AT. Dogs and human epilepsy. Vet Rec. 1993;132:337-8.

Edney AT. Dogs as predictors of human epilepsy. Vet Rec. 1991;129:251.

Ehmann R, Boedeker E, Friedrich U, Sagert J, Dippon J, Friedel G, Walles T. Canine scent detection in the diagnosis of lung cancer: revisiting a puzzling phenomenon. Eur Respir J. 2012;39:669-76.

Elenkov IJ, Chrousos GP. Stress system-organization, physiology and immunoregulation. Neuroimmunomodulation. 2006;13:257-67.

Elenkov IJ, Wilder RL, Chrousos GP, Vizi ES. The sympathetic nerve—an integrative interface between two supersystems: the brain and the immune system. Pharmacol Rev. 2000;52:595-638.

Elgier AM, Jakovcevic A, Barrera G, Mustaca AE, Bentosela M. Communication between domestic dogs (Canis familiaris) and humans: dogs are good learners. Behav Processes. 2009a;81:402-8.

Elgier AM, Jakovcevic A, Mustaca AE, Bentosela M. Learning and owner-stranger effects on interspecific communication in domestic dogs (Canis familiaris). Behav Processes. 2009b;81:44-9.

Engelman SR. Palliative care and use of animal-assisted therapy. Omega (Westport). 2013;67:63-7.

Enmarker I, Hellzén O, Ekker K, Berg AG. Health in older cat and dog owners: The Nord-Trondelag Health Study (HUNT)-3 study. Scand J Public Health. 2012;40:718-24.

Epilepsy Foundation [https://www.epilepsy.com/] (accessed on May 16, 2014)

Epstein TG, Bernstein DI, Levin L, Khurana Hershey GK, Ryan PH, Reponen T, Villareal M, Lockey JE, Lemasters GK. Opposing effects of cat and dog ownership and allergic sensitization on eczema in an atopic birth cohort. J Pediatr. 2011;158:265-71.

Ernst LS. Animal-assisted therapy: using animals to promote healing. Nursing. 2012;42:54-8.

Ernst LS. Animal-assisted therapy: paws with a cause. Nurs Manage. 2013;44:16-9.

Evans HE, de Lahunta A. Miller's Anatomy of the Dog. St. Louis, MO: Elsevier Saunders. 2013.

Ezell JM, Cassidy-Bushrow AE, Havstad S, Joseph CL, Wegienka G, Jones K, Ownby DR, Johnson CC. Prenatal dog-keeping practices vary by race: speculations on implications for disparities in childhood health and disease. Ethn Dis. 2014;24:104-9.

Faragó T, Andics A, Devecseri V, Kis A, Gácsi M, Miklósi A. Humans rely on the same rules to assess emotional valence and intensity in conspecific and dog vocalizations. Biol Lett. 2014;10:20130926.

Faragó T, Pongrácz P, Miklósi A, Huber L, Virányi Z, Range F. Dogs' expectation about signalers' body size by virtue of their growls. PLoS One. 2010;5:e15175.

Federico A, Morgillo F, Tuccillo C, Ciardiello F, Loguercio C. Chronic inflammation and oxidative stress in human carcinogenesis. Int J Cancer. 2007;121:2381-6.

Feldman R. Oxytocin and social affiliation in humans. Horm Behav. 2012;61:380-91.

Feng Z, Dibben C, Witham MD, Donnan PT, Vadiveloo T, Sniehotta F, Crombie IK, McMurdo ME. Dog ownership and physical activity in later life: A cross-sectional observational study. Prev Med. 2014;66:101-6.

Fike L, Najera C, Dougherty D. Occupational therapists as dog handlers: the collective experience with animal-assisted therapy in Iraq. US Army Med Dep J. 2012;Apr-Jun:51-4.

Filan SL, Llewellyn-Jones RH. Animal-assisted therapy for dementia: a review of the literature. Int Psychogeriatr. 2006;18:597-611.

Fine AH. Handbook on animal-assisted therapy: Theoretical Foundations and Guidelines for Practice. Academic Press, Elsevier. 2010; 3rd edition.

Finley R, Reid-Smith R, Ribble C, Popa M, Vandermeer M, Aramini J. The occurrence and antimicrobial susceptibility of salmonellae isolated from commercially available canine raw food diets in three Canadian cities. Zoonoses Public Health. 2008;55:462-9.

Fitzgerald CJ, Danner KM. Evolution in the office: how evolutionary psychology can increase employee health, happiness, and productivity. Evol Psychol. 2012;10:770-81.

Fogle B. Cocker Spaniel: English and American. New York: DK Publishing, Inc. 1996.

Fogle B. The Dog's Mind. Pelham Books. 1990.

Freeman ME, Kanyicska B, Lerant A, Nagy G. Prolactin: structure, function, and regulation of secretion. Physiol Rev. 2000;80:1523-31.

Freidin E, Putrino N, D'Orazio M, Bentosela M. Dogs' Eavesdropping from people's reactions in third party interactions. PLoS One. 2013;8:e79198.

Friedmann E, Galik E, Thomas SA, Hall PS, Chung SY, McCune S. Evaluation of a Pet-Assisted Living Intervention for Improving

Functional Status in Assisted Living Residents With Mild to Moderate Cognitive Impairment: A Pilot Study. Am J Alzheimers Dis Other Demen. 2014 Aug 11. pii: 1533317514545477. [Epub ahead of print – accessed May 2, 2015].

Friedmann E, Katcher AH, Lynch JJ, Thomas SA. Animal companions and one year survival of patients after discharge from a coronary care unit. Public Health Rep. 1980; 95: 307-12.

Friedmann E, Son H. The human-companion animal bond: how humans benefit. Vet Clin North Am Small Anim Pract. 2009;39:293-26.

Friedmann E, Thomas SA. Pet ownership, social support, and one-year survival after acute myocardial infarction in the cardiac arrhythmia suppression trial (CAST). Am J Cardiol. 1995;76:1213-7.

Friedmann E, Thomas SA, Son H. Pets, depression and long term survival in community living patients following myocardial infarction. Anthrozoos. 2011;24:273-85.

Fujimura KE, Demoor T, Rauch M, Faruqi AA, Jang S, Johnson CC, Boushey HA, Zoratti E, Ownby D, Lukacs NW, Lynch SV. House dust exposure mediates gut microbiome Lactobacillus enrichment and airway immune defense against allergens and virus infection. Proc Natl Acad Sci U S A. 2014;111:805-10.

Fujimura KE, Johnson CC, Ownby DR, Cox MJ, Brodie EL, Havstad SL, Zoratti EM, Woodcroft KJ, Bobbitt KR, Wegienka G, Boushey HA, Lynch SV. Man's best friend? The effect of pet ownership on house dust microbial communities. J Allergy Clin Immunol. 2010;126:410-2.

Furlan AD, Yazdi F, Tsertsvadze A, Gross A, Van Tulder M, Santaguida L, Cherkin D, Gagnier J, Ammendolia C, Ansari MT, Ostermann T, Dryden T, Doucette S, Skidmore B, Daniel R, Tsouros S, Weeks L, Galipeau J. Complementary and alternative therapies for back pain II. Evid Rep Technol Assess (Full Rep). 2010;194:1-764.

Gácsi M, Maros K, Sernkvist S, Faragó T, Miklósi A. Human analogue safe haven effect of the owner: behavioural and heart rate response to stressful social stimuli in dogs. PLoS One. 2013;8:e58475.

Gácsi M, McGreevy P, Kara E, Miklósi A. Effects of selection for cooperation and attention in dogs. Behav Brain Funct. 2009;5:31.

Gácsi M, Miklósi A, Varga O, Topál J, Csányi V. Are readers of our face readers of our minds? Dogs (Canis familiaris) show situation-dependent recognition of human's attention. Anim Cogn. 2004;7:144-53.

Gagnon J, Bouchard F, Landry M, Belles-Isles M, Fortier M, Fillion L. Implementing a hospital-based animal therapy program for children with cancer: a descriptive study. Can Oncol Nurs J. 2004;1:210-22.

Galibert F, Quignon P, Hitte C, André C. Toward understanding dog evolutionary and domestication history. C R Biol. 2011;334:190-6.

Gallace A, Spence C. The science of interpersonal touch: an overview. Neurosci Biobehav Rev. 2010;34:246-59.

Garcia DO, Wertheim BC, Manson JE, Chlebowski RT, Volpe SL, Howard BV, Stefanick ML, Thomson CA. Relationships between dog ownership and physical activity in postmenopausal women. Prev Med. 2015;70:33-8.

Gaunet F, Deputte BL. Functionally referential and intentional communication in the domestic dog: effects of spatial and social contexts. Anim Cogn. 2011;14:849-60.

Gee NR, Church MT, Altobelli CL. Preschoolers make fewer errors on an object categorization task in the presence of a dog. Anthrozoös. 2010a;23:223-30.

Gee NR, Crist EN, Carr DN. Preschool children require fewer instructional prompts to perform a memory task in the presence of a dog. Anthrozoös. 2010b;23:173-84.

Gee NR, Harris SL, Johnson KL. The role of therapy dogs in speed and accuracy to complete motor skills tasks for preschool children. Anthrozoos. 2007;20:375-86.

Geerdts MS, Van de Walle GA, LoBue V. Daily animal exposure and children's biological concepts. J Exp Child Psychol. 2015;130:132-46.

Geisler AM. Companion animals in palliative care: stories from the bedside. Am J Hosp Palliat Care. 2004;21:285-8.

Germonpré M, Láznicková-Galetová M, Sablin MV. Palaeolithic dog skulls at the Gravettian Predmostí site, the Czech Republic. J Archaeol Sci. 2012;39:184-202.

Germonpré M, Sablin MV, Stevens RE, Hedges REM, Hofreiter M, Stiller M, Despré VR. Fossil dogs and wolves from Palaeolithic sites in Belgium, the Ukraine and Russia: osteometry, ancient DNA and stable isotopes. J Archaeol Sci. 2009;36: 473–90.

Gern JE, Reardon CL, Hoffjan S, Nicolae D, Li Z, Roberg KA, Neaville WA, Carlson-Dakes K, Adler K, Hamilton R, Anderson E, Gilbertson-White S, Tisler C, Dasilva D, Anklam K, Mikus LD, Rosenthal LA, Ober C, Gangnon R, Lemanske RF Jr. Effects of dog ownership and genotype on immune development and atopy in infancy. J Allergy Clin Immunol. 2004;113:307-14.

Gervais H, Belin P, Boddaert N, Leboyer M, Coez A, Sfaello I. Abnormal cortical voice processing in autism. Nat Neurosc. 2004;7:801-2.

Goodavage M. Soldier Dogs: The Untold Story of America's Canine Heroes. New York: Dutton, Penguin Group. 2012.

Goodwin D, Bradshaw JWS, Wickens SM. Paedomorphosis affects agonistic visual signals of domestic dogs. Anim Behav. 1997;53:297-304.

Grandgeorge M, Hausberger M. Human-animal relationships: from daily life to animal-assisted therapies. Ann Ist Super Sanita. 2011;47:397-408.

Grandin T, Johnson C. Animals in translation: Using the mysteries of autism to decode animal behavior. New York: Scribner. 2005.

Green L, Fein D, Modahl C, Feinstein C, Waterhouse L, Morris M. Oxytocin and autistic disorder: alterations in peptide forms. Biol Psychiatry. 2001;50:609-13.

Greenberg D, Aminoff M, Simon R. Clinical Neurology. McGraw Hill Professional, 2012.

Grewen KM, Light KC. Plasma oxytocin is related to lower cardiovascular and sympathetic reactivity to stress. Biol Psychol. 2011;87:340-9.

Greyfriar's Bobby. [http://greyfriarsbobby.co.uk/story.html] (accessed April 19, 2014).

Grimm, D. Citizen Canine: our evolving relationship with cats and dogs. New York: PublicAffairs. 2014.

Gulick EE, Krause-Parello CA. Factors related to type of companion pet owned by older women. J Psychosoc Nurs Ment Health Serv. 2012;50:30-7.

Gutkowska J, Jankowski M. Oxytocin revisited: It is also a cardiovascular hormone. J Am Soc Hypertens. 2008;2:318-25.

Haeusler M, Schiess R, Boeni T. Evidence for juvenile disc herniation in a homo erectus boy skeleton. Spine (Phila Pa 1976). 2013;38:E123-8.

Handlin L. Human-human and human-animal interaction. Some common physiological and psychological effects. Doctoral Thesis. Acta Universitatis agriculturae Sueciae. 2010;98.

Handlin L, Hydbring-Sandberg E, Nilsson A, Ejdebäck M, Jansson A, Uvnäs-Moberg K. Short-term interaction between dogs and their owners: Effects on oxytocin, cortisol, insulin and heart rate - an exploratory study. Anthrozoos. 2011;24:301-15.

Hansen PB, Penkowa M, Kirk O, Skinhoj P, Pedersen C, Lisse I, Kiss K, Zhou X, Hamilton-Dutoit SJ. Human immunodeficiency virus-associated malignant lymphoma in eastern Denmark diagnosed from 1990-1996: clinical features, histopathology, and association with Epstein-Barr virus and human herpesvirus-8. Eur J Haematol. 2000;64:368-75.

Hare B, Brown M, Williamson C, Tomasello M. The domestication of social cognition in dogs. Science. 2002;298:1634-6.

Hare B, Woods V. The genius of dogs: Discovering the unique intelligence of man's best friend. London, UK: Oneworld Publications. 2013.

Hare B, Tomasello M. Human-like social skills in dogs? Trends in Cogn Sciences. 2005;9:439-44.

Hariri AR, Whalen PJ. The amygdala: inside and out. F1000 Biol Rep. 2011;3:2.

Harris CR, Prouvost C. Jealousy in dogs. PLoS One. 2014;9:e94597.

Hart V, Nováková P, Malkemper EP, Begall S, Hanzal V, Ježek M, Kušta T, Němcová V, Adámková J,

Benediktová K, Cerveny J, Burda H. Dogs are sensitive to small variations of the Earth's magnetic field.

Front Zool. 2013;10:80.

Hastings T, Burris A, Hunt J, Purdue G, Arnoldo B. Pet therapy: a healing solution. J Burn Care Res. 2008;29:874-6.

Hawkley LC, Cacioppo JT. Loneliness and pathways to disease. Brain Behav Immun. 2003;17:S98-105.

Hawkley LC, Cacioppo JT. Loneliness matters: a theoretical and empirical review of consequences and mechanisms. Ann Behav Med. 2010;40:218-27.

Headey B. Pet ownership: good for health? Med J Aust. 2003;179:460-1.

Headey B, Grabka M. Pets and human health in Germany and Australia: national longitudinal results. Soc Indic Res. 2007;80:297–311.

Headey B, Grabka M, Kelley J, Reddy P, Tseng YP. Pet ownership is good for your health and saves public expenditure too: Australian and German longitudinal evidence. Aust Social Monitor. 2002;4:93-9.

Helt MS, Eigsti IM, Snyder PJ, Fein DA. Contagious yawning in autistic and typical development. Child Dev. 2010;81:1620-31.

Hemsworth S, Pizer B. Pet ownership in immunocompromised children--a review of the literature and survey of existing guidelines. Eur J Oncol Nurs. 2006;10:117-27.

Henriksen BB, Sørensen KA, Sørensen I. Sværdborg I: Excavations 1943– 44: A Settlement of the Maglemose Culture. Copenhagen: Akademisk Forlag, København. 1976.

Herculano-Houzel S. The remarkable, yet not extraordinary, human brain as a scaled-up primate brain and its associated cost. Proc Natl Acad Sci USA. 2012;109:10661-8.

Herzog H. The Impact of Pets on Human Health and Psychological Well-Being: Fact, Fiction, or Hypothesis? Curr Dir Psychol Sci. 2011;20:236-9.

Hesselmar B, Aberg N, Aberg B, Eriksson B, Björkstén B. Does early exposure to cat or dog protect against later allergy development? Clin Exp Allergy. 1999;29:611-7.

Hidalgo J, Penkowa M, Espejo C, Martínez-Cáceres EM, Carrasco J, Quintana A, Molinero A, Florit S, Giralt M, Ortega-Aznar A. Expression of metallothionein-I, -II, and -III in Alzheimer disease and animal models of neuroinflammation. Exp Biol Med (Maywood). 2006;231:1450-8.

Hilgenberg E, Shen P, Dang VD, Ries S, Sakwa I, Fillatreau S. Interleukin-10-producing B cells and the regulation of immunity. Curr Top Microbiol Immunol. 2014;380:69-92.

Horn L, Virányi Z, Miklósi A, Huber L, Range F. Domestic dogs (Canis familiaris) flexibly adjust their human-directed behavior to the actions of their human partners in a problem situation. Anim Cogn. 2012;15:57-71.

Horowitz A. Domestic Dog Cognition and Behavior: The Scientific Study of Canis familiaris. Springer Verlag. 2014.

Horowitz A. Inside of a Dog: What Dogs See, Smell, and Know: What Dogs Think and Know. Simon & Schuster. 2010.

Horvath G, Andersson H, Paulsson G. Characteristic odour in the blood reveals ovarian carcinoma. BMC Cancer. 2010;10:643.

Houpt KA, Smith SL. Taste preferences and their relation to obesity in dogs and cats. Can Vet J. 1981;22:77-85.

Howard PJ. The Owner's Manual for the Brain (3rd Ed): Everyday Applications from Mind-Brain Research. Bard Press. 2006.

Howard PJ. The Owner's Manual for the Brain (4th Ed): The Ultimate Guide to Peak Mental Performance at All Ages. New York: HarperCollins Publishers. 2014.

Hubert G, Tousignant M, Routhier F, Corriveau H, Champagne N. Effect of service dogs on manual wheelchair users with spinal cord injury: a pilot study. J Rehabil Res Dev. 2013;50:341-50.

Hügler S. Diabetic alert dogs: A good nose for hypoglycemia. Dtsch Med Wochenschr. 2012;137:25.

Iezzoni LI, Rao SR, DesRoches CM, Vogeli C, Campbell EG. Survey shows that at least some physicians are not always open or honest with patients. Health Aff (Millwood). 2012;31:383-91.

Inbar S, Neeman E, Avraham R, Benish M, Rosenne E, Ben-Eliyahu S. Do stress responses promote leukemia progression? An animal study suggesting a role for epinephrine and prostaglandin-E2 through reduced NK activity. PLoS One. 2011;6:e19246.

Irani S, Mahler C, Goetzmann L, Russi EW, Boehler A. Lung transplant recipients holding companion animals: impact on physical health and quality of life. Am J Transplant. 2006;6:404-11.

Irwin MR. Human psychoneuroimmunology: 20 years of discovery. Brain Behav Immun. 2008;22:129-39.

Ishikawa-Takata K, Tabata I. Exercise and physical activity reference for health promotion (EPAR2006). J. Epidemiol. 2007;17:177.

Jakovcevic A, Elgier AM, Mustaca AE, Bentosela M. Breed differences in dogs' (Canis familiaris) gaze to the human face. Behav Processes. 2010;84:602-7.

Jalongo MR, Astorino T, Bomboy N. Canine Visitors: The Influence of Therapy Dogs on Young Children's Learning and Well-Being in Classrooms and Hospitals. Early Child Educ J. 2004;32:9-16.

Jankowski M, Gonzalez-Reyes A, Noiseux N, Gutkowska J. Oxytocin in the Heart Regeneration. Recent Pat Cardiovasc Drug Discov. 2012;7:81-7.

Javelot H, Antoine-Bernard E, Garat J, Javelot T, Weiner L, Mervelay V. Snoezelen and animal-assisted therapy in dementia patients. Soins Gerontol. 2012 Mar-Apr;(94):11-4.

Jenkins JL. Physiological effects of petting a companion animal. Psychol Rep. 1986;58:21-2.

Jeon A. German Shepherd? Belgian Malinois? Navy SEAL Hero Dog Is Top Secret. Global Animal. 2012; May 5. [http://www.globalanimal.org/2011/05/05/german-shepherd-belgian-malinois-bin-laden-hero-dog-is-top-secret/38799/] (accessed April 19, 2014).

Jezierski T, Sobczyńska M, Walczak M, Gorecka-Bruzda A, Ensminger J. Do trained dogs discriminate individual body odors of women better than those of men? J Forensic Sci. 2012;57:647-53.

Jia H, Pustovyy OM, Waggoner P, Beyers RJ, Schumacher J, Wildey C, Barrett J, Morrison E, Salibi N, Denney TS, Vodyanoy VJ, Deshpande G. Functional MRI of the olfactory system in conscious dogs. PLoS One. 2014;9:e86362.

Johansson E, Welinder-Olsson C, Gilljam M. Genotyping of Pseudomonas aeruginosa isolates from lung transplant recipients and aquatic environment-detected in-hospital transmission. APMIS. 2014;122:8591.

Johnson R, Beck AM, McCune S. The Health Benefits of Dog Walking for People and Pets: Evidence and Case Studies (New Directions in the Human-Animal Bond). Indiana: Purdue University Press. 2011.

Johnson RA, Meadows RL. Dog-walking: motivation for adherence to a walking program. Clin Nurs Res. 2010;19:387-402.

Johnson RA, Meadows RL, Haubner JS, Sevedge K. Animal-assisted activity among patients with cancer: effects on mood, fatigue, self-perceived health, and sense of coherence. Oncol Nurs Forum. 2008;35:225-32.

Johnson RA, Meadows RL, Haubner JS, Sevedge K. Human-animal interaction: a complementary/alternative medical (CAM) intervention for cancer patients. Am Behav Sci. 2003;47:55-69.

Johnson RA, Odendaal JS, Meadows RL. Animal-assisted interventions research: issues and answers. West J Nurs Res. 2002;24:422-40.

Joly-Mascheroni RM, Senju A, Shepherd AJ. Dogs catch human yawns. Biol. Lett. 2008;4:446-8.

Jones BM. Applied behavior analysis is ideal for the development of a land mine detection technology using animals. Behav Anal. 2011;34:55-73.

Jones AC, Josephs RA. Interspecies hormonal interactions between man and the domestic dog (Canis familiaris). Horm Behav. 2006;50:393-400.

Kameyama M, Fukuda M, Yamagishi Y, Sato T, Uehara T, Ito M, Suto T, Mikuni M. Frontal lobe function in bipolar disorder: a multichannel near-infrared spectroscopy study. Neuroimage. 2006;29:172-84.

Kaminski J, Schulz L, Tomasello M. How dogs know when communication is intended for them. Dev Sci. 2012;15:222-32.

Kamioka H, Okada S, Tsutani K, Park H, Okuizumi H, Handa S, Oshio T, Park SJ, Kitayuguchi J, Abe T, Honda T, Mutoh Y. Effectiveness of animal-assisted therapy: A systematic review of randomized controlled trials. Complement Ther Med. 2014;22:371-390.

Kanamori M, Suzuki M, Yamamoto K, Kanda M, Matsui Y, Kojima E, Fukawa H, Sugita T, Oshiro H. A day care program and evaluation of animal-assisted therapy (AAT) for the elderly with senile dementia. Am J Alzheimers Dis Other Demen. 2001;16:234-9.

Kandel ER, Schwartz JH, Jessell TM, Siegelbaum SA, Hudspeth AJ. Principles of Neural Science. The McGraw-Hill Companies Inc., McGraw-Hill Medical, Fifth Edition, 2013.

Kasparson AA, Badridze J, Maximov VV. Colour cues proved to be more informative for dogs than brightness. Proc Biol Sci. 2013;280:20131356.

Katcher AH, Beck AM. New perspectives on our lives with companion animals. Philadelphia: University of Pennsylvania Press, 1983.

Katsinas RP. The Use and Implications of a Canine Companion in a Therapeutic Day Program for Nursing Home Residents withDementia. Activ Adapt Aging. 2001;25:13-30.

Kerepesi A, Dóka A, Miklósi A. Dogs and their human companions: The effect of familiarity on dog-human interactions. Behav Processes. 2014;pii:S0376-6357(14)00041-2.

Kerepesi A, Kubinyi E, Jonsson GK, Magnusson MS, Miklósi A. Behavioural comparison of human-animal (dog) and human-robot (AIBO) interactions. Behav Processes. 2006;73:92-9.

Khan MA, Farrag N. Animal-assisted activity and infection control implications in a healthcare setting. J Hosp Infect. 2000;46:4-11.

Kirchhofer KC, Zimmermann F, Kaminski J, Tomasello M. Dogs (Canis familiaris), but not chimpanzees (Pan troglodytes), understand imperative pointing. PLoS One. 2012;7:e30913.

Kirsch I. The Emperor's New Drugs: Exploding the Antidepressant Myth. London, UK: The Random House Group Ltd. 2009.

Kirsch I, Low CB. Suggestion in the treatment of depression. Am J Clin Hypn. 2013;55:221-9.

Kirton A, Winter A, Wirrell E, Snead OC. Seizure response dogs: evaluation of a formal training program. Epilepsy Behav. 2008;13:499-504.

Kirton A, Wirrell E, Zhang J, Hamiwka L. Seizure-alerting and -response behaviors in dogs living with epileptic children. Neurology. 2004;62:2303-5.

Kis A, Bence M, Lakatos G, Pergel E, Turcsán B, Pluijmakers J, Vas J, Elek Z, Brúder I, Földi L, Sasvári-Székely M, Miklósi A, Rónai Z, Kubinyi E. Oxytocin receptor gene polymorphisms are associated with human directed social behavior in dogs (Canis familiaris). PLoS One. 2014;9:e83993.

Kis A, Topál J, Gácsi M, Range F, Huber L, Miklósi A, Virányi Z. Does the A-not-B error in adult pet dogs indicate sensitivity to human communication? Anim Cogn. 2012;15:737-43.

Kitch BT, Chew G, Burge HA, Muilenberg ML, Weiss ST, Platts-Mills TA, O'Connor G, Gold DR. Socioeconomic predictors of high allergen levels in homes in the greater Boston area. Environ Health Perspect. 2000;108:301-7.

Klonoff DC. Dirlotapide, a U.S. Food and Drug Administration-approved first-in-class obesity drug for dogs-will humans be next? J Diabetes Sci Technol. 2007;1:314-6.

Knight S, Edwards V. In the company of wolves: the physical, social, and psychological benefits of dog ownership. J Aging Health. 2008;20:437-55.

Knisely JS, Barker SB, Barker RT. Research on benefits of canine-assisted therapy for adults in nonmilitary settings. US Army Med Dep J. 2012;Apr-Jun:30-7.

Kogan LR, Schoenfeld-Tacher R, Simon AA. Behavioral effects of auditory stimulation on kenneled dogs. J Vet Behav. 2012;7:268-75.

Koizumi H. On innervation of taste-buds in larynx in dog. Tohoku J Exp Med. 1953;58:211-5.

Koivusilta LK, Ojanlatva A. To have or not to have a pet for better health? PLoS One. 2006;1:e109.

Kotrschal K, Ortbauer B. Behavioral effects of the presence of a dog in a classroom. Anthrozoös. 2003;16:147-59.

Krogh J, Nordentoft M, Sterne JA, Lawlor DA. The effect of exercise in clinically depressed adults:

systematic review and meta-analysis of randomized controlled trials. J Clin Psychiatry. 2011;72:529-38.

Krogh J, Videbech P, Thomsen C, Gluud C, Nordentoft M. DEMO-II trial. Aerobic exercise versus stretching exercise in patients with major depression-a randomised clinical trial. PLoS One. 2012;7:e48316.

Kovács Z, Kis R, Rózsa S, Rózsa L. Animal-assisted therapy for middle-aged schizophrenic patients living in a social institution. A pilot study. Clin Rehabil. 2004 Aug;18(5):483-6.

Kovalitskaya YA, Navolotskaya EV. Nonopioid effect of β-endorphin. Biochemistry. 2011;76:379-93.

Kotton CN. Zoonoses in solid-organ and hematopoietic stem cell transplant recipients. Clin Infect Dis. 2007;44:857-66.

Krause-Parello CA. Pet ownership and older women: the relationships among loneliness, pet attachment support, human social support, and depressed mood. Geriatr Nurs. 2012;33:194-203.

Krause-Parello CA. The mediating effect of pet attachment support between loneliness and general health in older females living in the community. J Community Health Nurs. 2008;25:1-14.

Krause-Parello CA, Tychowski J, Gonzalez A, Boyd Z. Human-canine interaction: exploring stress indicator response patterns of salivary cortisol and immunoglobulin A. Res Theory Nurs Pract. 2012;26:25-40

Kubinyi E, Miklósi A, Topál J, Csányi V. Social mimetic behaviour and social anticipation in dogs: Preliminary results. Anim Cogn. 2007;6:57-63.

Kumar M, Kumar J, Saxena I. The role of mental distraction on the pain response in healthy young Indian adults. J Clin Diagn Res. 2012;6:1648-52.

Kundey SM, De los Reyes A, Royer E, Molina S, Monnier B, German R, Coshun A. Reputation-like inference in domestic dogs (Canis familiaris). Anim Cogn. 2011;14:291-302.

Kurdek LA. Pet dogs as attachment figures. J Soc Pers Relat. 2008;25:247-66.

Kurdek LA. Pet dogs as attachment figures for adult owners. J Fam Psychol. 2009;23:439-46.

Kurth F, Narr KL, Woods RP, O'Neill J, Alger JR, Caplan R, McCracken JT, Toga AW, Levitt JG. Diminished gray matter within the hypothalamus in autism disorder: a potential link to hormonal effects? Biol Psychiatry. 2011;70:278-82.

Labinson PT, Giacco S, Gift H, Mansoor GA, White WB. The importance of the clinical observer in the development of a white-coat effect in African-American patients with hypertension. Blood Press Monit. 2008;13:139-42.

LaFrance C, Garcia LJ, Labreche J. The effect of a therapy dog on the communication skills of an adult with aphasia. J Commun Disord. 2007;40:215-24.

Lakatos G, Gácsi M, Topál J, Miklósi A. Comprehension and utilisation of pointing gestures and gazing in dog-human communication in relatively complex situations. Anim Cogn. 2012;15:201-13.

Lakatos G, Janiak M, Malek L, Muszynski R, Konok V, Tchon K, Miklósi A. Sensing sociality in dogs: what may make an interactive robot social? Anim Cogn. 2014;17:387-97.

Land of Pure Gold Foundation [http://landofpuregold.com/service-groups.htm] (accessed on April 26, 2015).

Larsen CS. Animal source foods and human health during evolution. J Nutr. 2003;133:3893S-97S.

Larsen CM, Grattan DR. Prolactin, neurogenesis, and maternal behaviors. Brain Behav Immun. 2012;26:201-9.

Larson G, Karlsson EK, Perri A, Webster MT, Ho SY, Peters J, Stahl PW, Piper PJ, Lingaas F, Fredholm M, Comstock KE, Modiano JF, Schelling C, Agoulnik AI, Leegwater PA, Dobney K, Vigne JD, Vilà C, Andersson L, Lindblad-Toh K. Rethinking dog domestication by integrating genetics, archeology, and biogeography. Proc Natl Acad Sci USA. 2012;109:8878-83.

Larson BR, Looker S, Herrera DM, Creagan ET, Hayman SR, Kaur JS, Jatoi A. Cancer patients and their companion animals: results from a 309-patient survey on pet-related concerns and anxieties during chemotherapy. J Cancer Educ. 2010;25:396-400.

Lawson MJ, Craven BA, Paterson EG, Settles GS. A computational study of odorant transport and deposition in the canine nasal cavity: implications for olfaction. Chem Senses. 2012;37:553-66.

Le Fanu J. How sniffer-dogs border on the supernatural. The Sunday Telegraph Review. 2001; Sept 23:4.

Lederbogen F, Kirsch P, Haddad L, Streit F, Tost H, Schuch P, Wüst S, Pruessner JC, Rietschel M, Deuschle M, Meyer-Lindenberg A. City living and urban upbringing affect neural social stress processing in humans. Nature. 2011;474:498-501.

Leeds J, Wagner S. Through a Dog's Ear. Colorado: Sounds True. 2008.

Lefebvre SL, Golab GC, Christensen E, Castrodale L, Aureden K, Bialachowski A, Gumley N, Robinson J, Peregrine A, Benoit M, Card ML, Van Horne L, Weese JS. Guidelines for animal-assisted interventions in health care facilities. Am J Infect Control. 2008a;36:78-85.

Lefebvre SL, Reid-Smith R, Boerlin P, Weese JS. Evaluation of the risks of shedding Salmonellae and other potential pathogens by therapy dogs fed raw diets in Ontario and Alberta. Zoonoses Public Health. 2008b;55:470-80.

Lentino C, Visek AJ, McDonnell K, Dipietro L. Dog walking is associated with a favorable risk profile independent of a moderate to high volume of physical activity. J Phys Act Health. 2012;9:414-20.

Lenz J, Joffe D, Kauffman M, Zhang Y, LeJeune J. Perceptions, practices, and consequences associated with foodborne pathogens and the feeding of raw meat to dogs. Can Vet J. 2009;50:637-43.

Leonard BC, Marks SL, Outerbridge CA, Affolter VK, Kananurak A, Young A, Moore PF, Bannasch DL, Bevins CL. Activity, expression and genetic variation of canine β-defensin 103: a multifunctional antimicrobial peptide in the skin of domestic dogs. J Innate Immun. 2012;4:248-59.

Leonard JA, Wayne RK, Wheeler J, Valadez R, Guillén S, Vilà C. Ancient DNA evidence for Old World origin of New World dogs. Science. 2002;298:1613-6.

Levine GN, Allen K, Braun LT, Christian HE, Friedmann E, Taubert KA, Thomas SA, Wells DL, Lange RA; on behalf of the American Heart Association Council on Clinical Cardiology and Council on Cardiovascular and Stroke Nursing. Pet ownership and cardiovascular risk: a scientific statement from the American Heart Association. Circulation. 2013;127:2353-63.

Levinson BM. Pet psychotherapy: use of household pets in the treatment of behavior disorder in childhood. Psychol Rep. 1965;17:695-8.

Levinson BM: The dog as co-therapist. Ment Hyg. 1962;46:59-65.

Le Roux MC, Kemp R. Effect of a companion dog on depression and anxiety levels of elderly residents in a long-term care facility. Psychogeriatrics. 2009;9:23-26.

Leuner B, Caponiti JM, Gould E. Oxytocin stimulates adult neurogenesis even under conditions of stress and elevated glucocorticoids. Hippocampus. 2012;22:861-8.

Li Q, Kawada T. Effect of forest environments on human natural killer (NK) activity. Int J Immunopathol Pharmacol. 2011;24:39S-44S.

Li Q, Kobayashi M, Inagaki H, Hirata Y, Li YJ, Hirata K, Shimizu T, Suzuki H, Katsumata M, Wakayama Y, Kawada T, Ohira T, Matsui N, Kagawa T. A day trip to a forest park increases human natural killer activity and the expression of anti-cancer proteins in male subjects. J Biol Regul Homeost Agents. 2010; 24:157-65.

Libet B. Reflections on the interaction of the mind and brain. Prog Neurobiol. 2006;78:322-6.

Linneberg A, Nielsen NH, Madsen F, Frølund L, Dirksen A, Jørgensen T. Pets in the home and the development of pet allergy in adulthood. The Copenhagen Allergy Study. Allergy. 2003;58:21-6.

Lim ML, Li D. Behavioural evidence of UV sensitivity in jumping spiders (Araneae: Salticidae). J Comp Physiol A Neuroethol Sens Neural Behav Physiol. 2006;192:871-8.

Lippi G, Cervellin G. Canine olfactory detection of cancer versus laboratory testing: myth or opportunity? Clin Chem Lab Med. 2012;50:435-9.

Lister SA. Raw meat poses risks to pets and owners. J Am Vet Med Assoc. 1997;211:698.

Little Angels Service Dogs. [http://www.littleangelsservicedogs.org/] (accessed on August 5, 2014).

Lowe LA, Woodcock A, Murray CS, Morris J, Simpson A, Custovic A. Lung function at age 3 years: effect of pet ownership and exposure to indoor allergens. Arch Pediatr Adolesc Med. 2004;158:996-1001.

Lust E, Ryan-Haddad A, Coover K, Snell J. Measuring clinical outcomes of animal-assisted therapy: impact on resident medication usage. Consult Pharm. 2007;22:580-5.

Lødrup Carlsen KC, Roll S, Carlsen KH, Mowinckel P, Wijga AH, Brunekreef B, Torrent M, Roberts G, Arshad SH, Kull I, Krämer U, von Berg A, Eller E, Høst A, Kuehni C, Spycher B, Sunyer J, Chen CM, Reich A, Asarnoj A, Puig C, Herbarth O, Mahachie John JM, Van Steen K, Willich SN, Wahn U, Lau S, Keil T; GALEN WP 1.5 'Birth Cohorts' working group. Does pet ownership in infancy lead to asthma or allergy at school age? Pooled analysis of individual participant data from 11 European birth cohorts. PLoS One. 2012;7:e43214.

Macauley BL. Animal-assisted therapy for persons with aphasia: A pilot study. J Rehabil Res Dev. 2006;43:357-66.

Maher LA, Stock JT, Finney S, Heywood JJN, Miracle PT, Banning EB. A Unique Human-Fox Burial from a Pre-Natufian Cemetery in the Levant (Jordan). PLoS ONE. 2011;6(1):e15815.

Mandhane PJ, Sears MR, Poulton R, Greene JM, Lou WY, Taylor DR, Hancox RJ. Cats and dogs and the risk of atopy in childhood and adulthood. J Allergy Clin Immunol. 2009;124:745-50.e4.

Marcus DA. Complementary Medicine in Cancer Care: Adding a Therapy Dog to the Team. Curr Pain Headache Rep. 2012a;16:289-91.

Marcus DA. Fibromyalgia: diagnosis and treatment options. Gend Med. 2009;6:139-51.

Marcus DA. The Power of Wagging Tails: A Doctor's Guide to Dog Therapy and Healing. New York: Demos Health. Demos Medical Publishing. 2011.

Marcus DA. The science behind animal-assisted therapy. Curr Pain Headache Rep. 2013a;17:322.

Marcus DA. The role of volunteer services at cancer centers. Curr Pain Headache Rep. 2013b;17:376.

Marcus DA. Therapy Dogs in Cancer Care: A Valuable Complementary Treatment. New York: Springer Publishing Company. 2012b.

Marcus DA, Bernstein CD, Constantin JM, Kunkel FA, Breuer P, Hanlon RB. Animal-assisted therapy at an outpatient pain management clinic. Pain Med. 2012;13:45-57.

Marcus DA, Bernstein CD, Constantin JM, Kunkel FA, Breuer P, Hanlon RB. Impact of animal-assisted therapy for outpatients with fibromyalgia. Pain Med. 2013;14:43-51.

Marcus DA, Bhowmick A. Survey of migraine sufferers with dogs to evaluate for canine migraine-alerting behaviors. J Altern Complement Med. 2013;19:501-8.

Marcus DA, Blazek-O'Neill B, Kopar JL. Symptom reduction identified after offering animal-assisted activity at a cancer infusion center. Am J Hosp Palliat Care. 2014;31:420-1.

Marshall-Pescini S, Passalacqua C, Barnard S, Valsecchi P, Prato-Previde E. Agility and search and rescue training differently affects pet dogs' behaviour in socio-cognitive tasks. Behav Processes. 2009;81:416-22.

Marshall-Pescini S, Passalacqua C, Ferrario A, Valsecchi P, Prato-Previde E. Social eavesdropping in the domestic dog. Anim Behav. 2011;81:1177-83.

Martin F, Farnum J. Animal-assisted therapy for children with pervasive developmental disorders. West J Nurs Res. 2002;24:657-70.

Martin KE, Wood L, Christian H, Trapp GS. Not Just "A Walking the Dog": Dog Walking and Pet Play and Their Association With Recommended Physical Activity Among Adolescents. Am J Health Promot. 2014 Aug 27. [Epub ahead of print – accessed May 2, 2015].

Marx MS, Cohen-Mansfield J, Regier NG, Dakheel-Ali M, Srihari A, Thein K. The impact of different dog-related stimuli on engagement of persons with dementia. Am J Alzheimers Dis Other Demen. 2010;25:37-45.

Maximilian AP. Travels in the interior of North America. Early Western Travels. 1906;22:5-393.

McConnell AR, Brown CM, Shoda TM, Stayton LE, Martin CE. Friends with benefits: on the positive consequences of pet ownership. J Pers Soc Psychol. 2011;101:1239-52.

McConnell PB. The Other end of The leash: Why We Do What We Do Around Dogs. New York: Ballantine's Books. 2002.

McConnell PB. For the Love of a Dog: Understanding Emotion in You and Your Best Friend. New York: Ballantine's Books. 2007.

McCulloch M, Jezierski T, Broffman M, Hubbard A, Turner K, Janecki T. Diagnostic accuracy of canine scent detection in early- and late-stage lung and breast cancers. Integr Cancer Ther. 2006;5:30-9.

McGregor BA, Antoni MH. Psychological intervention and health outcomes among women treated for breast cancer: a review of stress pathways and biological mediators. Brain Behav Immun. 2009;23:159-66.

McNicholas J, Gilbey A, Rennie A, Ahmedzai S, Dono JA, Ormerod E. Pet ownership and human health: a brief review of evidence and issues. BMJ. 2005;331:1252-4.

Mendl M, Brooks J, Basse C, Burman O, Paul E, Blackwell E, Casey R. Dogs showing separation-related behaviour exhibit a 'pessimistic' cognitive bias. Curr Biol. 2010;20:R839-40.

Meng H, Cao Y, Qin J, Song X, Zhang Q, Shi Y, Cao L. DNA Methylation, Its Mediators and Genome Integrity. Int J Biol Sci. 2015;11:604-17.

Meredith EJ, Holder MJ, Rosén A, Lee AD, Dyer MJ, Barnes NM, Gordon J. Dopamine targets cycling B cells independent of receptor/transporter for oxidative attack: Implications for non-Hodgkin's lymphoma. Proc Natl Acad Sci USA. 2006;103:13485-90.

Merola I, Prato-Previde E, Lazzaroni M, Marshall-Pescini S. Dogs' comprehension of referential emotional expressions: familiar people and familiar emotions are easier. Anim Cogn. 2014;17:373-85.

Merola I, Prato-Previde E, Marshall-Pescini S. Social referencing in dog-owner dyads? Anim Cogn. 2012a;15:175-85.

Merola I, Prato-Previde E, Marshall-Pescini S. Dogs' social referencing towards owners and strangers. PLoS One. 2012b;7:e47653.

Messent PR, Serpell JA. An historical and biological view of the pet-owner bond, In: Fogle B (Ed.) Interrelations between people and pets. Springfield: Charles C. Thomas. 1981.

Meyer-Lindenberg A, Domes G, Kirsch P, Heinrichs M. Oxytocin and vasopressin in the human brain: social neuropeptides for translational medicine. Nat Rev Neurosci. 2011;12:524-38.

Miklósi A. Dog Behaviour, Evolution, and Cognition. New York: Oxford University Press Inc. 2007.

Miklósi A, Kubinyi E, Topál J, Gácsi M, Virányi Z, Csányi V. A simple reason for a big difference: wolves do not look back at humans, but dogs do. Curr Biol. 2003;13:763-6.

Miklósi A, Topál J. What does it take to become 'best friends'? Evolutionary changes in canine social competence. Trends Cogn Sci. 2013;17:287-94.

Milberger SM, Davis RM, Holm AL. Pet owners' attitudes and behaviours related to smoking and second-hand smoke: a pilot study. Tob Control. 2009;18:156-8.

Miller J. Healing Companions: Ordinary Dogs and Their Extraordinary Power to Transform Lives. The Career Press: New Page Books. 2010.

Miller PE, Murphy CJ. Vision in dogs. J Am Vet Med Assoc. 1995;207:1623-34.

Miller SC, Kennedy C, DeVoe D, Hickey M, Nelson T, Kogan L. An examination of changes in oxytocin levels in men and women before and after interaction with a bonded dog. Anthrozoös. 2009;22:31-42.

Milton K. The critical role played by animal source foods in human (Homo) evolution. J Nutr. 2003;133:3886S-92S.

Mitsui S, Yamamoto M, Nagasawa M, Mogi K, Kikusui T, Ohtani N, Ohta M. Urinary oxytocin as a noninvasive biomarker of positive emotion in dogs. Horm Behav. 2011;60:239-43.

MNT Knowledge Center. [http://www.medicalnewstoday.com/info/parkinsons-disease/] (accessed April 29, 2014).

Molnár C, Pongrácz P, Faragó T, Dóka A, Miklósi A. Dogs discriminate between barks: the effect of context and identity of the caller. Behav Processes. 2009;82:198-201.

Moore KW, de Waal Malefyt R, Coffman RL, O'Garra A. Interleukin-10 and the interleukin-10 receptor. Annu Rev Immunol. 2001;19:683-765.

Morgan RJ. Thinking outside the box about screening for ovarian cancer: the nose knows! J Natl Compr Canc Netw. 2012;10:795-6.

Mormann F, Dubois J, Kornblith S, Milosavljevic M, Cerf M, Ison M, Tsuchiya N, Kraskov A, Quiroga RQ, Adolphs R, Fried I, Koch C. A category-specific response to animals in the right human amygdala. Nat Neurosci. 2011;14:1247-9.

Morris V, Esnayra J. Psychiatric Service Dog Work and Tasks. Psychiatric Service Dog Society. 2011. [http://psychdog.org/tasks.html] (accessed 20.04.2012).

Motooka M, Koike H, Yokoyama T, Kennedy NL. Effect of dog-walking on autonomic nervous activity in senior citizens. Med J Aust. 2006;184:60-3.

Müllersdorf M, Granström F, Sahlqvist L, Tillgren P. Aspects of health, physical/leisure activities, work and socio-demographics associated with pet ownership in Sweden. Scand J Public Health. 2010;38:53-63.

Mungan D, Celik G, Bavbek S, Misirligil Z. Pet allergy: how important for Turkey where there is a low pet ownership rate. Allergy Asthma Proc. 2003;24:137-42.

Muñoz Lasa S, Ferriero G, Brigatti E, Valero R, Franchignoni F. Animal-assisted interventions in internal and rehabilitation medicine: a review of the recent literature. Panminerva Med. 2011;53:129-36.

Muñoz Lasa S, Franchignoni F. The role of animal-assisted therapy in physical and rehabilitation medicine. Eur J Phys Rehabil Med. 2008;44:99-100.

Muñoz Lasa S, Máximo Bocanegra N, Valero Alcaide R, Atín Arratibel MA, Varela Donoso E, Ferriero G. Animal assisted interventions in neurorehabilitation: A review of the most recent literature.
Neurologia. 2013;pii:S0213-4853(13)00018-2.

Nagasawa M, Kawai E, Mogi K, Kikusui T. Dogs show left facial lateralization upon reunion with their owners. Behav Processes. 2013;98:112-6.

Nagasawa M, Kikusui T, Onaka T, Ohta M. Dog's gaze at its owner increases owner's urinary oxytocin during social interaction. Horm Behav. 2009a;55:434-41.

Nagasawa M, Mitsui S, En S, Ohtani N, Ohta M, Sakuma Y, Onaka T, Mogi K, Kikusui T. Social evolution. Oxytocin-gaze positive loop and the coevolution of human-dog bonds. Science. 2015;348:333-6.

Nagasawa M, Mogi K, Kikusui T. Attachment between humans and dogs. Jpn Psychol Res. 2009b;51:209-221.

Nagasawa M, Murai K, Mogi K, Kikusui T. Dogs can discriminate human smiling faces from blank expressions. Anim Cogn. 2011;14:525-33.

Nagengast SL, Baun MM, Megel M, Leibowitz JM. The effects of the presence of a companion animal on physiological arousal and behavioral distress in children during a physical examination. J Pediatr Nurs. 1997; 12:323-30.

Nahm N, Lubin J, Lubin J, Bankwitz BK, Castelaz M, Chen X, Shackson JC, Aggarwal MN, Totten VY. Therapy dogs in the emergency department. West J Emerg Med. 2012;13:363-5.

Nathans-Barel I, Feldman P, Berger B, Modai I, Silver H. Animal-assisted therapy ameliorates anhedonia in schizophrenia patients. A controlled pilot study. Psychother Psychosom. 2005;74(1):31-5.

Neal AJ, Hoskin PJ. Clinical Oncology Fourth Edition: Basic Principles and Practice. London UK: Hodder Arnold, 2009

New J, Cosmides L, Tooby J. Category-specific attention for animals reflects ancestral priorities, not expertise. Proc Natl Acad Sci USA. 2007;104:16598-603.

Nordqvist, J. What is a stroke? What causes a stroke? Medical News Today. 2014;May 15. [http://www.medicalnewstoday.com/articles/7624] (accessed June 1, 2014).

Nouhi Z, Chughtai N, Hartley S, Cocolakis E, Lebrun JJ, Ali S. Defining the role of prolactin as an invasion suppressor hormone in breast cancer cells. Cancer Res. 2006;66:1824-32.

Odendaal JS. Animal-assisted therapy - magic or medicine? J Psychosom Res. 2000;49:275-80.

Odendaal JS, Meintjes RA. Neurophysiological correlates of affiliative behaviour between humans and dogs. Vet J. 2003;165:296-301.

O'Haire ME. Animal-assisted intervention for autism spectrum disorder: a systematic literature review. J Autism Dev Disord. 2013;43:1606-22.

O'Haire M. Companion animals and human health: Benefits, challenges, and the road ahead. J Vet Behav. 2010;5:226-34.

O'Haire M. The benefits of companion animals for human mental and physical health. The annual Royal Society for the Prevention of Cruelty to Animals (RSPCA) Scientific Seminar, Canberra, ACT, Australia. 2009. [http://www.rspca.org.au/assets/files/Science/SciSem2009/seminars09_paper_ohaire.pdf] (accessed 20.04.2012).

Olmert MD. Made for Each Other: The Biology of the Human-Animal Bond. Merloyd Lawrence Books. 2009.

Onaka T, Takayanagi Y, Yoshida M. Roles of oxytocin neurones in the control of stress, energy metabolism, and social behaviour. J Neuroendocrinol. 2012;24:587-98.

Orlandi M, Trangeled K, Mambrini A, Tagliani M, Ferrarini A, Zanetti L, Tartarini R, Pacetti P, Cantore M. Pet therapy effects on oncological day hospital patients undergoing chemotherapy treatment. Anticancer Res. 2007;27:4301-3.

Osei-Bonsu PE, Bokhour BG, Glickman ME, Rodrigues S, Mueller NM, Dell NS, Zhao S, Eisen SV, Elwy AR. The role of coping in depression treatment utilization for VA primary care patients. Patient Educ Couns. 2014;94:396-402.

Ostrander EA, Beale HC. Leading the way: finding genes for neurologic disease in dogs using genome-wide mRNA sequencing. BMC Genet. 2012;13:56.

Ostrander EA, Wayne RK. The canine genome. Genome Res. 2005;15:1706-16.

Overall KL. That dog is smarter than you know: advances in understanding canine learning, memory, and cognition. Top Companion Anim Med. 2011;26:2-9.

Ovodov ND, Crockford SJ, Kuzmin YV, Higham TF, Hodgins GW, van der Plicht J. A 33,000-year-old incipient dog from the Altai Mountains of Siberia: evidence of the earliest domestication disrupted by the Last Glacial Maximum. PLoS One. 2011;6:e22821.

Ownby DR, Johnson CC, Peterson EL. Exposure to dogs and cats in the first year of life and risk of allergic sensitization at 6 to 7 years of age. JAMA. 2002;288:963-72.

Oyama MA, Serpell JA. General Commentary: Rethinking the role of animals in human well-being. Front Psychol. 2013;4:374.

Palley LS, O'Rourke PP, Niemi SM. Mainstreaming animal-assisted therapy. ILAR J. 2010;51:199-207.

Pante MC, Blumenschine RJ, Capaldo SD, Scott RS. Validation of bone surface modification models for inferring fossil hominin and carnivore feeding interactions, with reapplication to FLK 22, Olduvai Gorge, Tanzania. J Hum Evol. 2012;63:395-407.

Parish-Plass N. Animal-assisted therapy with children suffering from insecure attachment due to abuse and neglect: a method to lower the risk of intergenerational transmission of abuse? Clin Child Psychol Psychiatry. 2008;13:7-30.

Parker HG, Shearin AL, Ostrander EA. Man's best friend becomes biology's best in show: genome analyses in the domestic dog. Annu Rev Genet. 2010;44:309-36.

Parkinson's Association. [http://www.parkinsonsassociation.org/] (accessed May 1, 2014).

Parkinson's Association's Paws for Parkinson's. [http://www.parkinsonsassociation.org/resources/paws-for-parkinsons] (accessed May 4, 2014).

Parkinson's Disease Foundation. [http://www.pdf.org/en/index] (accessed April 29, 2014).

Parslow RA, Jorm AF. Pet ownership and risk factors for cardiovascular disease: another look. Med J Aust. 2003;179:466-68.

Paws for Parkinson's [http://www.sandiegopetsmagazine.com/view/full_story/17680504/article-Paws-for-Parkinson%E2%80%99s?instance=petpress] (accessed May 1, 2014).

Paws with a cause. [https://www.pawswithacause.org/what-we-do/service-dogs/] (accessed May 5, 2014).

Payne E, Bennett PC, McGreevy PD. Current perspectives on attachment and bonding in the dog-human dyad. Psychol Res Behav Manag. 2015;8:71-9.

Penkowa M. Metallothioneins are multipurpose neuroprotectants during brain pathology. FEBS J. 2006;273:1857-70.

Penkowa M. Inflammation and neuroregeneration. Ugeskr Laeger. 2010;172:1293-6.

Penkowa M. Hund på Recept. Copenhagen, Denmark: Dansk Psykologisk Forlag. 2012.

Penkowa M. Hund auf Rezept: Aktuelles aus Medizin und Forschung. Nerdlen, Germany: Kynos Verlag. 2014.

Penkowa M, Carrasco J, Giralt M, Moos T, Hidalgo J. CNS wound healing is severely depressed in metallothionein I- and II-deficient mice. J Neurosci. 1999 19:2535-45.

Penkowa M, Florit S, Giralt M, Quintana A, Molinero A, Carrasco J, Hidalgo J. Metallothionein reduces central nervous system inflammation, neurodegeneration, and cell death following kainic acid-induced epileptic seizures. J Neurosci Res. 2005;79:522-34.

Penkowa M, Hansen PB. AIDS-related non-Hodgkin lymphomas. Clinical picture and prognosis. Ugeskr Laeger. 1998;160:2685-88.

Penkowa M, Sørensen BL, Nielsen SL, Hansen PB. Metallothionein as a useful marker in Hodgkin lymphoma subclassification. Leuk Lymphoma. 2009

Feb;50(2):200-10. doi: 10.1080/10428190802699340. PubMed PMID: 19199157.

Pérez i de Lanuza G, Font E. Ultraviolet vision in lacertid lizards: evidence from retinal structure, eye transmittance, SWS1 visual pigment genes, and behaviour. J Exp Biol. 2014;217:2899-909.

Perkins J, Bartlett H, Travers C, Rand J. Dog-assisted therapy for older people with dementia: a review. Australas J Ageing. 2008;27:177-82.

Petersson M. Cardiovascular effects of oxytocin. Prog Brain Res. 2002;139:281-8.

Pinc L, Bartoš L, Reslová A, Kotrba R. Dogs discriminate identical twins. PloS One. 2011;6:e20704.

Pinto JM. Olfaction. Proc Am Thorac Soc. 2011;8:46-52.

Plummer T. Flaked stones and old bones: biological and cultural evolution at the dawn of technology. Am J Phys Anthropol. 2004;Suppl 39:118-64.

Podberscek AL, Serpell JA. Aggressive behaviour in English cocker spaniels and the personality of their owners. Vet Rec. 1997;141:73-6.

Prato-Previde E, Marshall-Pescini S, Valsecchi P. Is your choice my choice? The owners' effect on pet dogs' (Canis lupus familiaris) performance in a food choice task. Anim Cogn. 2008;11:167-74.

Prothmann A, Ettrich C, Prothmann S. Preference for, and responsiveness to, people, dogs and objects in children with autism. Anthrozoös. 2009;22:161-171.

Püllen R, Coy M, Hunger B, Koetter G, Spate M, Richter A. Animal-assisted therapy for demented

Patients in acute care hospitals. Z Gerontol Geriatr. 2013;46:233-6.

Quaranta A, Siniscalchi M, Vallortigara G. Asymmetric tail-wagging responses by dogs to different emotive stimuli. Curr Biol. 2007;17:R199-201.

Quignon P, Rimbault M, Robin S, Galibert F. Genetics of canine olfaction and receptor diversity. Mamm Genome. 2012;23:132-43.

Racca A, Guo K, Meints K, Mills DS. Reading faces: differential lateral gaze bias in processing canine and human facial expressions in dogs and 4-year-old children. PLoS One. 2012;7:e36076.

Raina P, Waltner-Toews D, Bonnett B, Woodward C, Abernathy T. Influence of companion animals on the physical and psychological health of older people: an analysis of a one-year longitudinal study. J Am Geriatr Soc. 1999;47:323-9.

Ramadour M, Guetat M, Guetat J, El Biaze M, Magnan A, Vervloet D. Dog factor differences in Can f 1 allergen production. Allergy. 2005;60:1060-4.

Range F, Horn L, Viranyi Z, Huber L. The absence of reward induces inequity aversion in dogs. Proc Natl Acad Sci U S A. 2009;106:340-5.

Ratcliffe VF, McComb K, Reby D. Cross-modal discrimination of human gender by domestic dogs. Anim Behav. 2014;91:126-34.

Räty LK, Wilde-Larsson BM. Patients' perceptions of living with epilepsy: a phenomenographic study. J Clin Nurs. 2011;20:1993-02.

Redefer LA, Goodman JF. Pet-facilitated therapy with autistic children. J Autism Dev Disord. 1989;19:461-7.

Reeves MJ, Rafferty AP, Miller CE, Lyon-Callo SK. The impact of dog walking on leisure-time physical activity: results from a population-based survey of Michigan adults. J Phys Act Health. 2011;8:436-44.

Rehn T, Handlin L, Uvnäs-Moberg K, Keeling LJ. Dogs' endocrine and behavioural responses at reunion are affected by how the human initiates contact. Physiol Behav. 2014;24:45–533.

Reiche EM, Nunes SO, Morimoto HK. Stress, depression, the immune system, and cancer. Lancet Oncol. 2004;5:617-25.

Reid PJ. Adapting to the human world: dogs' responsiveness to our social cues. Behav Processes. 2009;80:325-33.

Rennie RP. Current and future challenges in the development of antimicrobial agents. Handb Exp Pharmacol. 2012;211:45-65.

Richeson NE. Effects of animal-assisted therapy on agitated behaviors and social interactions of older adults with dementia. Am J Alzheimers Dis Other Demen. 2003;18:353-8.

Rintala DH, Matamoros R, Seitz LL. Effects of assistance dogs on persons with mobility or hearing impairments: a pilot study. J Rehabil Res Dev. 2008;45:489-503.

Rizzolatti G, Fabbri-Destro M, Cattaneo L. Mirror neurons and their clinical relevance. Nat Clin Pract Neurol. 2009;5:24-34.

Robin S, Tacher S, Rimbault M, Vaysse A, Dréano S, André C, Hitte C, Galibert F. Genetic diversity of canine olfactory receptors. BMC Genomics. 2009;10:21.

Rock C, Li Z, Roberg KA, Carlson-Dakes K, Tisler C, DaSilva D, Lemanske RF Jr., Gern JE. Effects of pet ownership on patterns of cytokine secretion and allergen sensitization in infancy. J Allergy Clin Immunol. 2003;111:S274.

Rojas Vega S, Hollmann W, Strüder HK. Influences of exercise and training on the circulating concentration of prolactin in humans. J Neuroendocrinol. 2012;24:395-402.

Romero T, Nagasawa M, Mogi K, Hasegawa T, Kikusui T. Oxytocin promotes social bonding in dogs. Proc Natl Acad Sci USA. 2014;111:9085-90.

Rondeau L, Corriveau H, Bier N, Camden C, Champagne N, Dion C. Effectiveness of a rehabilitation dog in fostering gait retraining for adults with a recent stroke: a multiple single-case study. NeuroRehabilitation. 2010;27:155-63.

Rook GA, Lowry CA, Raison CL. Microbial 'Old Friends', immunoregulation and stress resilience. Evol Med Public Health. 2013;1:46-64.

Rook GA, Raison CL, Lowry CA. Microbiota, immunoregulatory old friends and psychiatric disorders. Adv Exp Med Biol. 2014;817:319-56.

Rooney NJ, Morant S, Guest C. Investigation into the value of trained glycaemia alert dogs to clients with type I diabetes. PLoS One. 2013;8:e69921.

Roponen M, Hyvärinen A, Hirvonen MR, Keski-Nisula L, Pekkanen J. Change in IFN-gamma-producing capacity in early life and exposure to environmental microbes. J Allergy Clin Immunol. 2005;116:1048-52.

Rossetti J, King C. Use of animal-assisted therapy with psychiatric patients. J Psychosoc Nurs Ment Health Serv. 2010;48:44-8.

Rossi AP, Ades C. A dog at the keyboard: using arbitrary signs to communicate requests. Anim Cogn. 2008;11:329-38.

Roza MR, Viegas CA. The dog as a passive smoker: effects of exposure to environmental cigarette smoke on domestic dogs. Nicotine Tob Res. 2007;9:1171-6.

Rubí B, Maechler P. Minireview: new roles for peripheral dopamine on metabolic control and tumor growth: let's seek the balance. Endocrinology. 2010;151:5570-81.

Rugaas T. On Talking Terms With Dogs: Calming Signals. Washington: Dogwise Publishing. 2006.

Sablin MV, Khlopachev GA. The earliest ice age dogs: evidence from Eliseevichi 1. Curr. Anthropol. 2002;43:795-99.

Saetre P, Lindberg J, Leonard JA, Olsson K, Pettersson U, Ellegren H, Bergström TF, Vilà C, Jazin E. From wild wolf to domestic dog: gene expression changes in the brain. Brain Res Mol Brain Res. 2004;126:198-206.

Sahar NU. Assessment of psychological distress in epilepsy: perspective from pakistan. Epilepsy Res Treat. 2012;2012:171725.

Sakson S. Paws & Effect: The Healing Power of Dogs. New York: Spiegel & Grau. 2009.

Salazar I, Cifuentes JM, Sánchez-Quinteiro P. Morphological and immunohistochemical features of the vomeronasal system in dogs. Anat Rec (Hoboken). 2013;296:146-55.

Salmon PW, Salmon IM. A dog in residence. Melbourne: Joint Advisory Committee on Pets in Society (Australia). 1982.

Salo PM, Zeldin DC. Does exposure to cats and dogs decrease the risk of allergic sensitization and disease? J Allergy Clin Immunol. 2009;124:751-2.

Sarkar C, Basu B, Chakroborty D, Dasgupta PS, Basu S. The immunoregulatory role of dopamine: an update. Brain Behav Immun. 2010;24:525-8.

Sarkar DK, Murugan S, Zhang C, Boyadjieva N. Regulation of cancer progression by β-endorphin neuron. Cancer Res. 2012;72:836-40.

Scheider L, Grassmann S, Kaminski J, Tomasello M. Domestic dogs use contextual information and tone of voice when following a human pointing gesture. PLoS One. 2011;6:e21676.

Schantz P. Preventing potential health hazards incidental to the use of pets in therapy. Anthrozoös. 1990;4:14-23.

Scheede-Bergdahl C, Penkowa M, Hidalgo J, Olsen DB, Schjerling P, Prats C, Boushel R, Dela F. Metallothionein-mediated antioxidant defense system and its response to exercise training are impaired in human type 2 diabetes. Diabetes. 2005;54:3089-94.

Schleidt WM, Shalter MD. Co-evolution of humans and canids an alternative view of dog domestication: homo homini lupus? Evolution and cognition. 2003;9:57-72.

Schneider MS, Harley LP. How dogs influence the evaluation of psychotherapists. Anthrozoös. 2006;19:128-42.

Schreier HM, Schonert-Reichl KA, Chen E. Effect of volunteering on risk factors for cardiovascular disease in adolescents: a randomized controlled trial. JAMA Pediatr. 2013;167:327-32.

Servan-Schreiber D. Anticancer: A New Way of Life. London UK: Penguin Books Ltd. 2011

Searles H. The nonhuman environment in normal development and in schizophrenia. New York: International Universities Press. 1960.

Senju A. Developmental and comparative perspectives of contagious yawning. Front Neurol Neurosci. 2010;28:113-9.

Serpell JA. Beneficial aspects of pet ownership on some aspects of human health and behaviour. J R Soc Med. 1991;84:717-20.

Serpell JA. Evidence for long term effects of pet ownership on human health. In Pets, Benefits and Practice, Waltham Symposium 20, 1990. Ed.: Burger IH. BVA Publications. 1990:1-7.

Serpell JA. In the company of animals: A study of human-animal relationships. Cambridge: Cambridge University Press. 1996.

Service Dogs Europe. [http://www.servicedogseurope.com/] (accessed on August 5, 2014).

Service Dogs For America. [http://www.servicedogsforamerica.org/] (accessed on August 5, 2014).

Shelly S, Boaz M, Orbach H. Prolactin and autoimmunity. Autoimmun Rev. 2012;11:A465-70.

Shen G, Gao X, Gao B, Granger DE. Age of Zhoukoudian Homo erectus determined with (26)Al/(10)Be burial dating. Nature. 2009;458:198-200.

Shibata A, Oka K, Inoue S, Christian H, Kitabatake Y, Shimomitsu T. Physical activity of Japanese older adults who own and walk dogs. Am J Prev Med. 2012;43:429-33.

Shiloh S, Sorek G, Terkel J. Reduction of state-anxiety by petting animals in a controlled laboratory experiment. Anxiety Stress Copin. 2003;16:387-95.

Shintani M, Senda M, Takayanagi T, Katayama Y, Furusawa K, Okutani T, Kataoka M, Ozaki T. The effect of service dogs on the improvement of health-related quality of life. Acta Med Okayama. 2010;64:109-13.

Shipman P. How do you kill 86 mammoths? Taphonomic investigations of mammoth megasites. Quatern Int. 2015;359-360:38-46.

Shipman P. The Animal Connection and Human Evolution, Curr Anthropol. 2010;51:519-38.

Shipman P. The animal connection: A new perspective on what makes us human. 2011. New York: W.W. Norton & Company Inc.

Shubert J. Dogs and human health/mental health: from the pleasure of their company to the benefits of their assistance. US Army Med Dep J. 2012a;Apr-Jun:21-9

Shubert J. Therapy dogs and stress management assistance during disasters. US Army Med Dep J. 2012b;Apr-Jun:74-8.

Siegel JM. Stressful life events and use of physician services among the elderly: the moderating effects of pet ownership. J Pers Soc Psychol. 1990;58:1081-6.

Siegel JM, Angulo FJ, Detels R, Wesch J, Mullen A. AIDS diagnosis and depression in the Multicenter AIDS Cohort Study: the ameliorating impact of pet ownership. AIDS Care. 1999;11:157-70.

Silva K, Bessa J, de Sousa L. Auditory contagious yawning in domestic dogs (Canis familiaris): first evidence for social modulation. Anim Cogn. 2012;15:721-4.

Silva K, de Sousa L. 'Canis empathicus'? A proposal on dogs' capacity to empathize with humans. Biol Lett. 2011;7:489-92.

Simpson A. Effect of household pet ownership on infant immune response and subsequent sensitization. J Asthma Allergy. 2010;3:131-7.

Simpson A, Custovic A. Pets and the development of allergic sensitization. Curr Allergy Asthma Rep. 2005;5:212-20.

Simpson BS. Canine communication. Vet Clin North Am Small Anim Pract. 1997;27:445-64.

Siniscalchi M, Lusito R, Vallortigara G, Quaranta A. Seeing left- or right-asymmetric tail wagging produces different emotional responses in dogs. Curr Biol. 2013a;23:2279-82.

Siniscalchi M, Sasso R, Pepe AM, Vallortigara G, Quaranta A. Dogs turn left to emotional stimuli. Behav Brain Res. 2010;208:516-21.

Siniscalchi M, Sasso R, Pepe AM, Dimatteo S, Vallortigara G, Quaranta A. Sniffing with the right nostril: lateralization of response to odour stimuli by dogs. Anim Behav. 2011;82:399-404.

Siniscalchi M, Stipo C, Quaranta A. "Like owner, like dog": correlation between the owner's attachment profile and the owner-dog bond. PLoS One. 2013b;8:e78455.

Siniscalchi M, Quaranta A, Rogers LJ. Hemispheric specialization in dogs for processing different acoustic stimuli. PLoS One. 2008;3:e3349.

Smith CS. The Rosetta Bone: The Key to Communication Between Canines and Humans (Howell Dog Book of Distinction). Howell Book House. 2004.

Smith NL, Denning DW. Clinical implications of interferon gamma genetic and epigenetic variants. Immunology. 2014;143:499-511.

Snipelisky D, Burton MC. Canine-assisted therapy in the inpatient setting. South Med J. 2014;107:265-73.

Sobo EJ, Eng B, Kassity-Krich N. Canine visitation (pet) therapy: pilot data on decreases in child pain perception. J Holist Nurs. 2006;24:51-7.

Sonoda H, Kohnoe S, Yamazato T, Satoh Y, Morizono G, Shikata K, Morita M, Watanabe A, Morita M, Kakeji Y, Inoue F, Maehara Y.

Colorectal cancer screening with odour material by canine scent detection. Gut. 2011;60:814-9.

Spratt EG, Nicholas JS, Brady KT, Carpenter LA, Hatcher CR, Meekins KA, Furlanetto RW, Charles JM. Enhanced cortisol response to stress in children in autism. J Autism Dev Disord. 2012;42:75-81.

Stankiewicz AM, Swiergiel AH, Lisowski P. Epigenetics of stress adaptations in the brain. Brain Res Bull. 2013;98:76-92.

Stanley-Hermanns M, Miller J. Animal-Assisted Therapy: Domestic animals aren't merely pets. To some, they can be healers. Am J Nurs. 2002;102:69-76.

Steele RW. Should immunocompromised patients have pets? Ochsner J. 2008;8:134-9.

Steinman L. Elaborate interactions between the immune and nervous systems. Nat Immunol. 2004;5:575-81.

Steptoe A, Shankar A, Demakakos P, Wardle J. Social isolation, loneliness, and all-cause mortality in older men and women. Proc Natl Acad Sci USA. 2013;110:5797-801.

Sternberg EM. Neural regulation of innate immunity: a coordinated nonspecific host response to pathogens. Nat Rev Immunol. 2006;6:318-28.

Strachan DP. Family size, infection and atopy: the first decade of the "hygiene hypothesis". Thorax. 2000;55:S2-10.

Strachan DP. Hay fever, hygiene, and household size. BMJ. 1989;299:1259-60.

Strohmeyer RA, Morley PS, Hyatt DR, Dargatz DA, Scorza AV, Lappin MR. Evaluation of bacterial and protozoal contamination of commercially available raw meat diets for dogs. J Am Vet Med Assoc. 2006;228:537-42.

Strong V, Brown S, Huyton M, Coyle H. Effect of trained Seizure Alert Dogs on frequency of tonic-clonic seizures. Seizure. 2002;11:402-5.

Strong V, Brown SW, Walker R. Seizure-alert dogs--fact or fiction? Seizure. 1999;8:62-5.

Tamura T, Yonemitsu S, Itoh A, Oikawa D, Kawakami A, Higashi Y, Fujimooto T, Nakajima K. Is an entertainment robot useful in the care of elderly people with severe dementia? J Gerontol A Biol Sci Med Sci. 2004;59:83-5

Tanner CM, Chen B, Wang W, Peng M, Liu Z, Liang X, Kao LC, Gilley DW, Goetz CG, Schoenberg BS. Environmental factors and Parkinson's disease: a case-control study in China. Neurology. 1989;39:660-4.

Taverna G, Tidu L, Grizzi F, Torri V, Mandressi A, Sardella P, La Torre G, Cocciolone G, Seveso M, Giusti G, Hurle R, Santoro A, Graziotti P. Highly-Trained Dogs' Olfactory System Detects Prostate Cancer in Urine Samples. J Urol. 2014;pii: S0022-5347(14)04573-X.

Taylor AM, Reby D, McComb K. Cross modal perception of body size in domestic dogs (Canis familiaris). PLoS One. 2011;6:e17069.

Taylor AM, Reby D, McComb K. Human listeners attend to size information in domestic dog growls. J Acoust Soc Am. 2008;123:2903-9.

Téglás E, Gergely A, Kupán K, Miklósi Á, Topál J. Dogs' gaze following is tuned to human communicative signals. Curr Biol. 2012;22:209-12.

The Delaware Assistive Technology Initiative. [http://www.dati.org/newsletter/issues/1999n1/dogs.html] (accessed November 29, 2012).

The International Therapy Dog Association in Japan. [http://japanesepsychology.blogspot.dk/2012/06/international-therapy-dog-association.html] (accessed November 26, 2012).

The health benefits of pets. Workshop summary; 1987 Sep 10-11. Bethesda (MD): National Institutes of Health, Office of Medical Applications of Research. 1987.

The MIRA Foundation. [http://www.mira.ca/en/], [http://www.mirausa.org/], [http://www.miraeurope.org/] (accessed on August 10, 2014).

Therapy Dogs International. [http://www.tdi-dog.org/] (accessed November 26, 2012).

Thompson CD, Zurko JC, Hanna BF, Hellenbrand DJ, Hanna A. The therapeutic role of interleukin-10 after spinal cord injury. J Neurotrauma. 2013;30:1311-24.

Thorpe RJ Jr, Kreisle RA, Glickman LT, Simonsick EM, Newman AB, Kritchevsky S. Physical activity and pet ownership in year 3 of the Health ABC study. J Aging Phys Act. 2006a;14:154-68.

Thorpe RJ Jr, Simonsick EM, Brach JS, Ayonayon H, Satterfield S, Harris TB, Garcia M, Kritchevsky SB; Health, Aging and Body Composition Study. Dog ownership, walking behavior, and maintained mobility in late life. J Am Geriatr Soc. 2006b;54:1419-24.

Tirindelli R, Dibattista M, Pifferi S, Menini A. From pheromones to behavior. Physiol Rev. 2009;89:921-56.

Tomasello M, Kaminski J. Behavior. Like infant, like dog. Science. 2009;325:1213-4.

Topál J, Gergely G, Erdohegyi A, Csibra G, Miklósi A. Differential sensitivity to human communication in dogs, wolves, and human infants. Science. 2009;325:1269-72.

Toohey AM, McCormack GR, Doyle-Baker PK, Adams CL, Rock MJ. Dog-walking and sense of community in neighborhoods: implications for promoting regular physical activity in adults 50 years and older. Health Place. 2013;22:75-81.

Toohey AM, Rock MJ. Unleashing their potential: a critical realist scoping review of the influence of dogs on physical activity for dog-owners and non-owners. Int J Behav Nutr Phys Act. 2011;8:46.

Tota B, Angelone T, Cerra MC. The surging role of Chromogranin A in cardiovascular homeostasis. Front Chem. 2014;2:64.

Tran TH, Utama FE, Lin J, Yang N, Sjolund AB, Ryder A, Johnson KJ, Neilson LM, Liu C, Brill KL, Rosenberg AL, Witkiewicz AK, Rui H. Prolactin inhibits BCL6 expression in breast cancer through a Stat5a-dependent mechanism. Cancer Res. 2010;70:1711-21.

Tranah GJ, Bracci PM, Holly EA. Domestic and farm-animal exposures and risk of non-Hodgkin's lymphoma in a population-based study in the San Francisco Bay Area. Cancer Epidemiol Biomarkers Prev. 2008;17:2382-7.

Trasande L, Blustein J, Liu M, Corwin E, Cox LM, Blaser MJ. Infant antibiotic exposures and early-life body mass. Int J Obes (Lond). 2013;37:16-23.

Tribet J, Boucharlat M, Myslinski M. Animal-assisted therapy for people suffering from severe dementia. Encephale. 2008;34:183-6.

Tsai F, Coyle WJ. The microbiome and obesity: is obesity linked to our gut flora? Curr Gastroenterol Rep. 2009;11:307-13.

Tsanas A, Little MA, McSharry PE, Spielman J, Ramig LO. Novel speech signal processing algorithms for high-accuracy classification of Parkinson's disease. IEEE Trans Biomed Eng. 2012;59:1264-71.

Turcsán B, Szánthó F, Miklósi A, Kubinyi E. Fetching what the owner prefers? Dogs recognize disgust and happiness in human behaviour. Anim Cogn. 2015;18:83-94.

Uchino BN. Social support and health: a review of physiological processes potentially underlying links to disease outcomes. J Behav Med. 2006;29:377-87.

Uchino BN, Cacioppo JT, Kiecolt-Glaser JK. The relationship between social support and physiological processes: a review with emphasis on underlying mechanisms and implications for health. Psychol Bull. 1996;119:488-531.

Udell MA, Dorey NR, Wynne CD. What did domestication do to dogs? A new account of dogs' sensitivity to human actions. Biol Rev Camb Philos Soc. 2010;85:327-45.

Udell MA, Dorey NR, Wynne CD. Can your dog read your mind?: understanding the causes of canine perspective taking. Learn Behav. 2011;39:289-302.

Udell MA, Wynne CD. A review of domestic dogs' (Canis familiaris) human-like behaviors: or why behavior analysts should stop worrying and love their dogs. J Exp Anal Behav. 2008;89:247-61.

Udell MA, Wynne CD. Reevaluating canine perspective-taking behavior. Learn Behav. 2011;39:318-23.

Ulrich-Lai YM, Herman JP. Neural regulation of endocrine and autonomic responses. Nat Rev Neurosci. 2009;10:397-409.

Valavanidis A, Vlachogianni T, Fiotakis K, Loridas S. Pulmonary oxidative stress, inflammation and cancer: respirable particulate matter, fibrous dusts and ozone as major causes of lung carcinogenesis through reactive oxygen species mechanisms. Int J Environ Res Public Health. 2013;10:3886-907.

van Kerkhove W. A fresh look at the wolf-pack theory of companion-animal dog social behavior. J Appl Anim Welf Sci. 2004;7:279-85; discussion 299-300.

van Koppenhagen CF, Post MW, van der Woude LH, de Witte LP, van Asbeck FW, de Groot S, van den Heuvel W, Lindeman E. Changes and determinants of life satisfaction after spinal cord injury: a cohort study in the Netherlands. Arch Phys Med Rehabil. 2008;89:1733-40.

van Leeuwen CM, Post MW, van Asbeck FW, Bongers-Janssen HM, van der Woude LH, de Groot S, Lindeman E. Life satisfaction in people with spinal cord injury during the first five years after discharge from inpatient rehabilitation. Disabil Rehabil. 2012;34:76-83.

Vilà C, Maldonado J, Wayne RK. Phylogenetic relationships, evolution, and genetic diversity of the domestic dog. J. Hered. 1999;90:71-7.

Vilà C, Savolainen P, Maldonado JE, Amorim IR, Rice JE, Honeycutt RL, Crandall KA, Lundeberg J, Wayne RK. Multiple and ancient origins of the domestic dog. Science. 1997;276:1687-9.

Vincent C, Gagnon D, Routhier F, Leblond J, Boucher P, Blanchet M, Martin-Lemoyne V; the ADMI group. Service dogs in the province of Quebec: sociodemographic profile of users and the dogs' impact on functional ability. Disabil Rehabil Assist Technol. 2015;10:132-40.

Virués-Ortega J, Buela-Casal G. Psychophysiological effects of human-animal interaction: theoretical issues and long-term interaction effects. J Nerv Ment Dis. 2006;194:52-7.

VonHoldt BM, Pollinger JP, Earl DA, Knowles JC, Boyko AR, Parker H, Geffen E, Pilot M, Jedrzejewski W, Jedrzejewska B, Sidorovich V, Greco C, Randi E, Musiani M, Kays R, Bustamante CD, Ostrander EA, Novembre J, Wayne RK. A genome-wide perspective on the evolutionary history of enigmatic wolf-like canids. Genome Res. 2011;21:1294-305.

Voreades N, Kozil A, Weir TL. Diet and the development of the human intestinal microbiome. Front Microbiol. 2014;5:494.

Vormbrock JK, Grossberg JM. Cardiovascular effects of human-pet dog interactions. J Behav Med. 1988;11:509-17.

Vredegoor DW, Willemse T, Chapman MD, Heederik DJ, Krop EJ. Can f 1 levels in hair and homes of different dog breeds: lack of evidence to describe any dog breed as hypoallergenic. J Allergy Clin Immunol. 2012;130:904-9.e7.

Wagle Shukla A, Vaillancourt DE. Treatment and physiology in Parkinson's disease and dystonia: using transcranial magnetic stimulation to uncover the mechanisms of action. Curr Neurol Neurosci Rep. 2014;14:449.

Walker BR, Soderberg S, Lindahl B, et al. Independent effects of obesity and cortisol in predicting cardiovascular risk factors in men and women. J Intern Med. 2000;247:198-204.

Walsh F. Human-Animal Bonds I: The relational significance of companion animals. Fam Proc. 2009a;48:462-80.

Walsh F. Human-Animal Bonds II: The role of pets in family systems and family therapy. Fam Proc. 2009b;48:481-99.

Walsh P, Mertin P, Verlander D, Pollard CF. The effects of a "pets as therapy" dog on persons with dementia in a psychiatric ward. Aust Occup Ther J. 1995;42:161-6.

Warrior Canine Connection. [http://warriorcanineconnection.org/] (accessed on August 20, 2014).

Watanabe T, Abe O, Kuwabara H, Yahata N, Takano Y, Iwashiro N, Natsubori T, Aoki Y, Takao H, Kawakubo Y, Kamio Y, Kato N, Miyashita Y, Kasai K, Yamasue H. Mitigation of sociocommunicational deficits of autism through oxytocin-induced recovery of medial prefrontal activity: a randomized trial. JAMA Psychiatry. 2014;71:166-75.

Wayne RK, Ostrander EA. Lessons learned from the dog genome. Trends Genet. 2007;23:557-67.

Wayne RK, VonHoldt BM. Evolutionary genomics of dog domestication. Mamm Genome. 2012;23:3-18.

Wechsler ME. Getting Control of Uncontrolled Asthma. Am J Med. 2014;pii:S0002-9343(14)00392-1.

Weese JS, Rousseau J, Arroyo L. Bacteriological evaluation of commercial canine and feline raw diets. Can Vet J. 2005;46:513-6.

Wells D. The value of pets for human health. The Psychologist. 2011;24:172-6.

Wells DL. Dogs as a diagnostic tool for ill health in humans. Altern Ther Health Med. 2012;18:12-7.

Wells DL. Domestic dogs and human health. Br J Health Psychol. 2007;12:145-56.

Wells DL. The effects of animals on human health and well-being. J Soc Issues. 2009;65:523-43.

Wells DL, Graham L, Hepper PG. The influence of auditory stimulation on the behaviour of dogs housed in a rescue shelter. Animal Welfare. 2002;11:385-93.

Wells DL, Hepper PG. The discrimination of dog odours by humans. Perception. 2000;29:111-5.

Wells DL, Lawson SW, Siriwardena AN. Canine Responses to Hypoglycaemia in Patients with Type 1

Diabetes. J Altern Complement Med. 2008;14:1235-41.

Wells M, Perrine R. Critters in the cube farm: perceived psychological and organizational effects of pets in the workplace. J Occup Health Psychol. 2001;6:81-7.

Welsh JS. Olfactory detection of human bladder cancer by dogs: another cancer detected by "pet scan". BMJ. 2004;329:1286-7.

Wiggett C. Animal-assisted visitations, loneliness and depression among residents in old age homes. Doctoral Thesis. Department of Psychology, Stellenbosch University. 2003.

Williams H, Pembroke A. Sniffer dogs in the melanoma clinic? Lancet. 1989;1:734.

Willis CM, Church SM, Guest CM, Cook WA, McCarthy N, Bransbury AJ, Church MR, Church JC. Olfactory detection of human bladder cancer by dogs: proof of principle study. BMJ. 2004;329:712.

Wilson SM, Sato AF. Stress and paediatric obesity: what we know and where to go. Stress Health. 2014;30:91-102.

Wiltschko R, Dehe L, Gehring D, Thalau P, Wiltschko W. Interactions between the visual and the magnetoreception system: Different effects of bichromatic light regimes on the directional behavior of migratory birds. J Physiol Paris. 2013;107:137-46.

Winkle M, Crowe TK, Hendrix I. Service dogs and people with physical disabilities partnerships: a systematic review. Occup Ther Int. 2012;19:54-66.

Wisdom JP, Saedi GA, Green CA. Another breed of "service" animals: STARS study findings about pet ownership and recovery from serious mental illness. Am J Orthopsychiatry. 2009;79:430-6.

Wohlfarth R, Mutschler B, Beetz A, Kreuser F, Korsten-Reck U. Dogs motivate obese children for physical activity: key elements of a motivational theory of animal-assisted interventions. Front Psychol. 2013;4:796.

Wolf P. The role of nonpharmaceutic conservative interventions in the treatment and secondary prevention of epilepsy. Epilepsia. 2002;43 Suppl 9:2-5.

Wolf ME, Mosnaim AD. Phenylethylamine in neuropsychiatric disorders. Gen Pharmacol. 1983;14:385-90.

Wood B. Colloquium paper: reconstructing human evolution: achievements, challenges, and opportunities. Proc Natl Acad Sci U S A. 2010;107:8902-9.

Wood L, Giles-Corti B, Bulsara M, Bosch DA. More than a furry companion: the ripple effect of companion animals on neighborhood interactions and sense of community. Society and Animals. 2007;15:43-56.

World Health Organization (WHO) Neurological Disorders: Public Health Challenges. WHO. 2006.

Wrangham R, Carmody R. Human adaptation to the control of fire. Evol. Anthropol. 2010;19:187-199.

Wunderlich KA, Leveillard T, Penkowa M, Zrenner E, Perez MT. Altered expression of metallothionein-I and -II and their receptor megalin in inherited photoreceptor degeneration. Invest Ophthalmol Vis Sci. 2010;51:4809-20.

Yabroff KR, Troiano RP, Berrigan D. Walking the dog: Is pet ownership associated with physical activity in California? J. Phys. Act. Health. 2008;5:216–28.

Yamamoto Y, Atoji Y, Suzuki Y. Innervation of taste buds in the canine larynx as revealed by immunohistochemistry for the various neurochemical markers. Tissue Cell. 1997;29:339-46.

Yin S, McCowan B. Barking in domestic dogs: context specificity and individual identification. Anim Behav. 2004;68:343-55.

Yoshida M, Takayanagi Y, Inoue K, Kimura T, Young LJ, Onaka T, Nishimori K. Evidence that oxytocin exerts anxiolytic effects via oxytocin receptor expressed in serotonergic neurons in mice. J Neurosci. 2009;29:2259-71.

Yount RA, Olmert MD, Lee MR. Service dog training program for treatment of posttraumatic stress in service members. US Army Med Dep J. 2012;Apr-Jun:63-9.

Zahradnik E, Raulf M. Animal allergens and their presence in the environment. Front Immunol. 2014;5:76.

Zakeri N, Bain PG. Sustained improvement in a patient with young onset Parkinson's disease after the arrival of a pet dog. J Neurol. 2010;257:1396-7.

Zhang J, Pacifico R, Cawley D, Feinstein P, Bozza T. Ultrasensitive detection of amines by a trace amine-associated receptor. J Neurosci. 2013;33:3228-39.

Zilcha-Mano S, Mikulincer M, Shaver PR. Pet in the therapy room: an attachment perspective on Animal-Assisted Therapy. Attach Hum Dev. 2011;13:541-61.

Zilcha-Mano S, Mikulincer M, Shaver PR. Pets as safe havens and secure bases: The moderating role of pet attachment orientations. J Res Pers. 2012;46:571-80.

Ziemssen T, Kern S. Psychoneuroimmunology-cross-talk between the immune and nervous systems. J Neurol. 2007;254:II8-11.

RECOMMENDED BOOKS

Bekoff, M. *The Emotional Lives of Animals: A Leading Scientist Explores Animal Joy, Sorrow, and Empathy—and Why They Matter.* California: New World Library. 2007.

Fogle, B. *The Dog's Mind.* Pelham Books. 1990.

Horowitz, A. *Inside of a Dog: What Dogs See, Smell, and Know.* Simon & Schuster. 2010.

Howard, P.J. *The Owner's Manual for the Brain: The Ultimate Guide to Peak Mental Performance at All Ages.* New York: HarperCollins Publishers. 2014.

McConnell, P. B. *For the Love of a Dog: Understanding Emotion in You and Your Best Friend.* New York: Ballantine Books. 2007.

McConnell, P.B. *The Other end of The leash: Why We Do What We Do Around Dogs.* New York: Ballantine's Books. 2002.

Miklósi, A. *Dog Behaviour, Evolution, and Cognition.* New York: Oxford University Press Inc. 2007.

Olmert, M. D. *Made for Each Other: The Biology of the Human-Animal Bond.* Merloyd Lawrence Books. 2009.

Serpell, J. A. *In the Company of Animals: A Study of Human-Animal Relationships.* Cambridge University Press. 1996.

You can find the latest medical literature at this excellent free site:
Unbound MEDLINE
http://www.unboundmedicine.com/medline/ebm
I also recommend the following page:
http://www.unboundmedicine.com/medline/ebm/related/22333725/
Animal_assisted_therapy_

LINKS

- http://4pawsforability.org/mobility-assistance-dog/
- http://www.americanpetproducts.org/press_industrytrends.asp/
- http://www.assistancedogsinternational.org/
- http://caninecoaching.co.uk/working-cocker/
- http://www.caninepartners.co.uk/
- http://www.cdc.gov/
- http://www.cnbc.com/id/101396437
- http://www.dati.org/newsletter/issues/1999n1/dogs.html/
- http://www.dogchannel.com/dogsinreview/comparison-cocker-spaniel-english-cocker-spaniel.aspx
- http://en.wikipedia.org/wiki/English_Cocker_Spaniel#cite_note-darshama-40
- https://www.epilepsy.com/
- http://greyfriarsbobby.co.uk/story.html/
- http://japanesepsychology.blogspot.dk/2012/06/international-therapy-dog-association.html/
- http://laughingsquid.com/daughter-posts-video-catching-an-incredible-moment-between-non-verbal-father-with-alzheimers-and-loving-dog/
- http://www.littleangelsservicedogs.org/
- http://www.medicalnewstoday.com/info/parkinsons-disease/
- http://www.mentalhealthdogs.org/Psychiatric-Service-Dogs.html
- http://www.mira.ca/en/
- http://www.mirausa.org/
- http://www.miraeurope.org/
- http://www.parkinsonsassociation.org/

- http://www.parkinsonsassociation.org/resources/paws-for-parkinsons/
- http://www.pawsitivityservicedogs.com/ptsd.html
- https://www.pawswithacause.org/what-we-do/service-dogs/
- https://www.pawswithacause.org/what-we-do/service-dogs/
- http://www.petpartners.org/
- http://www.pdf.org/en/index/
- http://www.psychologytoday.com/blog/canine-corner/
- http://www.sandiegopetsmagazine.com/view/full_story/17680504/article-Paws-for-Parkinson%E2%80%99s?instance=petpress/
- http://www.servicedogseurope.com/3956-2/ptsd-anxiety-depression/
- http://www.servicedogseurope.com/mobility-service-dogs/
- http://www.servicedogsforamerica.org/
- http://www.tdi-dog.org/
- http://warriorcanineconnection.org/

Printed in the United States
By Bookmasters